Acute and Critical Care Nursing
at a Glance

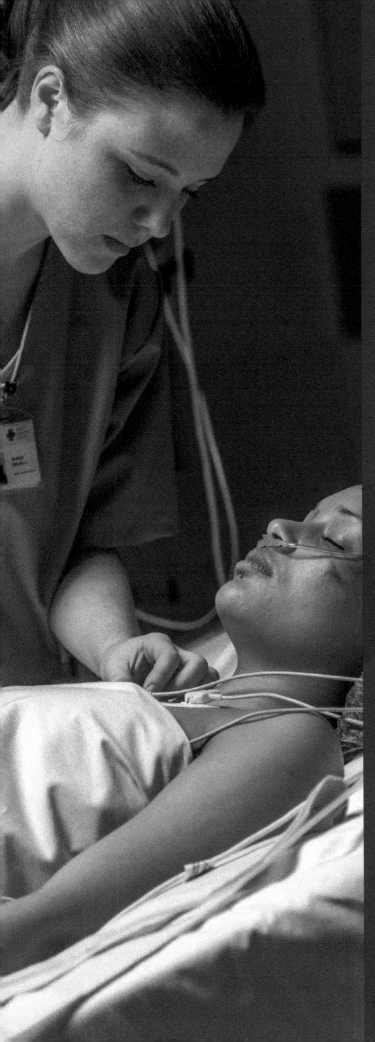

Acute and Critical Care Nursing
at a Glance

Edited by

Helen Dutton

MSc, BA, RNT, RGN
Senior Fellow, Higher Education Academy
Course Leader, BSc (Hons) Professional
Practice
Senior Lecturer, Critical Care
College of Nursing, Midwifery and Healthcare
University of West London, London, UK

Jacqui Finch

MSc, BSc (Hons), RGN, RNT, FHEA
Senior Lecturer/Course Leader, Intensive Care
College of Nursing, Midwifery and Healthcare
University of West London and The London
Northwest Healthcare NHS Trust, London, UK

Series Editor: Ian Peate OBE, FRCN

WILEY Blackwell

Registered Offices:
John Wiley & Sons, Inc., 111 River Street, Hoboken, NJ 07030, USA
John Wiley & Sons Ltd, The Atrium, Southern Gate, Chichester,
West Sussex, PO19 8SQ, UK

Editorial Office:
9600 Garsington Road, Oxford, OX4 2DQ, UK

For details of our global editorial offices, customer services, and more information about Wiley products visit us at www.wiley.com.

Wiley also publishes its books in a variety of electronic formats and by print-on-demand. Some content that appears in standard print versions of this book may not be available in other formats.

Library of Congress Cataloging-in-Publication Data

Names: Finch, Jacqui, 1961- editor. | Dutton, Helen, editor.
Title: Acute and critical care nursing at a glance / edited by Jacqui Finch, Helen Dutton.
Description: Hoboken, NJ : Wiley, 2017. | Series: At a glance series |
    Includes bibliographical references and index. |
Identifiers: LCCN 2017012986 (print) | LCCN 2017014342 (ebook) | ISBN
    9781118815151 (pdf) | ISBN 9781118815168 (epub) | ISBN 9781118815175 (pbk.)
Subjects: | MESH: Emergency Nursing—methods | Critical Care Nursing—methods
    | Handbooks
Classification: LCC RC86.8 (ebook) | LCC RC86.8 (print) | NLM WY 49 | DDC
    616.02/5--dc23
LC record available at https://lccn.loc.gov/2017012986

John Wiley & Sons Limited is a private limited company registered in England with registered number 641132. Registered office address: The Atrium, Southern Gate, Chichester, West Sussex, United Kingdom. PO19 8SQ.

Cover image: © simonkr/Gettyimages
Cover design by Wiley

Set in Minion Pro 9.5/11.5 by Aptara
Printed and bound by CPI Group (UK) Ltd, Croydon, CR0 4YY

C9781118815175_220224

Contents

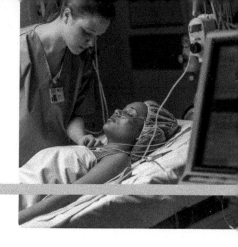

Contributors vii
Acknowledgements viii
Preface ix
Abbreviations x
About the companion website xii

Part 1 Nursing in acute and critical care   1
1   Critical care without walls 2
2   Recognising risk of deterioration: ABCDE assessment 4
3   Early warning tools and care escalation 6
4   Hospital-acquired infection: infection prevention and control 8
5   Pain management 10
6   Psychosocial issues 12
7   Safe transfer of the acutely unwell patient 14

Part 2 Airway: maintaining airway patency   17
8   Upper airway: assessment and management 18
9   Advanced airway management 20
10 Airway management: tracheostomy 22

Part 3 Breathing: patients with breathing problems   25
11 Respiratory physiology: oxygenation 26
12 Respiratory physiology: ventilation 28
13 Assessment of breathing 30
14 Respiratory investigations 32
15 Oxygen therapy 34
16 Respiratory failure 36
17 Breathing problems: obstructive disorders 38
18 Breathing problems: lung (parenchymal) disorders 40
19 Breathing problems: pleural disorders 42
20 Respiratory support: non-invasive ventilation 44
21 Principles of thoracic surgery 46

Part 4 Circulation: patients with circulatory problems   49
22 Circulatory physiology 1: circulation 50
23 Circulatory physiology 2: the heart and cardiac cycle 52
24 Circulatory physiology 3: control of circulation 54
25 Assessment of circulation 56
26 Cardiac investigations 58

27 Fluid, electrolytes and intravenous fluids 60
28 Haemodynamic monitoring 62
29 Acute chest pain 64
30 The 12-lead electrocardiogram 66
31 Altered heart rhythm 68
32 Physiology of the immune system 70
33 Acute circulatory failure 1: distributive (sepsis) 72
34 Acute circulatory failure 2: distributive (anaphylaxis and neurogenic) 74
35 Acute circulatory failure 3: hypovolaemia 76
36 Acute circulatory failure 4: obstructive 78
37 Acute circulatory failure 5: heart failure 80
38 Principles of cardiac surgery 82
39 Physiology of the gastrointestinal system 84
40 Acute medical and surgical gastrointestinal problems 86
41 Physiology of the renal system 88
42 Acute kidney injury 90
43 Burns: immediate care 92
44 Major trauma 94
45 Resuscitation 96

Part 5

Disability: patients with neurological impairment 99

46 Physiology of the brain 100
47 Neurological assessment 102
48 Neurological impairment 104
49 Drug overdose and poisoning 106
50 Acute endocrine problems 108

Part 6

Exposure 111

51 Skin integrity 112
52 Nutritional assessment and support 114

Part 7

Decision making in acute and critical care 117

53 Summary of decision making 118
54 Professional, legal and ethical considerations 120
55 Mental health concerns 122
56 Last days of life 124

Appendix 126
References and further reading 127
Glossary 136
Index 148

Contributors

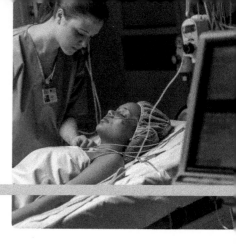

Sharon Elliot Chapters 8, 9, 37
Head of Pre-registration
University of West London, London, UK

Adrian Jugdoyal Chapter 55
Hepatology Advanced Nurse Practitioner
Northwick Park and St Mark's Hospital;
Associate Lecturer
University of West London, London, UK

Catherine Lynch Chapter 54
Senior Lecturer
University of West London, London, UK

Carl Margereson Chapters 11, 12, 53
Senior Lecturer
University of West London, London, UK

Caroline Smales Chapters 4, 32
Senior Lecturer
University of West London, London, UK

Sharon Smith Chapters 14, 26
Senior Lecturer
University of West London, London, UK

Renata Szczecinska Chapters 21, 30, 31, 38
Cardiac Practice Development Nurse
King's College Hospital NHS Foundation Trust
Associate Lecturer
University of West London, London, UK

Dean Whiting Chapter 44
Advanced Nurse Practitioner in Trauma and
    Orthopaedics
Buckinghamshire Healthcare NHS Trust;
Honorary Senior Lecturer in Trauma Science
Barts and the London School of Medicine and Dentistry
Queen Mary University of London, London, UK

Suzanne Whiting Chapter 43
Burn Care Advisor for the London and South East Burns
    Network
Buckinghamshire Healthcare NHS Trust, UK

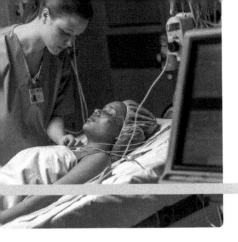

Acknowledgements

With grateful thanks to our academic and clinical colleagues who willingly shared their ideas, knowledge and experience to help in shaping many of the chapters in *Acute and Critical Care Nursing at a Glance*

Victoria Allen Chapter 35
Senior Lecturer, University of West London, London, UK

Kate Bradley Chapters 10, 20
Lecturer, University of West London, London, UK

Barry Hill Chapters 46, 47, 48
Lecturer, University of West London, London, UK

John Mears Chapters 5, 51
Senior Lecturer, University of West London, London, UK

Lyndsey Mears Chapter 56
Senior Lecturer, University of West London, London, UK

Trisha Mukherjee Chapters 28, 35
Modern Matron: Intensive Care
The London Northwest Healthcare NHS Trust, London, UK

Madhini Sivasubramanian Chapter 37
Lecturer, University of West London, London, UK

Liz Staveacre Chapters 1, 18
Senior Sister: Critical Care Outreach
The London Northwest Healthcare NHS Trust, London, UK

Preface

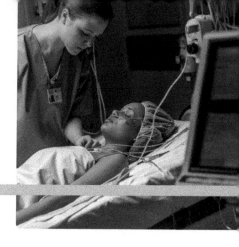

In 2000, the UK Department of Health's publication the *Comprehensive Critical Care – A Review of Adult Critical Care Services* classified patients according to the severity of their illness. This led to the concept of 'critical care without walls', identifying the presence of acutely unwell patients outside the Intensive Care Unit and acknowledging that specialist nurse education and training in recognition and preliminary management of acute deterioration, was now required in all areas of clinical practice. Since that time, society's growing, diverse and ageing population has augmented this need and an ever increasing use of technology in care settings has meant that practitioners are frequently required to plan, implement and evaluate care for patients with complex, multiple problems in a variety of clinical settings. Certainly, the expansion of community services has meant that many patients are successfully managed outside the hospital. However, the centralisation of acute services in healthcare, especially for emergency medicine, has seen a huge demand for in-hospital bed capacity in some areas. This has led to the increasing development of a wide range of assessment units designed to manage large numbers of patients presenting to hospital with acute problems. Over recent years the development of critical care outreach teams and the birth of track and trigger systems all assist with this, but there still remains a great need for nurses to further develop their assessment skills and their ability to promptly and appropriately respond to worsening clinical scenarios and life-threatening events. The 2015 Nursing and Midwifery Council Code of Conduct clearly states that registered nurses and midwives must, at all times, 'preserve safety'. Whilst acknowledging the limits of their competence, they have to be able to assess accurately the patients in their care, taking account of current evidence and knowledge and demonstrate the ability to make timely referral. Failure to achieve this standard is failure to act in the patients' best interests.

It has been suggested that nurses may possess differing perspectives on what clinical deterioration actually is. This may be irrespective of the scoring systems that exist to assist them and, of course, the tools themselves are sometimes subject to misinterpretation and misuse. One way to address this is to revisit the basic principles of normality and abnormality when considering how a patient might present, systematically collecting subjective and objective data in order to recognise when problems are occurring. Development of sound clinical reasoning like this, strongly founded in evidence-based knowledge, will vastly contribute to the provision of quality care, ensuring patient safety both now and in the future.

The chapters in the book are structured according to the systematic ABCDE framework.[1] This emphasises the priorities of care when faced with an acutely unwell patient and use of the 'at a glance' approach greatly facilitates this with its focus on immediacy. To complement this, in each chapter the text and accompanying diagrams present key information in a concise format, using current evidence gathered from local, national and international policies, protocols and guidelines. In addition, the inclusion of patient case studies and multiple choice questions covering a range of specialist content also serve to highlight significant issues in practice, enabling consolidation of learning by way of self-assessment. In summary, we hope this book will be a good reference source for our readers (be they registered or student practitioners), fostering their critical thinking. We also hope, in the interests of evidence-based quality care, that it creates a desire in our readers to learn more about critical care and that this knowledge is used to teach and support others who are providing care to the acutely ill.

Helen Dutton
Jacqui Finch

---

[1]Resuscitation Council UK (2015) The ABCDE approach. https://www.resus.org.uk/resuscitation-guidelines/abcde-approach/

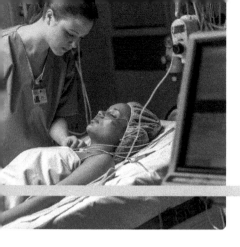

Abbreviations

A	Aorta
ABCDE	Airway, breathing, circulation, disability circulation
ABG	Arterial blood gas
ACEI	Angiotensin converting enzyme inhibitors
ACP	Advance care plan
ACS	Acute coronary syndrome
ACTH	Adrenocorticotrophic hormone
ADH	Antidiuretic hormone
AECOPD	Acute exacerbations of COPD
AF	Atrial fibrillation
AKI	Acute kidney injury
ALS	Adult advanced life support
AMI	Acute myocardial infarction
AMPLE	Allergies, Medications, Past medical history, Last ate and drank, Events leading (to injury)
AMTS	Abbreviated Mental Test Score
ANNT	Aseptic non-touch technique
ANS	Autonomic nervous system
ARB	Angiotensin receptor blockers
ARDS	Acute respiratory distress syndrome
ATOMFC	Airway, tension pneumothorax, open pneumothorax, massive haemothorax, flail chest, cardiac tamponade
ATP	Adenosine triphosphate
AV	Atrioventricular
AVN	Atrioventricular node
AVPU	Alert, voice, pain, unresponsive
BBB	Blood–brain barrier
BiPAP	Bi-level positive airways pressure
BMI	Body mass index
BMR	Basal metabolic rate
BNP	B-type natriuretic peptide
BP	Blood pressure
CA	Cardiac arrest
Ca⁺	Calcium ion
CABG	Coronary artery bypass grafting
CAM ICU	Confusion assessment method: Intensive care unit
CAP	Community-acquired pneumonia
CCF	Congestive cardiac failure
CCOT	Critical care outreach team
CHF	Chronic heart failure
CO	Cardiac output

COPD	Chronic obstructive pulmonary disease
CPAP	Continuous positive airways pressure
CPB	Cardiopulmonary bypass
CPR	Cardiopulmonary resuscitation
CQC	Care Quality Commission
CRBSI	Catheter-related blood stream infection
CRF	Chronic respiratory failure
CRP	C-reactive protein
CRT	Capillary refill time
CSF	Cerebrospinal fluid
CT	Computed tomography
CTPA	Computerised tomographic pulmonary angiography
CURB 65	Confusion, urea, respiratory rate, systolic blood pressure (age ≥65)
CVA	Cerebrovascular accident
CVC	Central venous catheter/cardiovascular centre
CVP	Central venous pressure
CXR	Chest X-ray
DDAVP	1- deamino-8-D-arginine vasopressin
DI	Diabetes insipidus
DINAMAP	Direct non-invasive automated mean arterial blood pressure measurement
DKA	Diabetic ketoacidosis
DNAR	Do not attempt to resuscitate
DVT	Deep vein thrombosis
ECG	Electrocardiogram
EPAP	End positive airways pressure
ERCP	Endoscopic retrograde cholangio-pancreatogram
ERV	Expiratory reserve volume
ETT	Endotracheal tube
EWS	Early warning systems
FBAO	Foreign body airway obstruction
FEV₁	Forced expiratory volume in one second
FRC	Functional residual capacity
FVC	Forced vital capacity
GABA	Gabba amino butyric acid
GAD-7	Generalised anxiety disorder assessment
GCS	Glasgow Coma Scale
GFR	Glomerular filtration rate
GI	Gastrointestinal
GTN	Glyceryl trinitrate
H⁺	Hydrogen ions

HADS	Hospital anxiety and depression scale	PCI	Percutaneous coronary intervention
HAP	Hospital-acquired pneumonia	PCT	Proximal convoluted tubule
HCO_3^-	Bicarbonate ion	PE	Pulmonary embolism
HCAI	Healthcare-associated infection	PEEP	Positive end expired pressure
HDU	High dependency unit	PEF	Peak expiratory flow
HF	Heart failure	PEFR	Peak expiratory flow rate
HFNC	High flow nasal cannula	PNS	Parasympathetic nervous system
HFPEF	Heart failure with preserved ejection fraction	PPCI	Primary percutaneous coronary intervention
HHS	Hyperglycaemic hyperosmolar syndrome	PPE	Personal protective equipment
HME	Heat and moisture exchanger	PS	Pressure support
HR	Heart rate	PSP	Primary spontaneous pneumothorax
I:E ratio	The ratio of inspiration to expiration	qSOFA	Quick Sequential (Sepsis Related) Organ Failure Assessment
ICD	Implantable cardioverter	RA	Right atrium
ICP	Intracranial pressure	RAAS	Renin-angiotensin-aldosterone system
ICU	Intensive care unit	REM	Rapid eye movement
IPAP	Inspiratory positive airways pressure	ROSC	Return of spontaneous circulation
IV	Intravenous	RR	Respiratory rate
JVD	Jugular venous distension	RV	Residual volume/Right ventricle
JVP	Jugular venous pressure	SAN	Sinoatrial node
K^+	Potassium ion	SAH	Subarachnoid haemorrhage
LMA	Laryngeal mask airway	SBAR	Situation, background, assessment, recommendation
LMWH	Low molecular weight heparin		
LOC	Level of consciousness	SBP	Systolic blood pressure
LPA	Lasting power of attorney	SIADH	Syndrome of inappropriate ADH
LV	Left ventricle	SNS	Sympathetic nervous system
LVF	Left ventricular failure	SOCRATES	Site, onset, character, radiation, associated symptoms, time course, exacerbating and relieving factors, severity
LVSD	Left ventricular systolic dysfunction		
mAChR	Muscarinic receptors		
MAP	Mean arterial pressure		
Mg^{++}	Magnesium ion	SP	Secondary pneumothorax
$MgSO_4$	Magnesium sulphate	SpO_2	Oxygen saturation of peripheral capillary blood
MI	Myocardial infarction		
MILS	Manual in-line stabilisation	SSP	Secondary spontaneous pneumothorax
MODS	Multiple organ dysfunction syndrome	SSRI	Selective Serotonin re-uptake inhibitor
MRI	Magnetic resonance imaging	STEMI	ST elevation myocardial infarction
MUST	Malnutrition universal screening tool	Sup.VC	Superior vena cava
Na^+	Sodium ion	SV	Stroke volume
NATMIST	Name, age, time of injury, mechanism of injury, injuries sustained, signs and symptoms, treatments given	SVR	Systemic vascular resistance
		SVT	Supraventricular tachycardia
		TBSA	Total body surface area
NC	Nasal cannula	TIA	Transient ischaemic attack
NEWS	National Early Warning Score	TIMI	Thrombolysis in myocardial infarction
NICE	The National Institute for Health and Care Excellence	TIPS	Trans intrahepatic portosystemic shunt
		TSH	Thyroid-stimulating hormone
NIV	Non-invasive ventilation	V/Q	Ventilation/perfusion
NSTEMI	Non-ST-segment elevated myocardial infarction	VATS	Video-assisted thoracoscopic surgery
		VBG	Venous blood gas
NPA	Nasopharyngeal airway	V_E	Minute ventilation
NSAID	Non-steroidal anti-inflammatory drugs	VF	Ventricular fibrillation
OPA	Oropharyngeal airway	VIP	Visual infusion phlebitis
PA	Pulmonary artery	V_T	Tidal volume
PAO_2	The partial pressure of oxygen in the alveoli	VT	Ventricular tachycardia
		VTE	Venous thromboembolism
PAINAD	Pain Assessment in Advanced Dementia	WBC	White blood cells
PaO_2	The partial pressure of oxygen in arterial blood	WCC	White cell count
		WHO	World Health Organization
PCA	Patient-controlled analgesia	WOB	Work of breathing

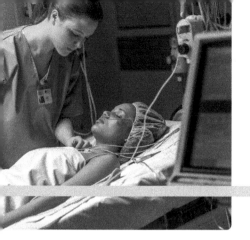

About the companion website

Don't forget to visit the companion website for this book:

www.ataglanceseries.com/nursing/acutecare

There you will find valuable material designed
to enhance your learning, including:

- Interactive multiple choice questions
- Nine patient case studies with questions and answers

Nursing in acute and critical care

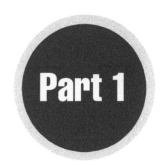

Part 1

Chapters

1 Critical care without walls   2
2 Recognising risk of deterioration:
   ABCDE assessment   4
3 Early warning tools and care escalation   6
4 Hospital-acquired infection: infection prevention
   and control   8
5 Pain management   10
6 Psychosocial issues   12
7 Safe transfer of the acutely unwell patient   14

1 Critical care without walls

Critical care without walls

Figure 1.1 Critical Care without walls

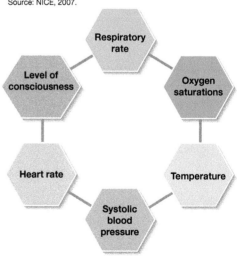

Emergency Care · Ward-based care · Critical Care Outreach · High-dependency care · Medical Emergency Team · Intensive Care · Coronary Care

Table 1.1 Selections from 'The Safer Nursing Care Tool', endorsed by NICE (2014), recommended staffing levels increase according to patient dependency.
Source: http://shelfordgroup.org[10]

Level of care	Descriptor
Level 1a Acutely ill patients requiring intervention or those who are **UNSTABLE** with a **GREATER POTENTIAL** to deteriorate	Care requirements may include the following: • Increased level of observations and interventions • Early Warning Score – trigger point • Postoperative care following complex surgery • Emergency admissions requiring immediate intervention • Oxygen therapy greater than 35% +/– • Post 24 hours following insertion of tracheostomy • Severe infection or sepsis
Level 1b Patients who are in a **STABLE** condition but are dependent on nursing care to meet most or all of the activities of daily living	Care requirements may include the following: • Complex wound management requiring more than one nurse or takes more than one hour to complete • Mobility or repositioning difficulties requiring assistance of two people • Patient and/or carers requiring enhanced psychological support • Patients on End of Life Care Pathway • Confused patients who are at risk or requiring constant supervision • Potential for self-harm, requiring observation
Level 2 May be managed within clearly identified, designated beds, resources with the required expertise and staffing level *OR* may require transfer to a dedicated level 2 facility/unit	• Deteriorating/compromised single organ system • Postoperative optimisation (preop invasive monitoring)/extended postop care • Patients requiring non-invasive ventilation/ respiratory support; CPAP/BiPAP in acute respiratory failure • First 24 hours following tracheostomy insertion • Requires: greater than 50% oxygen, continuous cardiac monitoring and invasive pressure monitoring • Drug infusions requiring more intensive monitoring e.g. vasoactive drugs (inotropes, GTN) or potassium, magnesium • CNS depression of airway and protective reflexes • Invasive neurological monitoring

Box 1.1 The Sepsis 6. Source: http://sepsistrust.org

To be initiated on suspicion of sepsis:

1. Administer high flow oxygen to meet target saturations
2. Take blood cultures and consider infective source
3. Administer intravenous antibiotics
4. Give intravenous fluid resuscitation
5. Check Hb and serial Lactates
6. Commence hourly urine measurements

Figure 1.2 Six key physiological parameters.
Source: NICE, 2007.

Respiratory rate · Level of consciousness · Oxygen saturations · Heart rate · Temperature · Systolic blood pressure

Acute and Critical Care Nursing at a Glance, First Edition. Edited by Helen Dutton and Jacqui Finch
© 2018 John Wiley & Sons, Ltd. Published 2018 by John Wiley & Sons, Ltd.
Companion website: www.ataglanceseries.com/nursing/acutecare

The last decade has seen a change in the environment in which care of the acutely unwell patient is delivered. Nurses working in acute care areas are increasingly exposed to patients who require more detailed assessment and monitoring. Nurses need to be competent in the skills required to care effectively for critically ill patients.

Changing patterns in acute care

The general population is ageing, with those requiring hospital admission older, sicker and generally more dependent. In 2010 the over-65 age group accounted for 10 million of the population in the UK, and by 2030 the number will be closer to 15.5 million. Emergency admissions for patients who have increasingly complex comorbidities requiring multidisciplinary and cross-speciality input are increasing. Meanwhile, greater emphasis has been placed on managing patients in their home environment for longer periods, meaning those who are admitted to hospital are sicker and require greater use of resources. Technological developments in healthcare means that treatments once thought too high a risk are now commonplace in hospitals.

With the increase in patient acuity it became evident that wards were not always able to cope effectively with the extra demands placed on them. Studies in the late 1990s identified that the deteriorating patient was not always recognised, and/or sufficient action was not taken prior to admission into the intensive care unit (ICU), adversely affecting patient outcome.

Reconfiguration of critical care services

In 2000 the Department of Health[1] published its report, *Comprehensive Critical Care*, recommending a systems approach was taken to deliver care for patients during acute and critical illness, and in the recovery period. Critical care emerged as a new speciality, addressing the severity of patient illness, regardless of their physical location within the hospital. The Department of Health introduced the concept of 'critical care without walls', to ensure acutely unwell patients nursed in a variety of environments, from ward-based care through to intensive care, come under the 'critical care umbrella' (Figure 1.1). A spectrum of dependency levels from levels 0 to 3, were outlined to encompass all those requiring critical care:[1]

• *Level 0*: Patients whose needs can be met through normal care in an acute hospital.
• *Level 1*: Patients at risk of their condition deteriorating, or those recently relocated from higher levels of care whose needs can be met on an acute ward with advice and support.
• *Level 2*: Patients requiring more detailed observation or interventions, including support for single organ failure, postoperative care, and those stepping down from a higher level of care.
• *Level 3*: Patients requiring advanced respiratory support or support of at least two organs, including all complex patients requiring support for multiorgan failure.

Workforce development, to ensure that staff caring for potentially critically ill patients receive education and training, is essential.[2] Key clinical competencies to be achieved have been identified.[3] Registered nurses are accountable for all aspects of care, even those tasks often delegated to others, such as the taking and recording of observations.[4]

Safe staffing levels

The Intensive Care Society (2013) and others published core standards for organisation of intensive care units (levels 2 and 3) and recommended safe staffing levels.[5] As acutely unwell patients are nursed across a range of environments, there are challenges for the provision of safe staffing levels on acute wards, which have been highlighted by the Francis Report (2013).[6] **NICE** (2014) issued guidance for safe staffing for nurses in acute hospitals supporting 'The Safer Nursing Care Tool' (Table 1.1).[2] This tool is based on the Department of Health classification, but adds an additional level, 1b, acknowledging the differing demands on nursing care activities, such as supporting the patient at risk of self-harm. It is designed to inform nursing establishments to be planned, linked to patient acuity both in ward-based care and critical care units.

Resuscitation to medical emergency

Cardiac arrests are predictable and preventable. Survival to discharge post cardiac arrest is as low as 15%.[7] Early recognition of deterioration is the first step in the chain of survival. Almost half of patients who die without a 'do not attempt resuscitation' (**DNAR**) order have serious, potentially reversible abnormalities in their vital signs in the 24 h preceding death. In fact, slow, progressive physiological deterioration with unrecognised and inadequately treated hypoxaemia and hypotension, can often be seen prior to admission to ICU and leads to poor survival. Delays in time to treatment have a profound effect on patient outcome. Specific intervention and timely instigation of organ support, via a medical emergency team or critical care outreach team (CCOT), is more important than getting the patient to the ICU.

Critical care outreach

Critical care outreach teams have evolved to provide expert input outside the environment of intensive and high dependency units. They aim to avert or ensure timely admissions to critical/intensive care and share critical care skills across the multidisciplinary team. Implementation of early therapies, for example, high flow oxygen, fluid resuscitation, or care bundles such as the 'Sepsis Six' (Box 1.1) can improve mortality and reduce rates of cardiac arrest. The CCOT's role in sharing critical care skills, improving early recognition of deterioration, has empowered nurses to escalate care appropriately and is now a widely adopted approach to maintaining patient safety.

Monitoring the acutely unwell patient

Recommendations to improve the recording of six key physiological observations (Figure 1.2), include the use of multiparameter Early Warning Scores to help identify patients at risk and escalate care appropriately.[8] The National Early Warning Score (**NEWS**)[9] (see Chapter 3) is a well-validated tool in the recognition and prevention of deterioration, and is now used widely in acute care trusts throughout the UK. Acutely unwell patients require competent and confident nurses to interpret clinical signs, recognise risk of deterioration and escalate care to the appropriate healthcare professional, ensuring senior medical input occurs in a timely manner to optimise patient outcome.

2 Recognising risk of deterioration: ABCDE assessment

Figure 2.1 The ABCDE approach to patient assessment

Airway assessment A
- Is the airway patent?
- Are there any signs of partial airway obstruction? (listen for stridor, snoring) If **YES**: then **call for help** and establish a clear airway
- Is the patient talking?
- Can they cough effectively?
- If **YES** move on to breathing assessment

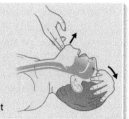

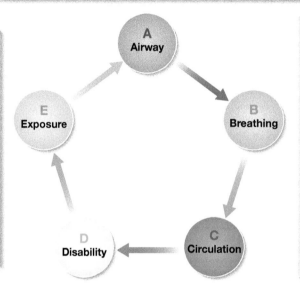

Exposure E
- Are there clues as to the reason for the patient's condition?
- Draw curtains to maintain privacy and dignity, and perform a top to toe assessment
- Look for signs of infection, trauma, rashes, swelling
- Assess pain

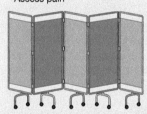

Breathing assessment B
- Is breathing adequate for patient's needs?
- Look at patient position, colour and movement of chest. Are they in distress?
- Measure oxygen saturations and respiratory rate. Treat by repositioning and giving oxygen as per target saturation and trust guidelines. Call for help as needed
- If critically ill give high flow oxygen until medical support arrives
- Move on to circulation

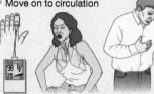

Disability assessment D
- Is the patient conscious and talking?
- Is the patient confused?
- Assess level of consciousness using AVPU
- **If V or below call for help**
- Look for signs of facial or limb weakness
- Assess blood glucose level, **correct hypoglycaemia**
  - If patient is conscious give oral glucose or hypostop
  - If unconscious consider administering 10% or 20% glucose IV, or glucagon 1 mg IM, according to trust guidelines
- If **hyperglycaemic**, alert medical staff and request review regarding need for sliding scale insulin
- To assess response to pain (**P**) try a **trapezius squeeze**: use thumb and two forefingers to twist and squeeze trapezius muscle

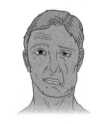

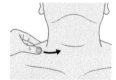

Circulatory assessment C
- Is circulation sufficient?
- Look for pallor, sweating, bleeding/fluid loss
- Measure heart rate, blood pressure and capillary refill time
- Urine output should be > 0.5 mL/kg/h
- Reposition patient: if hypovolaemic consider supine position, and elevating patient's legs
- Establish IV access and request medical assessment regarding need for fluid administration

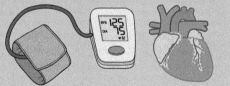

Acute and Critical Care Nursing at a Glance, First Edition. Edited by Helen Dutton and Jacqui Finch
© 2018 John Wiley & Sons, Ltd. Published 2018 by John Wiley & Sons, Ltd.
Companion website: www.ataglanceseries.com/nursing/acutecare

The acutely unwell patient

Most people in hospital are unlikely to become seriously unwell. If they should deteriorate, early detection through a detailed clinical assessment is essential so that nurses are able to identify the problem and ensure that appropriate care and treatments are given in a timely manner. When caring for an acutely unwell patient, the use of the Airway, Breathing, Circulation, Disability, Exposure (ABCDE) approach helps keep the focus on those aspects of deterioration that are most likely to be life threatening, thereby improving patient outcome. This chapter gives an overview of each area, but these are also considered in more detail in later chapters.

ABCDE

The ABCDE approach (Figure 2.1) is an excellent clinical tool for the assessment and treatment of patients who are acutely unwell.[1] This approach dictates that each element is assessed, then treated as necessary, before moving on to the next element. Early recognition and treatment of abnormal physiology in this progressive fashion initiates effective treatment, preventing further deterioration, whilst help can be sought from clinicians with specialist expertise. The process is used to reassess progress as treatments are instigated. Whilst nurses are familiar with taking and recording vital signs, assessment of the acutely unwell patient requires more detail, taking note and interpreting a range of clinical signs that assist in clinical decision making.

Assessment approach

A general impression when first approaching the patient is often the trigger for a more detailed assessment. The patient who does not respond to questions, has collapsed, or is perhaps severely distressed and sweating profusely, has clear markers of serious illness.

Airway (Figure 2.1A)

The airway is assessed for patency as a priority as **airway obstruction** is a **medical emergency**. If untreated it will rapidly lead to cardiac arrest, and so help is required immediately. An alert and chatty patient has a patent airway. A reduced level of consciousness is a common cause of both partial and complete airway obstruction, requiring the healthcare professional to perform the 'head tilt chin lift' manoeuvre, to keep the airway open. **Partial airway obstruction is noisy**, and requires **immediate management** (see also Chapters 8 and 9). Once the nurse is confident that the patient's airway is patent, they can move on to assessment of breathing.

Breathing assessment (Figure 2.1B)

Adequate oxygenation is essential. SpO_2 monitoring, available in all acute care environments, is measured promptly if deterioration is suspected. SpO_2 values outside the patient's target range (94–98% or 88–92% as prescribed) requires oxygen therapy to restore it to normal or near normal levels (also Chapter 15).[2]

Indicators of respiratory distress included:
- Use of accessory muscles.
- Central cyanosis.
- Paradoxical breathing.
- Leaning forward in tripod position.
- Inability to complete sentences in one breath.

- Audible wheeze (acute severe asthma/chronic obstructive pulmonary disease [COPD]).
- Rapid shallow breathing.
- Mouth breathing, purse-lipped breathing.

Respiratory rate has been shown to be a significant predictor of risk of deterioration.[3] This important observation should be counted for 1 min to ensure accuracy and will normally be between 12 and 20 breaths/min. The chest should be inspected for bilateral equal expansion. Failure of both sides of the chest to move equally on inspiration could suggest a collection of pleural fluid, or a chest infection. If the trachea is displaced from the midline, with unilateral chest expansion and respiratory distress, a **medical emergency** such as **tension pneumothorax**, may be present. **Urgent medical help** is required. A patient who has breathing difficulties should be repositioned in the upright position, given appropriate prescribed therapy promptly (such as oxygen or bronchodilators), and help should be summoned if necessary, before moving on to circulatory assessment.

Circulation (Figure 2.1C)

The circulatory system transports oxygenated blood to the tissues. Patient pallor as a result of vasoconstriction also causes hands and feet to cool if circulation is inadequate. Profuse sweating and changes in level of consciousness are also associated with decreased perfusion. A peripheral pulse should be palpated manually and assessed for rate, rhythm and strength. Any abnormalities should prompt an ECG recording. A fall in systolic blood pressure is a late sign and can be due to problems such as: hypovolaemia, cardiac failure, pulmonary embolism, sepsis or anaphylaxis. Most patients who are hypotensive require fluid therapy (after excluding cardiac causes), so intravenous access should be obtained as necessary. Blood and fluid losses should be noted, considering urine output (which should be greater than 0.5 mL/k/h) and overall fluid balance (see also Chapter 25).

Disability (Figure 2.1D)

Level of consciousness can be quickly assessed using an **AVPU** assessment to assesses neurological status (also Chapter 46):
- A: Alert: spontaneously talking and responding to questions.
- V: Unconscious but roused by voice.
- P: Unconscious but responds to painful stimuli, such as trapezius squeeze (see Figure 2.1D).
- U: Unresponsive.

If changes in AVPU are noted then a more detailed assessment using tools such as the Glasgow Coma Score is required. Changes in level of consciousness caused by either hypo- or hyperglycaemia should be treated promptly. Changes in face symmetry, unequal arm movement or speech alterations could indicate brain injury due to a stroke. Patients with deteriorating consciousness need their airway protected by appropriately skilled healthcare personnel.

Exposure (Figure 2.1E)

It is important to maintain patient dignity whilst performing a full body check. Looking 'under the sheets' ensures no essential clues are missed. Temperature is an important indicator for infection and may be assessed here, or under circulation. If the patient is pyrexial, look for the source of infection, checking all invasive lines/devices and inspecting wounds and lesions for signs of bleeding, oozing, inflammation or tenderness.

③ Early warning tools and care escalation

Figure 3.1 Ensure accurate recording of observations

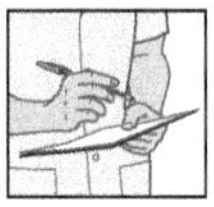

Recording observations as soon as they have been taken helps prevent errors occurring

Figure 3.4 Calculate NEWS

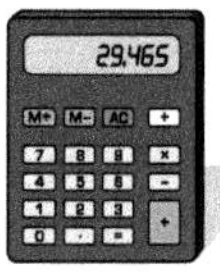

Check and recheck NEWS to ensure accuracy

Figure 3.5 NEWS thresholds and triggers

NEW scores	Clinical risk
0	Low
Aggregate 1 – 4	
RED score* (Individual parameter scoring 3)	Medium
Aggregate 5 – 6	
Aggregate 7 or more	High

© Royal College of Physicians 2012 — Royal College of Physicians — NHS Training for Innovation

Figure 3.2 National Early Warning Score (NEWS) Chart

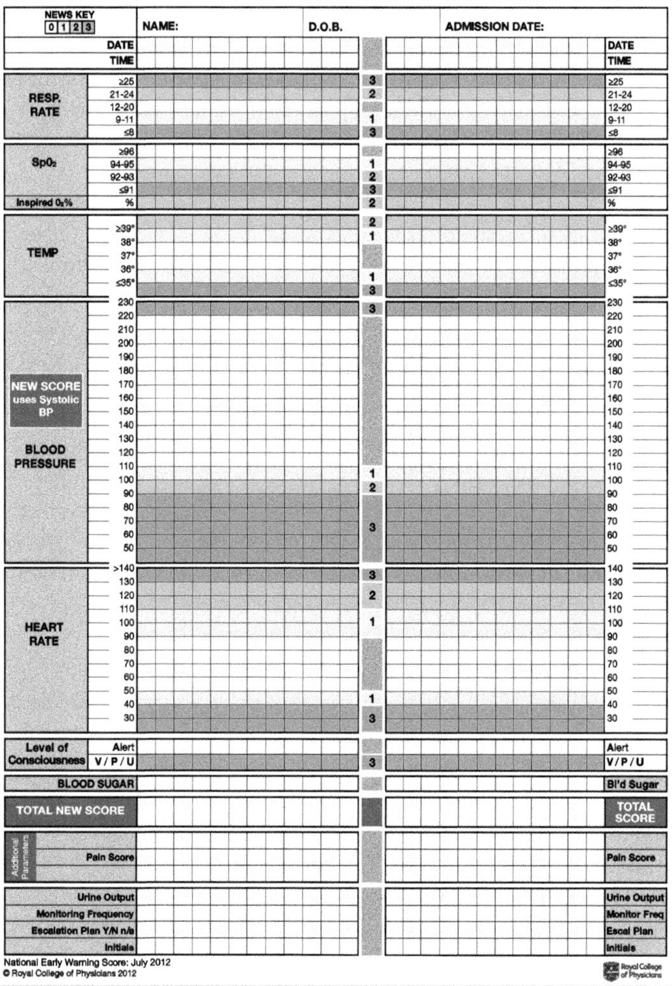

National Early Warning Score: July 2012
© Royal College of Physicians 2012

Figure 3.6 Care escalation according to clinical risk

Low risk
- 4–6 hourly monitoring
- Inform registered nurse (RN), who must assess patient
- RN to decide frequency of monitoring, and whether care escalation required

Medium risk
- Hourly monitoring
- RN to urgently inform medical team
- Urgent assessment by a clinician experienced in assessing acutely ill patients
- Clinical care to be delivered where patients can be monitored hourly

High risk
- Continuous monitoring
- RN to immediately inform medical team at Specialist Registrar level
- Emergency assessment by clinical team experienced in assessing acutely ill patients (with advanced airway skills)
- Consider transfer to level 2 or 3 care

Clinical red flags. Source: RCP, 2013.
- Cardiac chest pain lasting longer than 20 min
- Headache of dramatically sudden onset
- Recent onset headache with scalp tenderness and jaw claudication
- Palpitations associated with syncope
- Painful swollen red calf
- Cauda equina syndrome (compression of nerves in lower spine)

Figure 3.3 Score allocation for each observation with NEWS

PHYSIOLOGICAL PARAMETERS	3	2	1	0	1	2	3
Respiration Rate	≤ 8		9 – 11	12 – 20		21 – 24	≥ 25
Oxygen Saturations	≤ 91	92 – 93	94 – 95	≥ 96			
Any Supplemental Oxygen		Yes		No			
Temperature	≤ 35.0		35.1 – 36.0	36.1 – 38.0	38.1 – 39.0	≥ 39.1	
Systolic BP	≤ 90	91 – 100	101 – 110	111 – 219			≥ 220
Heart Rate	≤ 40		41 – 50	51 – 90	91 – 110	111 – 130	≥ 131
Level of Consciousness				A			V, P, or U

*The NEWS initiative flowed from the Royal College of Physicians' NEWS Development and Implementation Group (NEWSDIG) report, and was jointly developed and funded in collaboration with the Royal College of Physicians, Royal College of Nursing, National Outreach Forum and NHS Training for Innovation

Royal College of Physicians

Figure 3.7 Using SBAR

S
Your name and ward
Patient's name and age
Consultant
NEWS

B
Reason for admission
PMH, allergies, medication, recent results

A
ABCDE assessment
Reasons for concern
Actions taken and response

R
State what you need within a specified time
Make suggestions and clarify any instruction given

Source: Figures 3.2, 3.3 and 3.5 reproduced from the Royal College of Physicians. National Early Warning Score (NEWS): Standardising the assessment of acute-illness severity in the NHS. Report of a working party. London: RCP, 2012.

Acute and Critical Care Nursing at a Glance, First Edition. Edited by Helen Dutton and Jacqui Finch
© 2018 John Wiley & Sons, Ltd. Published 2018 by John Wiley & Sons, Ltd.
Companion website: www.ataglanceseries.com/nursing/acutecare

Recognising the deteriorating patient

Patients who are admitted into hospital with acute care needs have a right to receive reliable harm-free care. The recognition of clinical deterioration relies largely on nurses taking and recording vital signs, identifying where these are abnormal, communicating findings to skilled clinical personnel and ensuring appropriate interventions are given in a timely manner. Lack of recognition of physiological changes may lead to a delay in care, an extended hospital stay, ICU admission or even a premature death. Failure to rescue occurs when a patient's deterioration is not recognised and they suffer harm from a potentially treatable condition. Nurses are accountable for ensuring accurate clinical observations are recorded and acted upon (Figure 3.1), even if delegated to a non-registered healthcare professional.[1] Training, education and support for the healthcare team is essential in the delivery of harm-free care.

National Early Warning Score (NEWS)

In 2007 NICE recommended the use of 'aggregated weighted track and trigger systems'.[2] These are early warning systems (EWS) that consider a number of different clinical observations, generating an overall score to help evaluate risk of deterioration. The score gained is used to identify low, medium and high scoring groups, thereby determining frequency of observations and the need for review by the medical team and/or outreach. A number of EWS have been used across the UK, leading to a significant variation in trigger levels, and therefore a potential lack of understanding by clinical staff moving across the country to work in different clinical environments. A standardised National Early Warning Score (**NEWS**) developed by The Royal College of Physicians,[3] has been embraced by acute care trusts across the UK. A unified approach helps all clinical staff to understand the level of the risk of deterioration of patients. Using NEWS consists of a number of straightforward steps:

- Take each observation and record on NEWS chart (Figure 3.2).
- Use the chart(Figure 3.3), to identify the score for each measurement, add together to get the NEWS (Figure 3.4).
- Look at the **trigger thresholds** to determine whether the patient is at **low**, **medium** or **high** risk (Figure 3.5). Note that a score of 3 in any single parameter requires the doctor to be informed, even if they do not meet the medium trigger score of 5–6.
- Follow hospital/NEWS protocol as to frequency of observations and appropriate clinical personnel to call (Figure 3.6).
- Check for **clinical red flags**;[4] these may not score on NEWS but require urgent review (see red flags box).
- Use a communication tool such as SBAR to escalate care.

Recording clinical observations

The NEWS chart requires the recording and scoring of the six physiological parameters identified by NICE (2007) namely:[2]

- Respiratory rate.
- Oxygen saturations.
- Temperature.
- Systolic blood pressure.
- Heart rate.
- Level of consciousness.

Trust protocols vary as to whether numbers or dots are used to record observations, but it is recommended that respiratory rate and oxygen saturations are recorded as a number.[5] This enables changes in respiratory rate to be more clearly documented, especially when in the red zone at >25 breaths/min. The percentage of oxygen is recorded as either air, oxygen percentage, or in L/min (nasal specs), so response to oxygen therapy can be recorded.

NEWS and trigger thresholds

Figure 3.3 identifies scores for each physiological parameter, so there is no confusion between borderline values. For example, a heart rate of 110 beats/min scores 1; using the observation chart alone may not make this clear. The NEWS chart and the threshold and trigger chart have been made into pocket cards by some trusts, aiding accurate and consistent scoring.

An automatic **addition of 2** is made to the NEWS if the patient is receiving **oxygen therapy**, correctly highlighting that the hypoxaemic patient receiving supplemental oxygen is unwell, and is at increased risk of deterioration and death. An alternative trigger range of oxygen saturations for patients who have adapted to chronic disordered physiology such as COPD and are at risk of hypercapnia (target range SpO_2 of 88–92%), can be appropriate, but must be clearly marked and signed for by the doctor on the observation chart.

Trigger thresholds will define action to be taken at trust level. **NEWS >7** requires urgent action (within 15 min) at senior medical level, support from outreach, continuous observations, with the possibility of transfer to a higher level of care. This is an opportunity to ask the medical team to consider the 'ceiling of care' as not all patients benefit from receiving advanced levels of support, such as intubation and mechanical ventilation in an ICU environment.[3]

Care escalation using SBAR

Doctors and outreach nurses looking after a large number of patients have competing priorities for their time. Clear, precise and accurate information is needed to enable them to focus on those who are most unwell. NEWS conveys severity of illness. A communication tool such as **SBAR** (Situation, Background, Assessment, Recommendation) (Figure 3.7) supports structured communication and good clinical decision making to improve patient outcomes:

- **Situation**: state who you are, which ward you are on, patient's name, age, consultant and NEWS.
- **Background**: give a brief overview of the reason for admission, recent medical history, relevant past results, allergies, medication.
- **Assessment**: use the **ABCDE** mnemonic to outline current clinical assessment. State actions taken and any clinical response. For example, 'I have given 2 L oxygen via nasal specs and the SpO_2 has now risen from 91 to 94%'.
- **Recommendation**: explain what is worrying you, what you need from the doctor/outreach and in what time frame. Make sure you understand any actions required of you by repeating the instructions to ensure accuracy.

The accurate, consistent use of an early warning tool and escalation strategy such as NEWS, and a communication tool such as SBAR, contributes to ensuring care is focused on those patients who are at the greatest risk of deterioration.

4 Hospital-acquired infection: infection prevention and control

Figure 4.1 Healthcare-associated infections and antimicrobial use.
Source: English National Point Prevalence Survey on Healthcare-associated Infections and Antimicrobial Use, 2011.

This is the latest of four prevalence studies carried out since the 1980s. The latest survey gives a 'snap-shot' of the number of patients with an HCAI in English hospitals at the time of the study and reveals the six most common types of HCAI which account for more than 80% of all HCAIs.

The prevalence of antibiotic usage was 34.7% and was highest in the independent sector at 46.7% compared to NHS organisations at 34.3%.

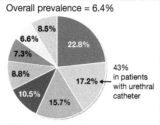

Overall prevalence = 6.4%

8.5%
6.6%
7.3%
8.8%
10.5%
22.8%
17.2%
15.7%

43% in patients with urethral catheter

- ■ Pneumonia
- □ UTI
- □ SSI
- ■ Sepsis
- □ Gastrointestinal
- ■ Bloodstream
- □ Unknown
- □ Other

Figure 4.2 Standard and transmission-based precautions.
Source: Centers for Diseases Control and Prevention, 2007.

Standard (routine) precautions
Precautions based on risk associated with task to be carried out and includes: hand hygiene, personal protective equipment, sharps management and disposal, safe waste management, principles of decontamination

Transmission-based precautions
May be used in addition to the above precautions for patients known, or suspected to be infected/colonised with epidemiologically important pathogens that can be transmitted by the following routes

Airborne transmission	Droplet transmission	Contact transmission
Microbes < 5 µm	Microbes > 5 µm	

Figure 4.3 Handwashing and alcohol handrub technique. Source: WHO, 2009.

How to Handwash?
WASH HANDS WHEN VISIBLY SOILED! OTHERWISE, USE HANDRUB

Duration of the entire procedure: 40-60 seconds

0 Wet hands with water;

1 Apply enough soap to cover all hand surfaces;

2 Rub hands palm to palm;

3 Right palm over left dorsum with interlaced fingers and vice versa;

4 Palm to palm with fingers interlaced;

5 Backs of fingers to opposing palms with fingers interlocked;

6 Rotational rubbing of left thumb clasped in right palm and vice versa;

7 Rotational rubbing, backwards and forwards with clasped fingers of right hand in left palm and vice versa;

8 Rinse hands with water;

9 Dry hands thoroughly with a single use towel;

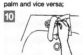
10 Use towel to turn off faucet;

11 Your hands are now safe.

How to Handrub?
RUB HANDS FOR HAND HYGIENE! WASH HANDS WHEN VISIBLY SOILED

Duration of the entire procedure: 20-30 seconds

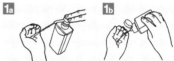
1a 1b 2
Apply a palmful of the product in a cupped hand, covering all surfaces;

Rub hands palm to palm;

3 Right palm over left dorsum with interlaced fingers and vice versa;

4 Palm to palm with fingers interlaced;

5 Backs of fingers to opposing palms with fingers interlocked;

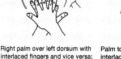
6 Rotational rubbing of left thumb clasped in right palm and vice versa;

7 Rotational rubbing, backwards and forwards with clasped fingers of right hand in left palm and vice versa;

8 Once dry, your hands are safe.

Figure 4.4 Areas commonly missed

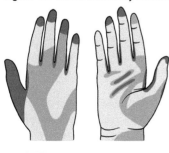

- ■ Most frequently missed
- ■ Frequently missed
- □ Less frequently missed

Box 4.1 Current high impact intervention care bundles that can be integrated into care plans and pathways and be used to set standards. Source: Department of Health High Impact Intervention Care Bundles, 2007.

1 Central venous catheter care
2 Peripheral intravenous cannula care
3 Renal dialysis catheter care
4 Prevention of surgical site infection
5 Care of ventilated patients
6 Urinary catheter care
7 Reducing the risk of *C. difficile*
8 Decontamination of environment
9 Enteral feeding
10 Chronic wounds
11 Blood cultures

Figure 4.5 Aseptic technique, aseptic field, micro critical aseptic field and key parts.
Source: www.antt.org Reproduced with permission of Stephen Rowley.

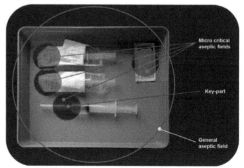

Micro critical aseptic fields

Key-part

General aseptic field

Acute and Critical Care Nursing at a Glance, First Edition. Edited by Helen Dutton and Jacqui Finch
© 2018 John Wiley & Sons, Ltd. Published 2018 by John Wiley & Sons, Ltd.
Companion website: www.ataglanceseries.com/nursing/acutecare

Infection prevention and control

Patients who are acutely unwell have increased susceptibility to infection due to accidental or surgical injuries, multiple invasive devices, decreased immunity, complex health problems and increased contact with healthcare staff. Therefore, **healthcare-associated infection** (HCAI), prevention and control in critical care is of paramount importance. Whilst twenty-first century healthcare can bring even the sickest and most traumatised patient back from the brink of death, a single infectious agent can enter the body and bring about death in a matter of hours. The National Point Prevalence Study (2011) on healthcare-associated infection,[1] gives a 'snapshot' of the overall HCAI prevalence rate (the number of people suffering from a HCAI during the time of the study); it shows a prevalence rate of 6.4, a reduction from 8.2. Figure 4.1 highlights the six most common types of HCAI which account for more than 80% of all HCAIs.

Standard and transmission-based precautions

Every single act or intervention has the potential to spread infection, as microorganisms invisible to the naked eye can be moved from place to place, and person to person, resulting in entry to a susceptible host (patients or staff) through any orifice or break in the skin. **Standard precautions** rely on staff assessing the risk of the 'task' they are carrying out and deciding on the appropriate precautions that should be taken and where these are considered insufficient, implement additional '**transmission-based precautions**' (Figure 4.2).[2] Following these recommended guidelines will not only prevent patients from becoming infected but also staff from occupationally acquired infections.

Evidence-based guidelines

Healthcare professionals have a professional, legal and ethical responsibility to follow recommended standard infection prevention and control guidelines and minimise any risk of infection. The Department of Health (2014) National Evidence-Based Guidelines for Preventing Healthcare-Associated Infections in NHS Hospitals in England (Epic 3)[3] consolidate the 'best available evidence currently available' informing current practice. These address the following areas and should be integrated into healthcare policies that are easily accessible for all staff:

1 Guidelines for standard precautions for preventing HCAIs in hospitals and other acute care settings:
- Hospital hygiene.
- Hand hygiene.
- Use of Personal Protective Equipment (PPE).
- Safe use and disposal of sharps.
- Asepsis.

2 Guidelines for preventing infections associated with the use of short-term indwelling urethral catheters.

3 Guidelines for preventing infections associated with the use of intravascular devices.

Hand hygiene

Hand hygiene, either hand washing or hand rubbing (Figure 4.3), is considered the single most important infection prevention activity[4, 5] and it is important that staff know: **how** to decontaminate their hands, **what** product to decontaminate with and **when** to decontaminate:[6]
- **What**: hand washing with liquid soap and running water are to be used routinely to cleanse hands, especially when hands are visibly soiled, and/or when specific microorganisms such as *Clostridium difficile* or *Norovirus* are suspected or confirmed. If a higher level of hand hygiene is required, such as prior to an aseptic technique, antiseptic soap should be used. Hand rubbing with an alcohol hand rub gel can be quicker and easier to use in place of hand washing on visibly clean hands and when *Clostridium difficile* and *Norovirus* are not suspected.
- **How**: the technique used is most important and in order for microorganisms to be removed from hands (Figure 4.3) the product being used, either soap or alcohol solution *must* cover all surfaces of the hands. Using a methodical, vigorous rubbing action which will lift up microorganisms from the skin surface to be washed away, or ensure the hand rub fluid has contact with all parts of the skin will enable it to assert its killing action on the microorganisms. Common areas missed are shown in Figure 4.4.
- **When**: staff must decontaminate their hands at the most crucial times:
  (i) Immediately before patient contact including aseptic procedures.
  (ii) Immediately after patient contact or care.
  (iii) Immediately after any exposure to body fluids.
  (iv) After contact with the patients surroundings.
  (v) After glove removal.

However, this is not exhaustive; additional hand hygiene opportunities include before and after starting a shift, after using the toilet, or before eating or preparing food.

A 'bare below the elbow' policy when providing direct patient care ensures sleeves do not impede access for regular hand washing and requires removal of wrist and hand jewellery. Any breaks in the skin need to be covered with a waterproof dressing and nails kept short and varnish free. Hand hygiene education and monitoring is important, in order to keep motivation high and ensure full compliance at all times.

High Impact Intervention Care Bundles

The Department of Health High Impact Intervention Care Bundles[7] integrate 'evidence' generated from sources such as Epic 3 and are regularly reviewed to enable best available evidence to be integrated into clinical practice. Care bundles 'bundle' together small, straightforward sets of evidence-based practices, usually about three to five. When performed consistently as a group or bundle, improved patient outcomes have been demonstrated. Care bundles can be used to inform staff, audit clinical practice, provide positive feedback and highlight areas for improvement (Box 4.1).

An integral part of High Impact Intervention Care Bundles is ensuring 'asepsis' by utilising the framework of ANTT (**aseptic non-touch technique**)[8] (Figure 4.5) which ensures 'key parts' and 'key sites' are protected from contamination, minimising the risk of infection.

HCAIs can result in significant morbidity and mortality, particularly in clinical areas that provide acute and critical care. Failure to prevent infection can be very costly in terms of lives affected and result in the closure of clinical services, delaying hospital admissions. Instigating all the measures mentioned above have contributed to a reduction in the prevalence of HCAIs. However, the challenge is ensuring ongoing improvement can be sustained.

5 Pain management

Box 5.1 Chemical mediators in nociceptive pain

- Bradykinin
- Histamine
- Substance P
- Prostaglandins, particularly PGE_2
- Protons (H^+)
- Adenosine triphosphate (ATP)
- 5-hydroxytryptamine (5-HT) (serotonin)
- Potassium (K^+)
- Lactic acid

Box 5.4 Pain assessment tool examples

- Visual analogue scale
- Numerical rating scale
- Verbal rating scale
- Baker and Wong faces
- Leeds assessment of neuropathic signs and symptoms for neuropathic pain
- McGill short form questionnaire
- PAINAD for dementia

Figure 5.1 Effects of untreated acute pain

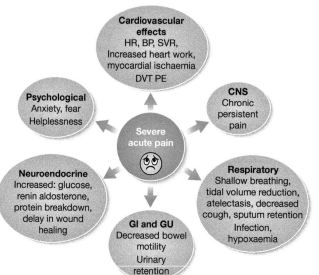

Cardiovascular effects
HR, BP, SVR,
Increased heart work,
myocardial ischaemia
DVT PE

Psychological
Anxiety, fear
Helplessness

CNS
Chronic persistent pain

Severe acute pain

Neuroendocrine
Increased: glucose,
renin aldosterone,
protein breakdown,
delay in wound healing

GI and GU
Decreased bowel motility
Urinary retention

Respiratory
Shallow breathing,
tidal volume reduction,
atelectasis, decreased
cough, sputum retention
Infection,
hypoxaemia

Box 5.2 Causes of neuropathic pain

- Phantom limb
- Ischaemic injury
- Painful diabetic neuropathy
- Trigeminal neuralgia

Box 5.3 Dimensions of pain

- Sensory: the physical sensations of having tissue damage
- Affective: influenced by anxiety and depression
- Cognitive: influenced by previous experience
- Social-cultural: influenced by cultural, spiritual and social factors

Figure 5.3 The pain ladder

Step 1
Non-opioid
(e.g. aspirin,
paracetamol
or NSAID)
± adjuvant

Step 2
Weak opioid
for mild to
moderate pain
(e.g. codeine)
± non-opioid
± adjuvant

Step 3
Strong opioid
for moderate
to severe pain
(e.g. morphine)
± non-opioid
± adjuvant

Pain persisting or increasing

Pain controlled

Pain persisting or increasing

Figure 5.4 Epidural catheter for epidural analgesia

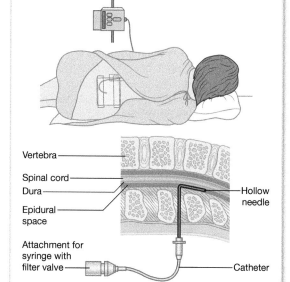

Vertebra

Spinal cord

Dura

Epidural space

Attachment for syringe with filter valve

Hollow needle

Catheter

Figure 5.2 SOCRATES to assist in ascertaining cause of pain

S	Site	Where exactly is the pain?
O	Onset	What were they doing when the pain started?
C	Character	What does the pain feel like?
R	Radiates	Does the pain go anywhere else?
A	Associated symptoms	e.g. nausea, vomiting
T	Time/duration	How long have they had the pain?
E	Exacerbating/relieving factors	Does anything make the pain better or worse?
S	Severity	Obtain an initial pain score

Box 5.5 Complications associated with PCA

- **Respiratory depression:** regular assessment of sedation and respiratory rate (RR) is required. Infusion is stopped if RR < 8. If RR < 5 naloxone in 100 µg increments may be given according to prescription and trust guidelines
- **Hypotension:** vasodilation may cause BP to drop. Intravenous fluids should be administered as prescribed. Assess fluid status
- **Nausea:** give anti-emetics as prescribed
- **Pruritus:** itching discomfort, give antihistamine as prescribed
- **Inadequate analgesia:** Check PCA is functioning correctly, seek pain team for further advice regarding pain relief. Non-opioid analgesics may be added as per prescription

Acute and Critical Care Nursing at a Glance, First Edition. Edited by Helen Dutton and Jacqui Finch
© 2018 John Wiley & Sons, Ltd. Published 2018 by John Wiley & Sons, Ltd.
Companion website: www.ataglanceseries.com/nursing/acutecare

Effectively managing pain remains a challenge for acute care nurses, with about 40% of hospital patients and 50% of surgical patients reporting pain, described as moderate or severe.[1] Pain should be anticipated in the acute care setting, although reports suggest that many nurses underestimate the levels of pain experienced. Poor pain relief has adverse physiological consequences (Figure 5.1) impacting on patient function, such as the ability to breathe deeply, cough, or mobilise sufficiently, and this affects patient outcome. To meet the challenges presented in the acute care setting, sufficient training and structured management guidelines are required to ensure effective pain relief, minimising complications and improving patient experience.[2]

Types of pain

Pain can be divided into two types:
- **Nociceptive pain** is associated with tissue damage and is one of the five features of the inflammatory process. This is also often referred to as protective pain.
- **Neuropathic pain** is associated with a primary lesion of the nervous system or damage to the nerves themselves.

The differences in the aetiology of the two types of pain are significant in terms of assessment, manifestation and treatment.[3]

Nociceptive pain

The primary event in the production of nociceptive pain is cell damage or necrotic death, which may be caused by trauma and ischaemia for example. The damage leads to the release of a range of chemicals which can stimulate the pain receptors (Box 5.1). The effect that these chemicals have can be modulated by the production of prostaglandins as a consequence of cell wall damage. The prostaglandins reduce the threshold of the pain receptors and are therefore **hyperalgesic**. The process of converting the chemical activity to electrical impulses (action potentials) is called transduction. The pain impulses follow the standard sensory pathway to the sensory cortex, where pain is perceived.

Neuropathic pain

Neuropathic pain is associated with damage to nerves. For example, damage to the blood vessels in patients with diabetes leads to nerve damage with changes in the stability of the nerve cell wall. Electrical discharges occur without any obvious stimulus, leading to intermittent pain or continuous unremitting pain such as the phantom pain of an amputated limb (Box 5.2).

Assessment of pain

Pain is multidimensional, having physical, emotional, cognitive, spiritual, psychological and sociocultural aspects (Box 5.3). Past experience also has a significant effect on pain perception. These various factors can modulate pain and therefore significantly affect pain experience. It is also now generally accepted that anxiety, often experienced by patients in acute care through activity in the hippocampus, has a significant effect by increasing focus on pain and therefore having a **hyperalgesic** effect. Nociceptive pain assessment tools are either **unidimensional** (usually measuring pain intensity) or **multidimensional** (measuring intensity, cognitive, psychological or emotional aspects). Whilst many pain assessment tools are available (Box 5.4) in the acute care setting it is often usual to use a unidimensional tool to measure pain intensity, such as the Wong Baker Face Scale. Self-report is the gold standard of any pain assessment tool, but

specialised tools such as the Pain Assessment in Advanced Dementia (PAINAD), a non-verbal pain assessment tool, designed for patients with dementia who are unable to clearly express their pain, is also useful for critically ill patients.[4] Tools developed to assess for neuropathic pain include a number of features such as sharpness, dullness, intensity and surface versus deep pain. Existing pain may also not be related to the current condition, or it may be incident pain, such as that arising in response to a specific stimulus, for example, coughing after abdominal surgery. The urgency of new chest pain, with the associated risks of life-threatening events, must be appreciated and acted upon. Tools using mnemonics such as **SOCRATES** (Figure 5.2) and PQRST explore both specific pain features and subjective experience, which can aid diagnosis.

Management of pain

Pharmacological interventions are the mainstay of nociceptive and neuropathic pain management, but different approaches are required for each.

Nociceptive pain management

In acute care, pain is often related to tissue injury (nociceptive) and a stepwise approach to management is taken. This is summed up in the WHO pain ladder which exists in a number of similar forms (Figure 5.3). The non-steroidal anti-inflammatory drugs (**NSAIDs**) act at the site of injury or damage reducing the inflammatory and pain-stimulating chemicals. It should be noted that paracetamol has a different mode of action to other NSAIDs. Opioids have a central action inhibiting the release of neurotransmitters in the central nervous system, thus preventing the signals reaching the sensory cortex. The nurse works with prescribers to ensure pain relief can be escalated/de-escalated as appropriate.

Neuropathic pain

Neuropathic pain does not respond well to NSAIDs or opioids. The drugs of choice are pregabalin and gabapentin. Both drugs are related to gamma amino butyric acid (GABA) which is an inhibitory neurotransmitter. Amitriptyline, a tricyclic antidepressant, has also been used in reduced doses, with good effect for many.

Patient-controlled analgesia and epidural analgesia

Small doses of opiates, such as intravenous morphine are very effective at pain relief, but if repeated doses are needed this places heavy demands on nursing time. Patient-controlled analgesia (**PCA**) enables patients to deliver their own opioid analgesia via a volumetric pump, delivering an intravenous dose when a control button is pressed. The pump has a 'lockout' safety period to prevent overmedication or an inadvertent drug bolus. PCA is highly effective for pain relief in postoperative care, burns and even emergency care.[5] Complications of PCA are outlined in Box 5.5.

Many postoperative patients benefit from an epidural catheter (Figure 5.4) which is inserted into the epidural space so continuous analgesia can be given via a volumetric pump. Managed by trained competent nursing staff and anaesthetists, good pain relief is achieved. This increases mobility and reduces some postoperative complications such as deep vein thrombosis (DVT) and chest infection.

6 Psychosocial issues

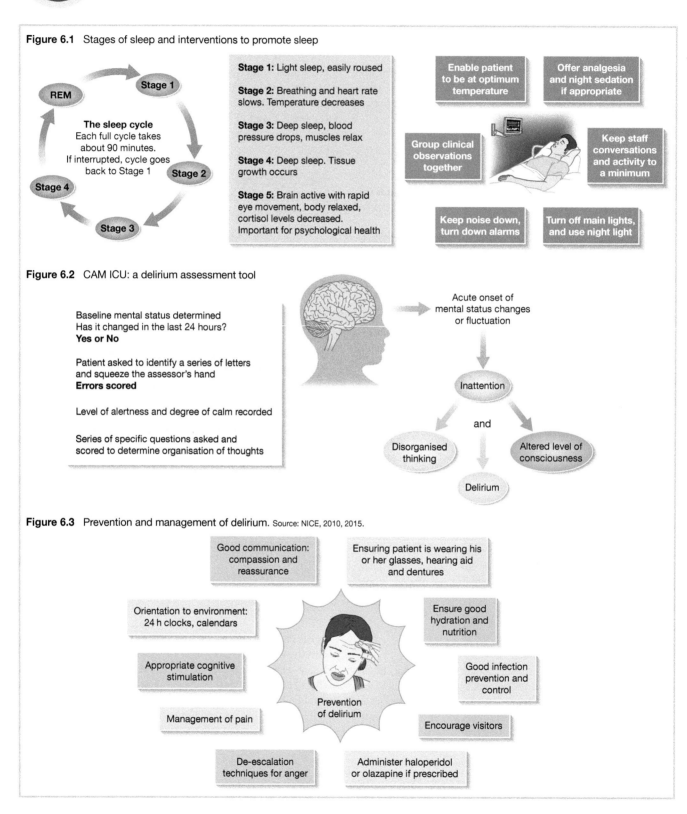

Figure 6.1 Stages of sleep and interventions to promote sleep

The sleep cycle
Each full cycle takes about 90 minutes. If interrupted, cycle goes back to Stage 1

REM · Stage 1 · Stage 2 · Stage 3 · Stage 4

Stage 1: Light sleep, easily roused

Stage 2: Breathing and heart rate slows. Temperature decreases

Stage 3: Deep sleep, blood pressure drops, muscles relax

Stage 4: Deep sleep. Tissue growth occurs

Stage 5: Brain active with rapid eye movement, body relaxed, cortisol levels decreased. Important for psychological health

Enable patient to be at optimum temperature

Offer analgesia and night sedation if appropriate

Group clinical observations together

Keep staff conversations and activity to a minimum

Keep noise down, turn down alarms

Turn off main lights, and use night light

Figure 6.2 CAM ICU: a delirium assessment tool

Baseline mental status determined
Has it changed in the last 24 hours?
Yes or No

Patient asked to identify a series of letters and squeeze the assessor's hand
Errors scored

Level of alertness and degree of calm recorded

Series of specific questions asked and scored to determine organisation of thoughts

Acute onset of mental status changes or fluctuation

Inattention

Disorganised thinking · and · Altered level of consciousness

Delirium

Figure 6.3 Prevention and management of delirium. Source: NICE, 2010, 2015.

Good communication: compassion and reassurance

Ensuring patient is wearing his or her glasses, hearing aid and dentures

Orientation to environment: 24 h clocks, calendars

Ensure good hydration and nutrition

Appropriate cognitive stimulation

Good infection prevention and control

Management of pain

Prevention of delirium

Encourage visitors

De-escalation techniques for anger

Administer haloperidol or olazapine if prescribed

Acute and Critical Care Nursing at a Glance, First Edition. Edited by Helen Dutton and Jacqui Finch
© 2018 John Wiley & Sons, Ltd. Published 2018 by John Wiley & Sons, Ltd.
Companion website: www.ataglanceseries.com/nursing/acutecare

Acute illness or injury usually has a major impact on patients' lives and on those of family and friends. People are at their most vulnerable in these circumstances, often with little experience to guide them through the process.[1] In addition to the physical, may be life-threatening problems, the patient will find themselves in the uncomfortable and unfamiliar environment of acute care. The nurse therefore has a crucial role in providing care that ensures that the psychological and social needs of patients and their families are assessed and appropriate, with timely measures put in place to address them. Failure to do so may have consequences long after the patient's initial illness or injury.

Anxiety

In most cases the environment in which acutely ill patients are being cared for is unfamiliar and strange to them (as it is for their visitors). There are several factors that may contribute to the patient becoming anxious and disorientated: the presence of many unknown people, the use of technical monitoring equipment creating a noisy, foreign setting and invasive lines limiting mobility. Rest may also be difficult. The many social roles and responsibilities that patients have in their lives, such as husband, mother or employee are absent. Together these contribute to a sense of isolation and powerlessness and may well be exacerbated by pain, fear of the unknown and absence of family and friends. The acute care nurse needs to be aware of these potential stressors. Anxiety is an uncomfortable feeling which precedes signs of physical stress. Asking patients specific questions about their anxieties and fears gives an opportunity to address concerns and establish trusting relationships.

Transfer or relocation anxiety

Transfer from the ICU or high-dependency unit (HDU) to a ward environment can cause a variety of emotions for the patient. Some feel positive and relieved to recover, especially as part of a planned recovery process, but many experience distress, fear and nervousness that are part of relocation anxiety. Good patient preparation for ICU discharge, with clear explanations and good communication with patients as well as receiving wards and relatives, is associated with more positive patient outcomes. Daytime transfers evoke less anxiety, and have reduced rates of ICU readmission, than those occurring at night. Ward nurses can support the process by ensuring they receive a detailed handover from ICU staff, and allow time to address any fears the patient may have. Social support from trusted relatives can help in this transition period.

Sleep deprivation

Lack of sleep is a common problem for acutely ill patients. Their presenting complaint may have unpleasant side effects such as anxiety, pain and nausea. A restful sleep for physiological and psychological repair requires the repeated completion of stages 1–5 in the sleep cycle (Figure 6.1), and absence of this results in sleep deprivation. Interruption to stages 1–4 (non-rapid eye movement sleep) results in physiological problems and to stage 5 (rapid eye movement sleep), psychological disturbances. The acutely ill patient requires frequent interventions, increasing the possibility of sleep interruption. If even the very early stages of the sleep cycle are disrupted, both physical and psychological problems could occur.

Confusion and delirium

Those most at risk of becoming confused include:
- Patients over 65 years of age.
- Those with pre-existing mental impairment such as dementia.
- Patients who have been hospitalised for a long period.

Delirium has been defined as an acute cognitive dysfunction associated with critical illness. It may have both serious short- and long-term consequences. The patient's altered physiology may be exacerbated by the release of stress substances such as noradrenaline and vasopressin, activated as a result of a psycho-immunological response. These can override the body's 'coping' agents such as melatonin and oxytocin, precipitating an overall inflammatory reaction leading to cellular dysfunction. Longer term effects include the development of profound psychological disturbance, such as post-traumatic distress disorder. These effects are felt long after discharge, leading to ongoing problems such as relationship difficulties and mental health issues. Delirium presents in different ways: *hyperactive*, with agitated or aggressive behaviour; *hypoactive*, appearing withdrawn and non-communicative.

Auditory and visual hallucinations often feature, causing great distress to patients. Occasionally these may lead to paranoia, with the conviction that people are trying to harm them. A recommended diagnostic algorithm for determining the presence or absence of delirium is the **Confusion Assessment Method: Intensive Care Unit** (CAM-ICU). This tool, established by Ely *et al.* (2001)[2] (which in spite of the name can be used with acutely ill patients outside the ICU), measures the existence or absence of cognitive impairment according to four key features:
- Acute change or a fluctuation in mental status.
- Inattention.
- Disorganised thinking.
- Altered level of consciousness.

The patient is scored as either 'CAM positive' or 'CAM negative' (Figure 6.2). The nurse can ensure that this assessment process is fully carried out (usually by medical staff) with the result clearly documented, so that a record of the patient's mental status is available. Care delivery to prevent and treat delirium (whilst individualised to meet the patient's needs), follows NICE (2010) guidelines (revalidated 2015) on delirium management (Figure 6.3).[3]

Ethical concerns

Care should always comply with ethical and legal requirements. Acutely ill patients sometimes lack autonomy and cannot give informed consent for investigations and treatments. Factors such as delirium and hypoxaemia can significantly impair judgement, leading some patients to refuse life-saving interventions. The multidisciplinary team in urgent situations adhere to ethical principles of beneficence and non-maleficence. Clinical intervention is always delivered with the individual patient's best interests in mind, in consultation, where possible, with relatives. The Mental Capacity Act (2005)[4] and the supplementary Deprivation of Liberty Safeguards (DOLS 2009)[5] clearly state that all care must be perceived to be of benefit, be of a proportionate response to the existing problem and be the least restrictive to the patient's liberty as possible.

Safe transfer of the acutely unwell patient

7

Acute and Critical Care Nursing at a Glance, First Edition. Edited by Helen Dutton and Jacqui Finch
© 2018 John Wiley & Sons, Ltd. Published 2018 by John Wiley & Sons, Ltd.
Companion website: www.ataglanceseries.com/nursing/acutecare

Types of patient transfer

Patients who are acutely unwell often need to be moved from one clinical environment to another, as their clinical condition changes, or additional tests/investigations are required. The transfer may be an **intrahospital transfer**, where the patient is moved between departments in the same building (for example, from the Accident and Emergency Department to the HDU), or it may be an **interhospital transfer**, where the patient is moved to another hospital for specialist investigations or treatment.

Decision making and professional accountability

Legally, the decision to transfer a patient is ultimately the responsibility of the attending consultant. From an ethical perspective, this should be an act of beneficence and made in the best interests of the patient. Occasionally, transfer may occur for non-clinical reasons, but ideally no patient should be moved on the grounds of bed capacity alone. Whatever the circumstances, the same principles of care apply. Whilst a multidisciplinary approach to patient transfer should always be adopted, the nurse has a key role in facilitating the meticulous preparation of the patient, the accompanying staff, the equipment to be taken and the documentation to be completed. Healthcare professionals are accountable for their own actions and have a responsibility to ensure that they are clinically competent to undertake a transfer. Nurses, however, owing to their close proximity to the patient, are in a unique position to take overall responsibility for the transfer process, effectively liaising with other members of the multidisciplinary team and safely coordinating all events.

Assessment, medical and nursing management

Optimisation of the patient's clinical condition prior to and during transfer is an essential requirement if physiological complications are to be avoided or at least minimised.[1] Using the **ABCDE** format,[2] a **systematic assessment** of the patient's physical condition, taking into account any previous medical history, should be carried out by medical and nursing staff. Vital signs need to be taken, recorded and monitored throughout the transfer process (Box 7.1). Trust transfer **documentation** throughout the transfer procedure. Thorough assessment and planning is required to prevent complications of transfer (Figure 7.1).

Firstly, **airway** assessment and maintenance is of primary importance. If airway patency or respiratory gas exchange is considered to be at all at risk, early measures should be taken to enhance the patient's clinical condition prior to moving. **Airway adjuncts**, including Guedel airway, nasopharyngeal airway and endotracheal intubation equipment, might be required and transportable suction apparatus should always be available.

Breathing: gravitational forces during transfer lead to volume displacement and maldistribution of blood flow which could affect lung perfusion and lead to poor oxygenation. Oxygen therapy may be required and, if so, the level should be titrated to achieve target saturations depending on clinical condition and medical history.[3] SpO_2 requires continuous monitoring to enable prompt response to deteriorating respiratory status. A sufficient amount of oxygen must also be taken for the transfer (see oxygen requirements box).

Circulation must also be continuously assessed. Maldistribution of circulating volume can also lead to cardiovascular compromise, with changes in blood pressure and cardiac arrhythmias occurring in patients being transported. These problems will be exacerbated in the patient with low blood pressure, or the 'shocked' patient, and may lead to other systemic complications such as renal failure and gastrointestinal impairment. Continuous electrocardiogram (ECG) and intermittent blood pressure measurement will be required for a patient of level 2 dependency.

Disability: neurological problems such as raised intracranial pressure secondary to impaired perfusion may also be a possibility. In such circumstances, prompt therapeutic intervention may be necessary. Gravitational forces cause fluid shifts, the effects of which are reduced with adequate volume in the circulation. As noted by Handy and Zwanenberg (2009) 'full patients travel better', so fluid therapy may be required.[4] If seriously unwell, vasopressors, inotropic agents, antiarrhythmics and antihypertensives may also be necessary depending on the nature of the patient's haemodynamic instability. Venous access is also essential before moving the patient.

Finally, **exposure** should be reviewed carefully. The patient needs to be protected against any environmental temperature changes. Alterations in temperature change metabolic requirements, so this should be monitored carefully. Wounds, intravenous cannulae, invasive monitoring and catheters all require close attention as they may be destabilised during transit.

Equipment required for transfer

Assembly of equipment is an important aspect of transfer preparation. It is best practice for nursing staff to keep a checklist of what will be required (Box 7.2) and this should include a designated '**transfer bag**' to carry the smaller items. All of this equipment should be in **good working order**, **checked daily** and ready for immediate use. This avoids hasty gathering of materials, with the ever present risk of a significant omission and one that might only be discovered when a piece of equipment is needed urgently during the transfer process. All staff accompanying the acutely unwell patient during a transfer should be trained and competent in the use of the clinical equipment taken. In cases of malfunction, all problems experienced should be reported via clinical risk and auditing processes.

Communication

For all transfer procedures **effective communication** is of great importance and the nurse should ensure that the **patient**, **the family** and all **clinical personnel** involved are fully informed of events, including the specific reason for the transfer and the relevant timings such as departure and expected arrival. The transferring team will continue to have full responsibility for the patient until they have given the receiving team a detailed **verbal handover** accompanied by all the **relevant documentation**. SBAR, a recommended tool for a systematic clinical handover, should be used. A **don't forget** summary is included as a useful final checklist.

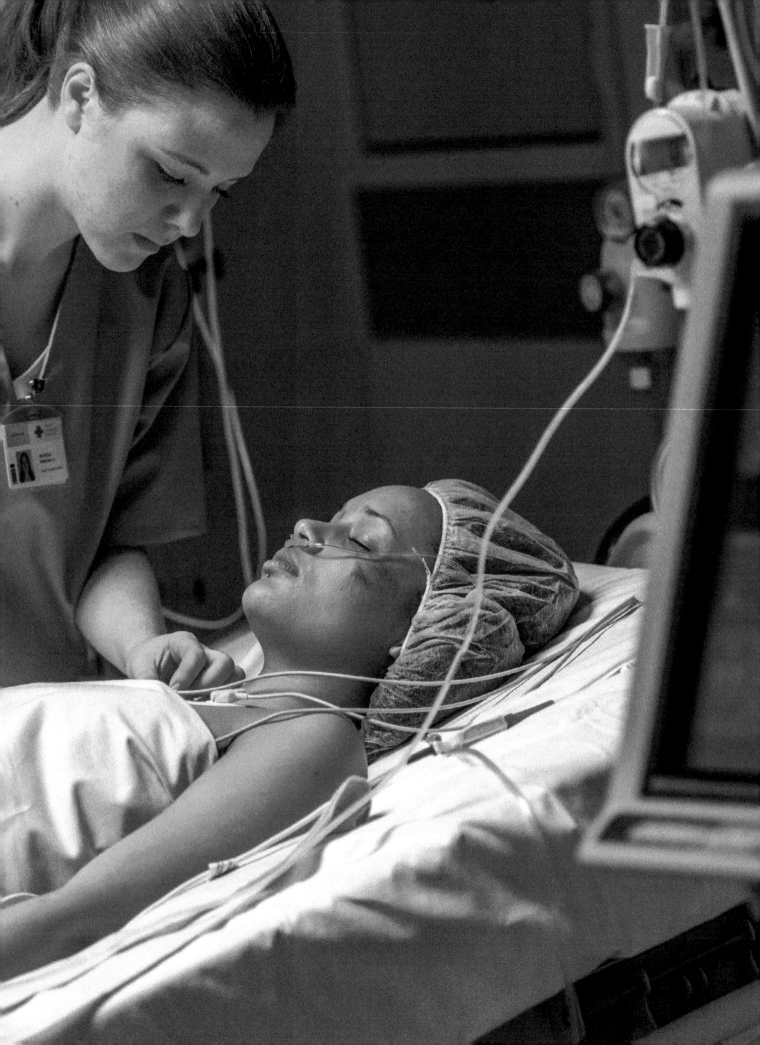

Airway: maintaining airway patency

Part 2

Chapters

8   Upper airway: assessment and management   18
9   Advanced airway management   20
10   Airway management: tracheostomy   22

8 Upper airway: assessment and management

Figure 8.1 The respiratory tract, showing the upper and lower airway structures. Source: Peate I. and Nair M., 2011. Reproduced with permission of John Wiley & Sons.

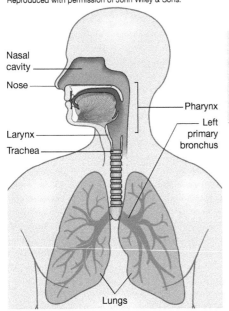

Nasal cavity
Nose
Pharynx
Larynx
Trachea
Left primary bronchus
Lungs

Upper airway: consists of the nasopharynx, oropharynx and laryngopharynx (nose, oral cavity, pharynx and larynx)

Lower airways: consist of the trachea, bronchi and bronchioles

Pharyngeal tonsil
Nasopharynx
Palatine tonsil
Oropharynx
Epiglottis
Laryngopharynx
Oesophagus
Trachea
External naris
Tongue
Lingual tonsil
Hyoid bone
Thyroid cartilage
Larynx
Cricoid cartilage
Thyroid gland

Figure 8.2 Upper airway obstruction. Source: Leach R.M., 2014. Reproduced with permission of John Wiley & Sons.

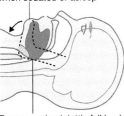

Chin (mandible) falls back when sedated or asleep

Tongue and epiglottis fall back to the posterior pharyngeal wall occluding the airway

Figure 8.3 Opening the airway (a) head tilt chin lift and (b) jaw thrust

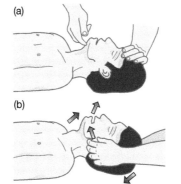

(a)

(b)

Figure 8.4 Recovery position

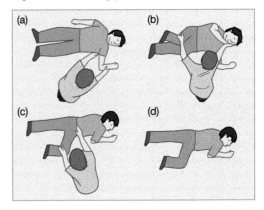

(a)   (b)

(c)   (d)

Figure 8.5 RCUK choking algorithm. Source: Resuscitation Council (UK). Reproduced with the kind permission of the Resuscitation Council (UK).

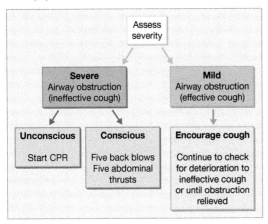

Assess severity

Severe
Airway obstruction (ineffective cough)

Mild
Airway obstruction (effective cough)

Unconscious
Start CPR

Conscious
Five back blows
Five abdominal thrusts

Encourage cough
Continue to check for deterioration to ineffective cough or until obstruction relieved

Figure 8.6 Removal of foreign body obstruction. Source: Leach R.M., 2014. Reproduced with permission of John Wiley & Sons.

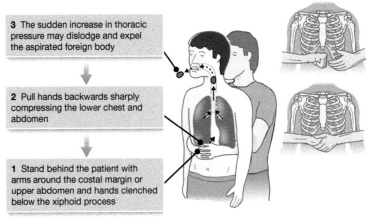

3 The sudden increase in thoracic pressure may dislodge and expel the aspirated foreign body

2 Pull hands backwards sharply compressing the lower chest and abdomen

1 Stand behind the patient with arms around the costal margin or upper abdomen and hands clenched below the xiphoid process

Acute and Critical Care Nursing at a Glance, First Edition. Edited by Helen Dutton and Jacqui Finch
© 2018 John Wiley & Sons, Ltd. Published 2018 by John Wiley & Sons, Ltd.
Companion website: www.ataglanceseries.com/nursing/acutecare

Upper airway structure and function

The upper airway is the route by which air first travels from the environment into the trachea, then through the lower airways into the lungs, in order for gaseous exchange to occur (Figure 8.1). Assessment of the upper airway is A of the ABCDE assessment and has priority as airway problems can quickly lead to deterioration, with complete airway obstruction leading to death within a few minutes. Any airway problems must be recognised and dealt with promptly by appropriately trained and competent healthcare practitioners. The upper airway (Figure 8.1) comprises the nose, oral cavity, pharynx and larynx. The primary functions of the upper airway are:

- To conduct air from the environment to the lower airways.
- To warm and humidify inspired air.
- To prevent foreign particles from entering the lower airways.

Airway assessment

If the **upper airway** becomes obstructed due to swelling or the presence of a foreign body, hypoxia, respiratory arrest and death will occur quickly unless prompt action is taken. Assessment of the airway is always the first procedure to be carried out in any acute situation. The airway may become partially obstructed or completely obstructed. Accurate assessment and recognition of the problem will determine the appropriate and effective action to take.

The best approach to airway assessment is first of all to **look** at the person: their pattern of breathing and whether they are conscious. If they are conscious, are they able to speak? Ability to speak indicates the airway is patent as air is able to pass over the vocal cords. Whilst reassuring, the ability to speak does not necessarily mean all is well, as there may be a degree of partial obstruction. Similarly, a lack of verbal response does not always indicate an obstructed airway. Take note of any abnormal skin colour and use of accessory muscles that could indicate partial obstruction. Assess further for partial obstruction and presence of normal breathing by **listening** for breath sounds.

Partial airway obstruction is *noisy* and could include:

- Inspiratory stridor – caused by obstruction at, or above, the larynx.
- Gurgling – suggests liquid in the upper airway.
- Snoring – the pharynx is semi-occluded by the tongue.
- Crowing or stridor – caused by laryngeal spasm or obstruction.
- Expiratory wheeze – suggests constriction or spasm of the lower airways.

Complete airway obstruction is *silent* and may result in paradoxical or 'see-saw' breathing, as attempts are made to draw in air: the chest is drawn in and the abdomen distends. The opposite occurs on exhalation.

Causes of airway obstruction

The airway can become obstructed either by external pressure or internal blockage of some kind, often requiring surgery. These more uncommon causes of external obstruction include:

- Swelling of the soft tissues of the neck.
- Tumours of the neck.
- Enlarged thyroid or local lymph glands.
- Physical pressure on the neck (strangulation).

It is more usual for the cause of the acute obstruction to be internal for example:

- Blockage by vomit, blood secretions or an inhaled foreign body (removed by suctioning, removal of foreign body and/or positioning).

- Swelling of the airway such as in allergic responses.
- Blockage by the tongue in the unconscious casualty.

One of the most common causes of acute airway obstruction is the patient's tongue. When unconscious, if the patient is supine the tongue will slip backwards occluding the airway (Figure 8.2) due to the fact that the muscles which hold the tongue in place are completely relaxed and the normal reflex responses which protect the airway are absent. In this situation the airway can be maintained by simple airway manoeuvres.

Maintaining the airway

With any upper airway problems, whether complete or partial obstruction, help must be summoned urgently as this is a medical emergency.

The unconscious patient

The head-tilt-chin-lift manoeuvre is the easiest to perform. Bringing the head back, and the chin up as shown (Figure 8.3a), results in the tongue moving away from the back of the throat. This action opens the airway enabling the patient to breathe spontaneously, or for rescue breaths to be performed.

By moving the lower jaw forward, the jaw thrust technique has the same effect (Figure 8.3b), but is achieved without flexing the neck. It is therefore the technique of choice in suspected neck injuries. Two people will be required to perform the jaw thrust technique and rescue breaths, whereas one person can perform rescue breaths and maintain the airway with the head-tilt-chin-lift manoeuvre.

Maintaining an open airway with these techniques is effective but needs to be applied continuously to the unconscious breathing casualty. The risk of regurgitation of stomach contents with secondary airway blockage and/or aspiration remains. Therefore, in a conscious but breathing casualty, in absence of any other injury or contraindication, the recovery position is the safest way to protect the airway (Figure 8.4). The recovery position allows maintenance of the airway whilst at the same time allowing drainage of any fluid from the mouth.

Airway obstruction due to a foreign body

The inhalation of a foreign body, causing a physical obstruction, is another acute cause of airway obstruction. With foreign body airway obstruction (FBAO) the correct response is outlined in the Resuscitation Council UK's choking algorithm (Figure 8.5).[1] This involves assessing the severity of the problem initially. If the patient is able to cough, the first action should be to encourage coughing with the person sitting or standing upright and leaning slightly forward. If the casualty is unable to cough, but is still conscious, then up to five back blows should be given. If these do not relieve the obstruction then abdominal thrusts should be performed as shown in Figure 8.6. This inward and upward motion with the fists positioned just underneath the diaphragm increases intrathoracic pressure and hopefully results in the foreign body being forcibly expelled. If at any stage the patient is unconscious then immediate help should be summoned, and if breathing also ceases, cardiopulmonary resuscitation should be commenced.

Advanced airway management

Figure 9.1 Oral suction using a wide bore suction device

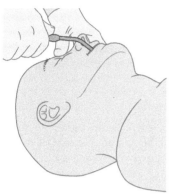

Figure 9.2 Oropharyngeal airway

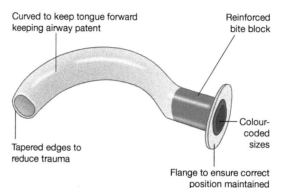

Curved to keep tongue forward keeping airway patent

Reinforced bite block

Colour-coded sizes

Tapered edges to reduce trauma

Flange to ensure correct position maintained

Figure 9.3 Nasopharyngeal airway

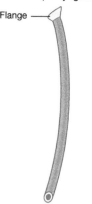

Flange

Figure 9.4 Sizing of oropharyngeal airway

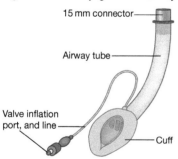

Figure 9.5 Oropharyngeal airway (OPA) insertion

(a)

(b)

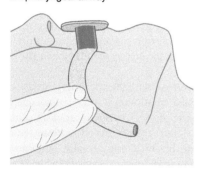
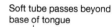
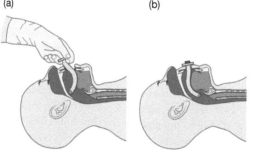

Open patient's mouth Insert OPA with the tip facing the roof of the mouth

Guide OPA past the tongue rotating 180° so the tip faces downwards

Figure 9.6 The nasopharyngeal airway (NPA) sits just above the epiglottis. Source: Leach R.M., 2014. Reproduced with permission of John Wiley & Sons.

Soft tube passes beyond base of tongue

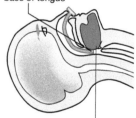

Tongue held forward providing a channel for air passage or air can pass through the airway

Figure 9.7 The laryngeal mask airway

15 mm connector

Airway tube

Valve inflation port, and line

Cuff

Figure 9.8 The laryngeal mask airway *in situ*

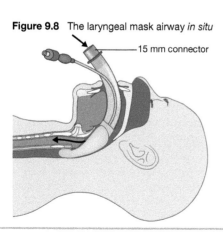

15 mm connector

Figure 9.9 Endotracheal tube (ETT) *in situ*

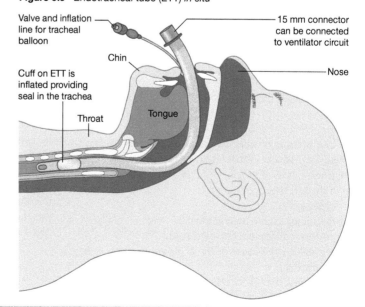

Valve and inflation line for tracheal balloon

Chin

Cuff on ETT is inflated providing seal in the trachea

Throat

Tongue

15 mm connector can be connected to ventilator circuit

Nose

Acute and Critical Care Nursing at a Glance, First Edition. Edited by Helen Dutton and Jacqui Finch
© 2018 John Wiley & Sons, Ltd. Published 2018 by John Wiley & Sons, Ltd.
Companion website: www.ataglanceseries.com/nursing/acutecare

Assessment and maintenance of a safe and open airway remains the top priority in all acute situations.[1] Systematic assessment continues throughout the acute phase of deterioration and beyond, to enable recognition and prioritise management of ongoing and new problems. Once the airway is open it must be maintained effectively in order to ensure adequate ventilation for oxygenation of vital organs and tissues.

Ensuring a clear airway

If the patient is unable to maintain a clear or safe airway independently, it should be opened using the techniques described in Chapter 8. If the airway is obstructed or at risk of obstruction due to blood, vomit or secretions, gentle oral suction should be applied using a wide bore oral suction device (Figure 9.1). When carrying out this procedure do not advance the catheter into the oropharynx as this causes gagging and vomiting, further compounding the problem.

Maintaining the airway with adjuncts

Simple airway adjuncts such as the oropharyngeal airway (OPA) (Figure 9.2) and nasopharyngeal airway (NPA) (Figure 9.3) can be helpful in maintaining an open airway, but should only be inserted by healthcare staff who are trained and competent to do so. Once inserted they help maintain airway patency and are used in conjunction with the pocket mask or bag valve mask devices as an aid to ventilation as necessary.

Oropharyngeal airway

Oropharyngeal airways come in a variety of sizes from infant to adult and ensuring the correct size is important. If it is too big it can obstruct the airway or cause trauma. OPAs should only be used in an unconscious patient, as in a conscious person their insertion can stimulate the gag reflex and induce vomiting.

To ensure the correct size, the bite block should be placed at the level of the incisors and it should reach to the angle of the jaw (Figure 9.4). The airway is inserted upside down and then turned 180° once contact has been made with the back of the throat (Figure 9.5). Once in situ the OPA can assist with the maintenance of the airway and enables access to the oropharynx with a fine bore flexible suction catheter, to clear secretions if required.

Nasopharyngeal airway

The NPA is useful for awake or conscious patients as it does not stimulate the gag reflex. It is inserted into the nasal passageway and sits just above the epiglottis, separating the soft palate from the wall of the oropharynx and maintaining airway patency (Figure 9.6).
• Select the correct size of NPA by measuring from the patient's earlobe to the tip of the nostril.
• The nostril should be inspected for polyps prior to insertion, and if necessary the other nostril used.
• A water-based lubricant is used prior to insertion.
• Insert gently, as trauma and bleeding can occur in around 30% of insertions. If resistance is felt do not continue, try the other nostril.
• When inserted the flange should rest just below the patient's nostril.

NPAs can facilitate removal of secretions in patients who have a weak cough, as a suction catheter can be passed down into the lower airway. NPAs should not be used in the case of head trauma until the possibility of a fractured base of skull has been ruled out. **Even with an OPA or NPA in situ the airway can obstruct if the head is not correctly positioned.**

Artificial airways

It is sometimes necessary to insert a more long-term device if airway maintenance and management is likely to be prolonged or there is a need to overcome an airway obstruction. OPAs ensure a patent airway, but give no protection from aspiration of vomit or secretions. Aspiration is defined as the inhalation of either oropharyngeal or gastric contents into the lower airways. Gastric acid causes inflammation of the lung tissue or pneumonitis. Bacteria aspirated from the oropharynx cause a bacterial pneumonia. Both of these lung problems are associated with significant mortality. The insertion of an artificial airway ensures a secure airway and protection from aspiration. Artificial airways enable tracheobronchial suction, removal of secretions and artificial ventilation.

Laryngeal mask airway

The laryngeal mask airway (LMA) is a supraglottic airway device (Figure 9.7). This means it is placed above the level of the **glottis** (Figure 9.8). It is often used in the emergency setting to enable establishment of a secure airway relatively quickly and easily. It is also used for more prolonged airway management, in addition to tracheal suction to remove secretions, and effective ventilation. The LMA consists of a large tube with an elliptical mask on the distal end. This mask's inflatable cuff covers the tracheal opening covering the supraglottic structures and allows isolation of the trachea from the oesophagus, reducing risk of aspiration. There are a number of benefits of LMAs:
• They are relatively easy to use and quick to place, even for the less experienced clinician. Despite this they should only be inserted by healthcare staff trained and competent in their use.
• LMA use results in less gastric distension when used in conjunction with bag-valve-mask as opposed to a facemask for ventilation.
• Due to the isolation of the trachea, the risk of aspiration is significantly reduced although not entirely eliminated.

LMAs are used in patients who are unconscious or heavily sedated.

Endotracheal tube intubation

The placement of an **endotracheal tube** (ETT) is considered the 'gold standard' in terms of establishing a secure artificial airway (Figure 9.9). The inflated cuff on the ETT provides a seal to prevent gastric or oropharyngeal contents entering the lung, so the airway is kept patent and protected from the risk of aspiration. Endotracheal suction removes secretions. ETTs may be inserted nasally or orally. The oral route is common in an acute situation but may be contraindicated in situations of oral trauma. Nasal intubation is used when required over a longer period of time, as it enables effective oral hygiene to be carried out. Intubation with an ETT enables positive pressure ventilation to be established. Intubated patients will be cared for in an ICU by staff who are competent in caring for ventilated patients.

Insertion of an ETT is highly skilled and should only be attempted by those trained and experienced in the technique. Both LMAs and ETTs are used in patients who are unconscious or heavily sedated. Therefore, the long-term management of both requires specialist skills and knowledge to ensure patient safety.

10 Airway management: tracheostomy

Figure 10.1 Location of tracheostomy site, tube and anatomical landmarks

- Epiglottis
- Larynx
- Vocal cords
- Thyroid cartilage
- Cricoid cartilage
- Trachea
- Oesophagus
- Tracheostomy site
- Tracheostomy tube

Flange of trache tube: ties attached here to secure tube in place

Cricothyroid membrane: mini tracheostomy may be formed here

Tracheal tube inflated cuff to prevent aspiration

Box 10.1 Common reasons for a tracheostomy

- Airway maintenance
- Airway protection
- To enable suctioning of secretions
- Weaning from ventilation

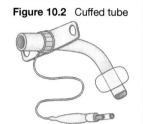

Figure 10.2 Cuffed tube

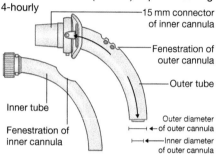

Figure 10.3 Fenestrated tube with inner cannula. Inner tube (cannula) requires cleaning 4-hourly

- 15 mm connector of inner cannula
- Fenestration of outer cannula
- Outer tube
- Inner tube
- Fenestration of inner cannula
- Outer diameter of outer cannula
- Inner diameter of outer cannula

Figure 10.4 Emergency tracheostomy management – patent upper airway.
Source: McGrath B.A., et al., 2012. Reproduced with permission from Blackwell Publishing Ltd.

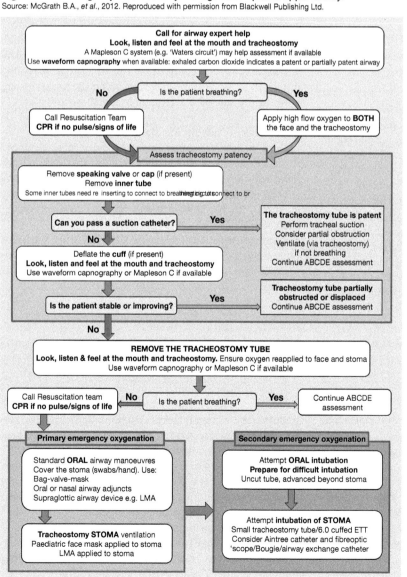

Call for airway expert help
Look, listen and feel at the mouth and tracheostomy
A Mapleson C system (e.g. 'Waters circuit') may help assessment if available
Use **waveform capnography** when available: exhaled carbon dioxide indicates a patent or partially patent airway

Is the patient breathing?

No → Call Resuscitation Team **CPR if no pulse/signs of life**

Yes → Apply high flow oxygen to **BOTH** the face and the tracheostomy

Assess tracheostomy patency

Remove **speaking valve** or **cap** (if present)
Remove **inner tube**
Some inner tubes need re inserting to connect to breathing circuit

Can you pass a suction catheter?

Yes → The tracheostomy tube is patent
Perform tracheal suction
Consider partial obstruction
Ventilate (via tracheostomy)
if not breathing
Continue ABCDE assessment

No ↓

Deflate the **cuff** (if present)
Look, listen and feel at the mouth and tracheostomy
Use waveform capnography or Mapleson C if available

Is the patient stable or improving?

Yes → Tracheostomy tube partially obstructed or displaced
Continue ABCDE assessment

No ↓

REMOVE THE TRACHEOSTOMY TUBE
Look, listen & feel at the mouth and tracheostomy. Ensure oxygen reapplied to face and stoma
Use waveform capnography or Mapleson C if available

Call Resuscitation team **CPR if no pulse/signs of life** ← No — **Is the patient breathing?** — Yes → Continue ABCDE assessment

Primary emergency oxygenation

Standard **ORAL** airway manoeuvres
Cover the stoma (swabs/hand). Use:
Bag-valve-mask
Oral or nasal airway adjuncts
Supraglottic airway device e.g. LMA

Tracheostomy STOMA ventilation
Paediatric face mask applied to stoma
LMA applied to stoma

Secondary emergency oxygenation

Attempt **ORAL** intubation
Prepare for difficult intubation
Uncut tube, advanced beyond stoma

Attempt **intubation of STOMA**
Small tracheostomy tube/6.0 cuffed ETT
Consider Aintree catheter and fibreoptic 'scope/Bougie/airway exchange catheter

Box 10.2 Bedside equipment for all tracheostomy patients (and for patient transfer). Source: Intensive Care Society, 2014.

- Suction unit, Yankauer sucker and suction catheters
- Tracheostomy disconnection wedge
- Non-powdered latex free gloves, aprons and eye protection
- Rebreathe bag and tubing, catheter mount or connector
- Spare tracheostomy tubes, same size and size smaller
- 10 mL syringe if tube cuffed
- Tracheal dilators
- Resuscitation equipment

Ongoing care equipment
- Humidification equipment
- Scissors if tube sutured
- Call bell
- Clean pot for spare cannula
- Water-soluble lubricating jelly
- Communication aids
- Sterile water for cleaning suction tube
- Sterile dressing pack
- Bedside equipment checklist

Hints and tips: tracheostomy wound care

- Secretions that collect above the cuff ooze out of the stoma site leading to possible excoriation and infection. The site should be assessed an stoma cleaned once a day using a clean technique
- Red, excoriated or exuding stomas should have swabs sent for culture

Red flag events

- Pain at tracheostomy site
- Visibly displaced tube
- Bleeding
- Suction catheter not passing easily into trachea
- Cuffed tracheostomy patient being able to talk, or bubbles coming from upper airways
- Frequent need to reinflate cuff to prevent air leaks
- Respiratory distress, difficulty in breathing
- Surgical emphysema (air in the soft tissues)
- Aspirating feed from trachea (cuff not functioning)

Acute and Critical Care Nursing at a Glance, First Edition. Edited by Helen Dutton and Jacqui Finch
© 2018 John Wiley & Sons, Ltd. Published 2018 by John Wiley & Sons, Ltd.
Companion website: www.ataglanceseries.com/nursing/acutecare

Atracheostomy is a surgical procedure to create an artificial opening (stoma) in the anterior wall of the trachea, just below the cricoid cartilage. A small and curved tracheostomy tube is placed into the trachea, via the newly created stoma, sitting just above the level of the **carina** (Figure 10.1). Up to 15 000 tracheostomies are performed each year in England with common indications given in Box 10.1. Most patients have their tracheal tubes removed (known as decannulation) prior to discharge from ITU/HDU to the ward environment. However, this is not always possible. The Intensive Care Society (2014)[1,] informed by the National Confidential Enquiry into Patient Outcome and Death (NCEPOD) (2014)[2,] published standards and guidelines for the care of adult patients with a temporary tracheostomy, to inform safe practice in any care setting.

Tracheostomies

The majority of tracheostomies will be planned, using a variety of approaches, depending on the reasons for tracheostomy formation:

• A **surgical tracheostomy** is performed in a theatre environment by a surgeon for patients with difficult anatomy who require permanent or long-term airway protection. This type of tracheostomy can be permanent or temporary.

• A **percutaneous tracheostomy** is temporary. This procedure is usually performed in critical care by an anaesthetist. A small hole is made and dilated using specialised equipment, until the tracheostomy tube can be inserted. Usually the site heals more quickly and with less scarring than surgical tracheostomy.

A **cricothyroid/mini-tracheostomy** is formed in the relatively avascular cricothyroid membrane (Figure 10.1). A small diameter tube, which is uncuffed, is inserted using a guidewire and dilator. A mini tracheal tube is sufficient to remove excessive bronchial secretions with a narrow 10F suction catheter, thereby relieving sputum retention.

Types of tracheostomy tubes

Staff caring for a patient with a tracheostomy **must know the type of tube in place** and this should be **clearly documented in the patient's notes** and care plan. **Cuffed tracheostomy tubes** (Figure 10.2), when inflated, provide a seal in the trachea to protect the lungs. Air does not pass through the upper airway, but through the tube. An **uncuffed tracheostomy tube** allows air to move through and around the tracheostomy tube. **Fenestrated tracheostomy tubes** have holes in the outer cannula (Figure 10.3) allowing air to pass through vocal cords in the upper airway, and the patient to speak. Most tracheostomy tubes will have an inner tube that is regularly removed for cleaning (Figure 10.3).

Tracheostomy tube: care issues

• **Emergency protocols must be in place to maintain a patent upper airway: nurses must be familiar and competent with guidelines (Figure 10.4)** in the case of a blocked upper airway or tracheostomy tube.[3]

• **Essential tracheostomy equipment** must be at the patient's bedside at all times (Box 10.2).

• **Humidification is essential** for patients with a temporary tracheostomy, using regular nebulisers, humidifier systems or heat moisture exchanger (HME). Inadequate humidification may lead to **life-threatening blockage** of **the tracheostomy tube**.

• **Inner cannulae** must be regularly changed and cleaned 4-hourly (Figure 10.3) according to trust guidance, to maintain patency.

• **Cuff pressure** should not exceed 25 cm H_2O, as above this permanent damage to the trachea can occur. An air leak may be heard as a squeaking sound. If this occurs with the cuff pressure at 25 cm H_2O, the tube may have become displaced or require changing, and immediate expert review is required.

• **Communication**. Following a tracheostomy procedure, the patient will be temporarily unable to speak. Communication boards and signing can be frustrating and tiring, so time and encouragement is required. Verbal communication is possible with a speaking valve placed on either an uncuffed tube, or a fenestrated tube with the cuff down. It is essential that the **cuff is deflated prior to speaking valve placement** as failure to do so will cause airway occlusion. If the patient exhibits **signs of respiratory distress** or they are unable to vocalise, the **speaking valve must be removed immediately** and the cause of the problem identified.

• **Regular suction** removes secretions which can be aspirated from the end of the tube in shallow suctioning. Deeper tube suction requires an appropriately trained and competent practitioner.

• The **tracheostomy site** must be cleaned and dressed daily (see hints and tips box).

• **Tracheostomy tube change** must occur as necessary as a planned procedure; those with inner tubes can remain for a maximum of 30 days. Only **staff trained and competent to change tracheostomy tubes** should do so. Nurses must adhere to trust policies and procedures when carrying out any clinical procedures.

Cuff deflation

An inflated cuff compresses the oesophagus making swallowing difficult. The decision to allow feeding with a deflated cuff should be made after a swallowing assessment, with the patient monitored for any evidence of aspiration. Before cuff deflation, the patient is warned about the alterations in tracheal airflow sensation and that they may need to cough. If coughing persists, and is not resolved with suction and reassurance, the cuff must be re-inflated. On cuff deflation the tracheostomy tube should be occluded briefly with a clean, gloved finger to check that air is flowing around the tube.

Tracheostomy red flags

Red flags are used as a warning signal that a problem needs to be urgently dealt with (see red flag box). All staff caring for patients with a tracheostomy need to be aware of these signs.

Weaning

Weaning is a planned process completed under the instruction of a clinical expert, involving increasing the periods of time the cuff is deflated. A **decannulation cap** is placed on a fenestrated tracheostomy tube with deflated cuff, effectively blocking the tracheostomy tube opening. The decannulation cap should only to be used with a fenestrated inner tube in place. The decision to remove the tube is made by the multidisciplinary team, with one person having overall responsibility. This is very important for ward-based patients who may not always be under the direct care of the critical care team.

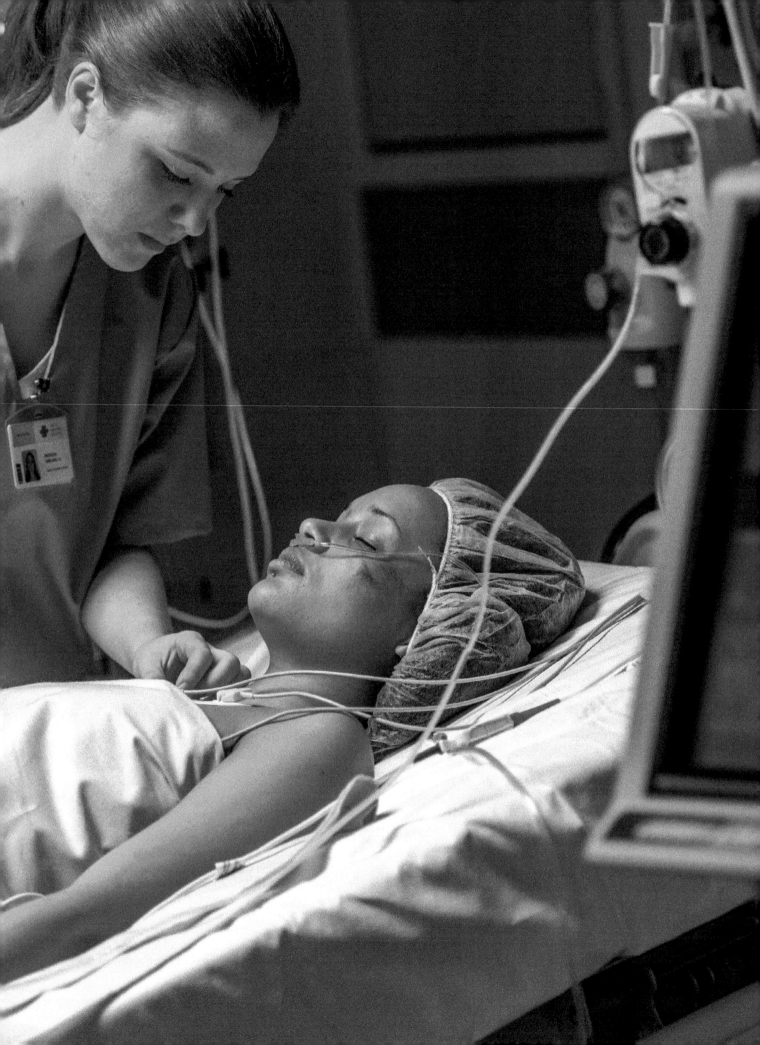

Breathing: patients with breathing problems

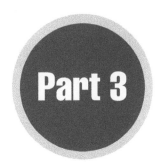

Part 3

Chapters

11 Respiratory physiology: oxygenation   26
12 Respiratory physiology: ventilation   28
13 Assessment of breathing   30
14 Respiratory investigations   32
15 Oxygen therapy   34
16 Respiratory failure   36
17 Breathing problems: obstructive disorders   38
18 Breathing problems: lung (parenchymal)
    disorders   40
19 Breathing problems: pleural disorders   42
20 Respiratory support: non-invasive ventilation   44
21 Principles of thoracic surgery   46

11 Respiratory physiology: oxygenation

Figure 11.1 The movement of oxygen

Atmosphere
PO_2 = 5.3 kPa

Alveoli
PAO_2 = 14 kPa

Remember:
PAO_2 : partial pressure of oxygen in the alveoli
PaO_2 : partial pressure of oxygen in arterial blood
PvO_2 : partial pressure of oxygen in venous blood

Venous blood
PvO_2 = 5.3 kPa
14.5 mL/100 mL

Oxygen moves down pressure gradient from atmosphere to cells

Arterial blood
PaO_2 = 13.5 kPa
19.5 mL/100 mL

19.5 mL – 5 mL/100 mL

Cells
PO_2 = 5.3 kPa

Mitochondrion
Ribosomes
Nucleus
Cell membrane
Nuclear membrane
Cytoplasm

Oxygen is used by the **mitochondria** in the cell to produce ATP. CO_2 and water are waste products of this metabolism

Table 11.1 Partial pressures of atmospheric and alveolar gases (approximate)

Atmospheric air composition Atmospheric pressure 101 kPa at sea level			Alveolar air
Gas	%	Partial pressure	Partial pressure
Oxygen (O_2)	21	21.2 kPa	14 kPa
Nitrogen (N_2)	76	76.7 kPa	77 kPa
Carbon dioxide (CO_2)	0.04	0.04 kPa	5.3 kPa
Water vapour			6.0 kPa

Figure 11.5 Ventilation perfusion relationships

1 Normal V̇/Q̇ — Well ventilated / Well perfused

2 High V̇/Q̇ Alveolar dead space — Well ventilated / Poorly perfused

3 Low V̇/Q̇ Right to left shunt — Poorly ventilated / Well perfused

4 Silent unit — Poorly ventilated / Poorly perfused

Figure 11.2 Gaseous exchange across the alveolar capillary membrane

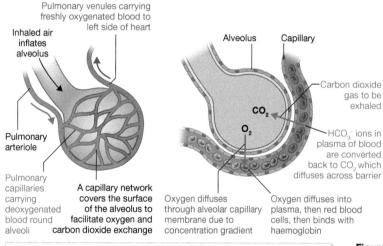

Pulmonary venules carrying freshly oxygenated blood to left side of heart

Inhaled air inflates alveolus

Alveolus
Capillary

Pulmonary arteriole

CO_2
O_2

Carbon dioxide gas to be exhaled

HCO_3^- ions in plasma of blood are converted back to CO_2 which diffuses across barrier

Pulmonary capillaries carrying deoxygenated blood round alveoli

A capillary network covers the surface of the alveolus to facilitate oxygen and carbon dioxide exchange

Oxygen diffuses through alveolar capillary membrane due to concentration gradient

Oxygen diffuses into plasma, then red blood cells, then binds with haemoglobin

Figure 11.3 The red blood cell, haemoglobin and oxygen transport

O_2 molecule

Haem unit with iron atom

Red blood cells contain haemoglobin (Hb). One molecule of Hb carries four molecules of oxygen when fully saturated

Deoxygenated haemoglobin is blue in colour

Haemoglobin fully saturated with oxygen (oxyhaemoglobin) is bright red in colour

Figure 11.4 Transport of carbon dioxide

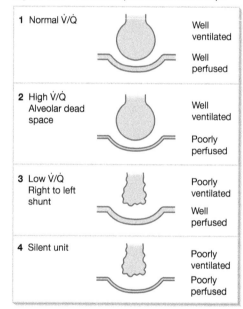

$$CO_2 + H_2O \longleftrightarrow H_2CO_3 \longleftrightarrow HCO_3^- + H^+$$

Carbon dioxide + water   **Carbonic acid**   **Bicarbonate + hydrogen ion**

CO_2 from cellular metabolism dissolves in plasma

Equation moves to the right

Once in the pulmonary capillary the equation moves to the left

CO_2 is transported as carbonic acid and bicarbonate in the red blood cell, and some in the plasma which is transported to the lung

CO_2 is reformed and diffuses into alveoli, where it is exhaled (see Figure 11.2)

Most of the CO_2 is carried in the red blood cells, due to the enzyme carbonic anhydrase which speeds up the reaction

Acute and Critical Care Nursing at a Glance, First Edition. Edited by Helen Dutton and Jacqui Finch
© 2018 John Wiley & Sons, Ltd. Published 2018 by John Wiley & Sons, Ltd.
Companion website: www.ataglanceseries.com/nursing/acutecare

The respiratory system's function is to ensure that oxygen enters the arterial blood so that it can be transported to tissues and organs. Oxygen (O_2) is required for the breakdown of glucose into the energy essential for cellular function. This process of **aerobic metabolism** occurs in the mitochondria of the cell, producing energy in the form of **adenosine triphosphate (ATP)**. Carbon dioxide (CO_2) is the waste product of this metabolism and is removed by the lungs in the process of ventilation. Some cells can cope with periods of **anaerobic metabolism** (without O_2) (e.g. skeletal muscle), but even short periods without O_2 is detrimental for other cells (brain/myocardium). The principles described in this chapter can seem a little complex, but if understood can greatly enhance understanding of the factors that influence effective oxygen delivery to the tissues. Acutely unwell patients experience physiological stress, often with increased oxygen requirements that require prompt treatment, to prevent clinical deterioration.

Transport of oxygen

Atmospheric air is a mixture of gases (Table 11.1) with each gas exerting a partial pressure in kilopascals (kPa) contributing to the total atmospheric pressure of 101 kPa at sea level. Atmospheric air moves through the upper and lower airways on inspiration, arriving at the alveoli, where gaseous exchange takes place. Alveolar air composition alters due to mixing with expired CO_2 and the addition of water vapour in the moist lung environment.

Gases move down a pressure gradient by **diffusion**; this is from an area of higher partial pressure, to an area of lower partial pressure. Oxygen moves from the atmosphere to the alveoli by bulk flow, then diffuses into the blood and body cells (Figure 11.1). The partial pressure of O_2 in venous blood (PvO_2), returning via the right side of the heart to the pulmonary capillary, is lower than the alveolar partial pressure of oxygen (PAO_2). Oxygen diffuses across the alveolar capillary membrane until **equilibrium** is reached. CO_2 moves by similar principles from pulmonary capillary blood to alveolar air (Figure 11.2). Given the millions of alveoli, each having a pulmonary capillary, there is an extensive surface area for diffusion of gases across the alveolar capillary membrane. Note that the partial pressure of oxygen in arterial blood (PaO_2) is at slightly lower pressure than PAO_2 (alveolar air), as some bronchial venous blood is drained into the left ventricle (this is a normal anatomical shunt). Diffusion across the alveolar capillary membrane is mainly influenced by oxygen percentage/partial pressure of alveoli air and the surface area of the lung. Diffusion is reduced when the alveolar membrane is thickened, the alveoli have filled with fluid/pus (as in pneumonia) or have collapsed (as in pneumothorax or atelectasis).

Oxyhaemoglobin

Once in the blood, oxygen is carried as **oxyhaemoglobin**. One molecule of **haemoglobin (Hb)** can carry four molecules of oxygen (Figure 11.3) and when this is so, the Hb is fully saturated. This is measured by pulse oximetry (SpO_2), which measures oxygen saturation of capillary blood. Normal values lay between 94 and 98%. Although oxygen has a great affinity for Hb the nurse must ensure that breathing is effective, and consider adding supplemental oxygen according to prescription if SpO_2 falls below the normal range identified for the patient.

Oxygen capacity

It is strange to think of oxygen in terms of millilitres, but this gives an accurate picture of the oxygen content of the blood, so important for tissue oxygenation. Each gram of Hb can carry 1.39 mL of oxygen; in an adult with an Hb of 150 g/L (or 15 g per 100 mL of arterial blood), approximately 20 mL of oxygen is carried (1.39 × 15) in each 100 mL (Figure 11.1). This is the oxygen capacity of arterial blood. Given a cardiac output of 5000 mL per minute, this is a delivery of 1000 mL of oxygen per minute (DO_2). In health and at rest only 250 mL is extracted by the cells each minute.

Oxygen delivery

Oxygen delivery will depend not only on oxygen saturation, but on Hb levels and cardiac output for each individual. Hb needs to be measured, as a low Hb (e.g. from blood loss) reduces the amount of oxygen in arterial blood, reducing oxygen delivery to the tissues, even with a normal SpO_2. The cardiac output is the means of delivering oxygen; if this is reduced (e.g. as a result of hypovolaemia or heart failure), oxygen delivery will be impaired. Patients with breathing difficulties, anaemia, or reduced cardiac output will all have compromised oxygen delivery, with potential organ damage occurring due to lack of oxygen (tissue hypoxia).

Transport of carbon dioxide

CO_2 is produced at cellular level, as a by-product of metabolism. It also moves down a pressure gradient and is transported in the blood, dissolved in the plasma as carbonic acid (10%), carbamino protein (20%) and bicarbonate (70%), and in the red blood cells. The reversible equation (Figure 11.4) illustrates how CO_2 moves from cells to pulmonary capillary and how once in the pulmonary capillary, the equation moves from right to left so that CO_2 is then exhaled. Where **alveolar ventilation** is reduced, **hypercapnia** develops, as the CO_2 cannot be expelled sufficiently.

Ventilation and perfusion

The relationship between the amount of air reaching the alveoli or alveolar ventilation (V) and pulmonary capillary perfusion (Q) can influence oxygenation significantly. Effective alveolar ventilation is about 4 L/min, and perfusion (dependent on cardiac output), about 5 L/min. This facilitates good oxygenation across the alveolar capillary membrane. However, there can be significant changes to V/Q as a result of disease (Figure 11.5):
- Example 1: a normal V/Q relationship so that saturations will be within a normal range.
- Example 2: a high V/Q ratio with good ventilation but poor perfusion, possibly due to low cardiac output or pulmonary embolism.
- Example 3: a low V/Q ratio with poor ventilation and good perfusion. This is commonly seen where there are respiratory problems such as obstructive pulmonary disease, pneumonia or atelectasis. The blood which flows through a poorly ventilated unit returns to the left-side heart with a reduced oxygen saturation. **V/Q mismatch** usually responds well to supplemental oxygen therapy, as even though ventilation is reduced, the higher PAO_2, increases the diffusion gradient. A **right to left shunt** (no ventilation with blood bypassing the lung unit) does not respond well to oxygen therapy, as ventilation of that lung unit is absent.
- Example 4: poor ventilation and perfusion, occurring in critically ill patients with cardiac and pulmonary problems.

If risk of cellular hypoxia is to be avoided health care professionals need to consider the following:
- Pulmonary ventilation (maximising saturations).
- Haemoglobin levels and correction where necessary.
- Ensuring adequate cardiac output so oxygen is delivered effectively.

12 Respiratory physiology: ventilation

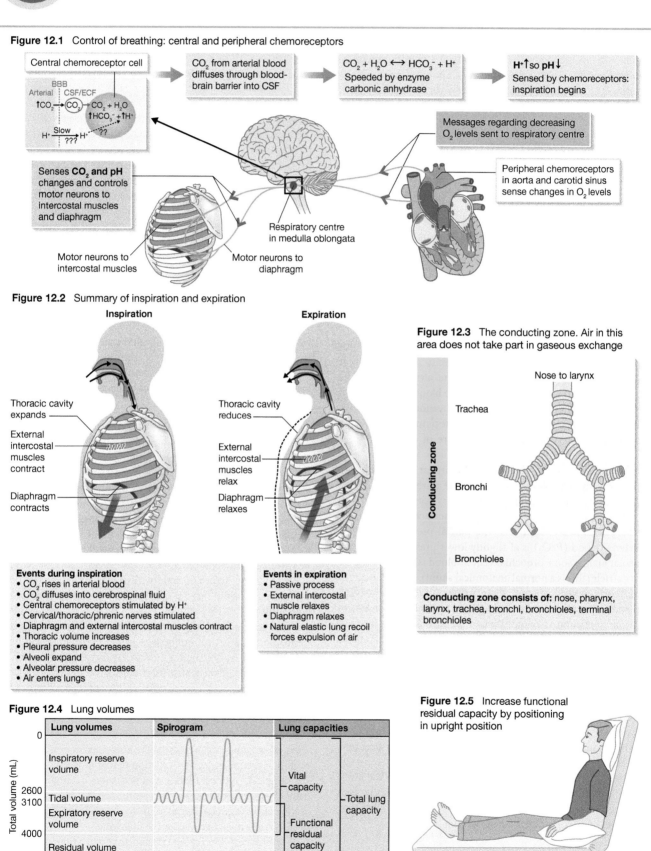

Figure 12.1 Control of breathing: central and peripheral chemoreceptors

Central chemoreceptor cell

BBB
Arterial | CSF/ECF
↑CO_2 → (CO_2) → CO_2 + H_2O
↑HCO_3^- +↑H^+
H^+ → Slow → H^+
??? ??

CO_2 from arterial blood diffuses through blood-brain barrier into CSF

CO_2 + H_2O ⟷ HCO_3^- + H^+
Speeded by enzyme carbonic anhydrase

H^+↑so pH↓
Sensed by chemoreceptors: inspiration begins

Messages regarding decreasing O_2 levels sent to respiratory centre

Senses **CO_2 and pH** changes and controls motor neurons to intercostal muscles and diaphragm

Peripheral chemoreceptors in aorta and carotid sinus sense changes in O_2 levels

Respiratory centre in medulla oblongata

Motor neurons to intercostal muscles

Motor neurons to diaphragm

Figure 12.2 Summary of inspiration and expiration

Inspiration

Expiration

Thoracic cavity expands

External intercostal muscles contract

Diaphragm contracts

Thoracic cavity reduces

External intercostal muscles relax

Diaphragm relaxes

Figure 12.3 The conducting zone. Air in this area does not take part in gaseous exchange

Nose to larynx

Trachea

Bronchi

Bronchioles

Conducting zone

Conducting zone consists of: nose, pharynx, larynx, trachea, bronchi, bronchioles, terminal bronchioles

Events during inspiration
• CO_2 rises in arterial blood
• CO_2 diffuses into cerebrospinal fluid
• Central chemoreceptors stimulated by H^+
• Cervical/thoracic/phrenic nerves stimulated
• Diaphragm and external intercostal muscles contract
• Thoracic volume increases
• Pleural pressure decreases
• Alveoli expand
• Alveolar pressure decreases
• Air enters lungs

Events in expiration
• Passive process
• External intercostal muscle relaxes
• Diaphragm relaxes
• Natural elastic lung recoil forces expulsion of air

Figure 12.4 Lung volumes

Lung volumes	Spirogram	Lung capacities
Inspiratory reserve volume		
Tidal volume		Vital capacity
Expiratory reserve volume		Total lung capacity
Residual volume		Functional residual capacity

Total volume (mL)
0
2600
3100
4000
5200

Figure 12.5 Increase functional residual capacity by positioning in upright position

Acute and Critical Care Nursing at a Glance, First Edition. Edited by Helen Dutton and Jacqui Finch
© 2018 John Wiley & Sons, Ltd. Published 2018 by John Wiley & Sons, Ltd.
Companion website: www.ataglanceseries.com/nursing/acutecare

Ventilation refers to the cyclical exchange of air in the lungs during inspiration and expiration and is crucial for gaseous exchange to occur. If ventilation is inadequate, then carbon dioxide can accumulate in the blood (hypercapnia) and oxygen levels fall (hypoxaemia). The nurse must be able to appreciate the factors that determine effective ventilation to be able to recognise when this is compromised, and take appropriate action.

Inspiration and expiration

Inspiration is a mechanical event clearly visible when counting respirations. Whilst this can be voluntary, breathing is regulated unconsciously by the **respiratory centre** situated in the **medulla oblongata** (Figure 12.1). Inspiration is initiated by rising levels of CO_2 in arterial blood. CO_2 diffuses into the cerebrospinal fluid (CSF) of the brain (cerebral ventricles), generating hydrogen (H) ions (Figure 12.1). Hydrogen ions stimulate the **central chemoreceptors** in the respiratory centre of the medulla oblongata. Peripheral chemoreceptors in the carotid artery and aorta also stimulate breathing but are more sensitive to falling PaO_2. Motor impulses generated by the respiratory centre travel along cervical, thoracic and diaphragmatic nerves initiating contraction of the diaphragm and external intercostal muscles, initiating inspiration (Figure 12.1). Thoracic expansion occurs as the rib cage is pulled upwards and outwards and the diaphragm descends (Figure 12.2). As intrapulmonary volume is increased the pressure becomes less than atmospheric pressure (<101 kPa) and air moves into the lungs by bulk flow. Expiration is passive as muscles relax and the lungs recoil inwards (Figure 12.2). In breathless patients, muscle contraction becomes excessive both during both inspiration and expiration.

Pulmonary ventilation (V_E) airways

Pulmonary or **minute volume** is expired total ventilation (V_E) per minute. At rest the volume inhaled with each breath is approximately 500 mL and is called the **tidal volume** (V_T). With a respiratory rate of around 12/min at rest, then the V_E is 6000 mL/min (500 × 12). However, not all this air is available for gaseous exchange as the last 150 mL of the V_T remains in the anatomical dead space (V_D) (**conducting zone,** Figure 12.3), **airway generations 0–16**. V_E can be increased considerably when required (to as much as 70 L) by increasing respiratory rate and V_T, but this utilises more energy and therefore more oxygen.

Alveolar ventilation (V_A)

This is the volume of air which is available for gaseous exchange in the respiratory bronchioles, where alveolar ducts and sacs are found. This **respiratory zone** consists of airway generations 17–23. V_A is calculated by first subtracting from the V_T the anatomical dead space volume (500 – 150 mL = 350 mL) and then multiplying by the respiratory rate (12):

$$\text{e.g. } (500 - 150 \text{ mL}) \times 12 = 4200 \text{ mL (or 4.2 L)}$$

Effective V_A ensures $PaCO_2$ and PaO_2 remain within normal range. Changes in tidal volume and/or respiratory rate will alter V_A. Where tidal volume decreases, for example as in hypoventilation, increased $PaCO_2$ will contribute to a fall in PaO_2. When V_A is halved then $PaCO_2$ doubles! Additional dead space may occur where, despite air entering an alveolus, there is no corresponding perfusion (no pulmonary capillary blood) in the area. This is called alveolar dead space and represents wasted ventilation and added to the **anatomical dead space** is called **physiological dead space**. This may increase considerably in pathological states such as pulmonary embolus or shock

Work of breathing

Normal breathing in health, with diaphragmatic contraction, requires very little ventilatory effort, accounting for only 3% of total energy expenditure. **Work of breathing** refers to the work/effort requires to breathe, and is made up of:

- **Resistance work.**
- **Compliance work.**

During inspiration, work is needed to drive air through the airways from the nose to respiratory bronchioles. Air flow through the airways meets varying degrees of **resistance** where narrowed airway lumen (reduced diameter/increased resistance) requires greater muscular effort to drive air through. Although airway resistance is lower in the small bronchioles (generations 12–23) due to the large cross-sectional area, resistance can be increased by mucus, inflammation and bronchoconstriction. Airway narrowing can cause problems during both inspiration and expiration. **Compliance** is defined as the volume change per unit of pressure change across the lungs. During inspiration, effort is needed to overcome the density of the lung tissue and chest wall. The greater the compliance the easier it is to move the chest wall and lungs outwards making inspiration easier. Conversely, a reduction in compliance results in stiffness restricting ability of the chest wall and/or lung tissue to expand. Where resistance is increased and/or compliance reduced then the work of breathing is increased. This results in accessory muscle use (e.g. sternocleidomastoid, pectorals, trapezius, internal intercostal and abdominal) with increased energy expenditure and possible muscle fatigue leading to ventilatory failure.

Lung volumes

In clinical practice, a knowledge and sometimes measurement of various lung volumes can be helpful both in diagnosis and to evaluate therapeutic interventions (Figure 12.4). Volumes such as tidal volume, vital capacity (maximal inspiration followed by maximum expiration) can be easily measured at the bedside with spirometry and peak expiratory flow rate (**PEFR**) with a peak flow meter (Chapter 14). Alveolar ventilation, residual volume (volume at the end of forced expiration) and function residual capacity (FRC) requires more elaborate methods in a laboratory.

Functional residual capacity

Functional residual capacity (FRC) is the volume in the lungs at the end of normal expiration. It is made up of the expiratory reserve volume (ERV) and residual volume (RV). FRC is important in maintaining good oxygenation; if this reduces due to poor lung expansion or positioning, SpO_2 will fall. Practitioners should take steps to maximise FRC to minimise alveolar collapse and optimise effective oxygenation. FRC can be reduced by as much as 30% when patients are lying down. Therefore positioning is important; sitting the patient upright (Figure 12.5), or high side-lying, or sitting in a chair are preferable positions. Early mobilisation is effective at helping maintain lung volumes and maximise respiratory status. In high-dependency areas nurses and physiotherapists work collaboratively to ensure that FRC is optimised.

13 Assessment of breathing

Figure 13.1 Factors for consideration in a respiratory assessment

Patient history

- Smoking
- Recent viral infection
- COPD: target saturations (88–82%)
- CO_2 retention?
- Malnutrition
- Swallowing difficulties
- Asthma
- Pneumothorax
- Pleural effusion
- Empyema
- Neuromuscular problems
- Chest deformity
- Hypertension
- Sleep apnoea
- Medication: long-term oxygen therapy
- Bronchodilators
- Steroids
- Recent antibiotics

Look

- Tripod position
- Use of accessory muscles
- Cyanosis of lips and oral mucosa
- Nasal flaring
- Paradoxical breathing
- Mouth breathing
- Pursed lip breathing
- Unequal lung expansion
- Ratio of inspiration to expiration altered
- Rhythm of breathing altered

Listen

- To sounds of breathing from upper airway
- For audible wheeze
- To what the patient is telling you
- Auscultate lung fields

Any signs of new confusion can indicate hypoxaemia, or the development of cerebral hypoxia

I'm feeling more breathless

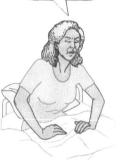

Feel

- Peripheral warmth
- Diaphoresis (sweating)
- Check for midline trachea
- Check for equal chest expansion

Measure

- Oxygen saturations (SpO_2) – check with specified target range
- 94–98% for most patients
- 88–92% for those at risk of hypercapnia
- Altered respiratory rate, depth and/or pattern
- Altered heart rate and/or blood pressure

Investigate

- Arterial blood gas analysis
- Chest X-ray
- Wheeze: peak flow as able, compare predicted to current best of three
- Pyrexia (> 38.3°):
  - sample of sputum, for MC&S (septic screen)
  - bloods: check WCC and CRP

Further investigations
- Lung function tests/spirometry
- MRI
- Computerised tomography

Figure 13.2 Clubbing of fingernails

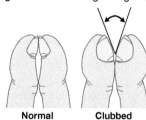

Normal   **Clubbed**

Clubbing of the nail beds is seen as a loss of the normal angle at the nail bed. Tip of nails when backs of hands placed together do not touch

Possible causes:
- COPD
- lung cancer
- any disease featuring chronic hypoxia
- endocarditis

Figure 13.3 Changes in I:E ratio

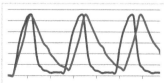

Normal breathing pattern I:E ratio is around 1:2 (blue)
I:E ratio with obstructive airways disease, prolonged expiratory phase (red)

Figure 13.4 Kussmaul breathing and Cheyne–Stokes respirations

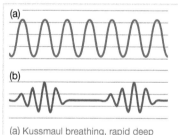

(a) Kussmaul breathing, rapid deep breaths seen in diabetic ketoacidosis, uraemia, sepsis, lactic acidosis
(b) Cheyne–Stokes respiration, periodic breathing with episodes of apnoea. Seen in hypoperfusion of respiratory centre in the brain, hypoxaemia

Figure 13.7 Signs of hypercapnia

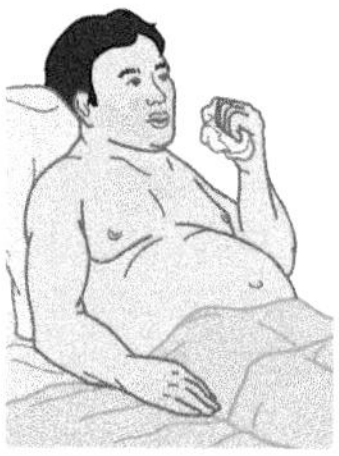

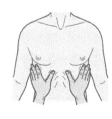

Mild hypercapnia
- Flushed skin
- Muscle twitches
- Elevated HR
- Minor confusion

Moderate hypercapnia
- Lethargy/drowsy
- Dizziness
- Sweaty

Severe hypercapnia
- Unconscious
- Seizures
- Respiratory arrest
- Cardiac arrest, death

Figure 13.5 Pattern of lung auscultation

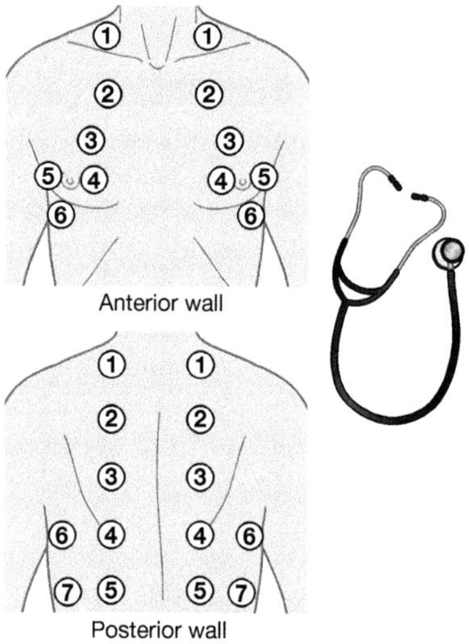

Anterior wall

Posterior wall

Figure 13.6 Palpation of chest expansion

Place hands on costal angle of the anterior thorax.

Both sides should be felt moving equally as the patient breathes in and out. If one side moves less than the other, this suggests problems such as chest infection, atelectasis, pleural effusion or pneumothorax

Acute and Critical Care Nursing at a Glance, First Edition. Edited by Helen Dutton and Jacqui Finch
© 2018 John Wiley & Sons, Ltd. Published 2018 by John Wiley & Sons, Ltd.
Companion website: www.ataglanceseries.com/nursing/acutecare

Assessment of breathing is the second step of the ABCDE approach. In order to obtain an accurate assessment and interpret clinical findings, the nurse needs to be familiar with basic respiratory physiology, understanding oxygenation with concepts of gaseous exchange and ventilation (Chapters 11 and 12). Respiratory disease comprises a significant percentage of hospital admissions and acute respiratory problems may develop as a secondary problem whilst in hospital. A knowledge of pre-existing conditions that place the individual at risk of respiratory problems is helpful for early identification. It is important to be familiar with the patient history (Figure 13.1), as knowledge of underlying chronic respiratory problems will inform the assessment and subsequent action taken. The respiratory system is responsive to problems in cardiac, neurological and renal status, and even subtle changes can be an early indicator of deterioration. A systematic approach to data collection, using the 'look, listen, feel, measure, investigate' approach, contributes to a comprehensive assessment and has been summarised in Figure 13.1.

Breathing assessment: look

Visual clues to a patient's clinical status are required to augment information from routine observations. Examining fingers for signs of nail bed clubbing infers chronic lung disease (Figure 13.2). Normal quiet breathing is effortless whether supine or sitting, but a patient experiencing respiratory distress may initially make small changes such as mouth breathing as the work of breathing increases, or moving to an upright position. The use of accessory muscles (scalene, trapezius and sternocleidomastoid) are indicative of more severe distress, especially when accompanied by pursed lip breathing (closing lips to prevent air movement briefly, on expiration). This action increases pressure in the alveoli, holding them open through the respiratory cycle, increasing functional residual capacity and therefore oxygenation. Conversational ability is reduced to a few words at a time, a key marker of respiratory distress.

Observing the respiratory pattern gives clues to respiratory status. The ratio of inspiration to expiration (I:E ratio) in health will vary from about 1:2 when at rest, to 1:1 during exertion. As respiratory rate rises expiratory time will generally shorten, but in those with obstructive airways disease, such as asthma or **chronic obstructive pulmonary disease** (COPD), the I:E ratio changes, with the expiratory time lengthening as air squeezes through the narrowed airways (Figure 13.3). Altered breathing patterns also include:

• **Kussmaul breathing**: a very deep and rapid breathing pattern, possibly a response to a severe metabolic acidosis caused by problems such as diabetic ketoacidosis.

• **Cheyne–Stoke's breathing**: periods of breathing during which the tidal volume is initially shallow, gets progressively deeper, and then progressively shallow again. Apnoea follows, which can continue for some time. This may indicate traumatic brain injury, stroke, or may occur following a large dose of morphine (Figure 13.4)!

Breathing assessment: listen

Listening to the patient's story is essential in understanding the development of the symptoms experienced. Assess features relating to cough such as, is it productive or has it changed in frequency from the 'usual morning cough'? Explore exacerbating and relieving factors. Sputum needs to be observed for colour, amount and consistency, with a sample being sent for culture if green, purulent or accompanied by a pyrexia. Check for added features such as wheeze or chest pain, assessing the type, location and severity.

Sounds associated with breathing can often be heard by the bedside. Rattling airway noises indicate the presence of airway secretions, usually caused by the inability of the patient to cough sufficiently or to take a deep breath. An asthmatic patient may be heard wheezing, a polyphonic musical sound, heard most clearly on expiration. This requires further assessment of PEFR to assess severity and prompt intervention such as bronchodilators.

Additional skills of lung auscultation are used by more experienced nurses, medical staff and physiotherapists to aid diagnosis. Figure 13.5 identifies areas for placement of the diaphragm of the stethoscope on the anterior and posterior thorax. A ladder pattern is used to listen for breath sounds, comparing one side of the chest to the other. Normal breath sounds are:

• Vesicular: soft and low pitched with a long inspiratory phase.
• Bronchial: higher pitched, with a shorter inspiratory phase.
• Bronchovesicular.
  Adventitious, or abnormal sounds include:
• Wheezes: polyphonic musical sounds, a result of air flowing through narrowed airways.
• Crackles: discontinuous popping sounds caused by air moving through fluid in small airways or alveoli.

Breathing assessment: feel

Feel for equal and bilateral chest expansion, as changes can identify breathing problems (Figure 13.6). Tension pneumothorax is a rare life-threatening condition, recognised by severe respiratory distress, unequal lung expansion and a shift in the trachea from the midline position (normally aligned with the suprasternal notch). The pressure in the thorax prevents lung expansion and immediate help is required.

Breathing assessment: measure

Accurate recording of the respiratory rate over one full minute is essential. Deviations of as few as four breaths per minute at rest are associated with clinical deterioration.[1] Rates of over 25 or under 8 per minute require urgent medical review.[2] The pulse oximeter measures the saturation of Hb with oxygen in peripheral capillary blood (SpO_2). Normal Hb oxygen saturations fall between 94 and 98%, when breathing room air. A decrease in SpO_2 of >3% requires additional assessment, considering the need for **arterial blood gas** (ABG) analysis.[3] Hypoxaemia should be treated with prescribed supplemental oxygen to maintain SpO_2 within target saturations. In patients with chronic underlying problems such as COPD, 88–92% may be identified as a target SpO_2. These patients are particularly vulnerable to retaining CO_2 as they may be unable to move sufficient volumes of air (minute ventilation) for its excretion. Signs of CO_2 retention are described (Figure 13.7), but ABG analysis is essential to ascertain exact $PaCO_2$ (see Chapter 14).

Breathing assessment: investigate

Additional investigations such as chest X-ray, lung function tests, magnetic resonance imaging and computerised tomography are performed as necessary to guide treatment and aid diagnosis.

14 Respiratory investigations

Figure 14.1 Examples of chest X-ray. (a) Normal, showing key structures. (b) Right lower lobe pneumonia. (c) Pulmonary oedema with enlarged failing heart (LVF). Source: (a) Clarke C. and Dux A., 2011. (b) Leach R.M., 2014. (a, b) Reproduced with permission of John Wiley & Sons.

(a)

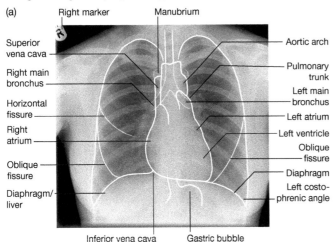

Right marker
Manubrium
Superior vena cava
Right main bronchus
Horizontal fissure
Right atrium
Oblique fissure
Diaphragm/ liver
Inferior vena cava
Gastric bubble
Aortic arch
Pulmonary trunk
Left main bronchus
Left atrium
Left ventricle
Oblique fissure
Diaphragm
Left costo- phrenic angle

Important items to check when viewing a chest X-ray
- Is it the correct patient?
- Check the date and time it was taken.
  Can this be compared to previous dates?
- Type of film – PA or AP, erect or supine
- Is the marker for the Left or Right in the correct place?
- For what reason was the CXR taken, what is being considered?

(b)

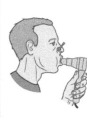

Consolidation right lower lobe

(c)

Prominent upper lobe vessels
Alveolar oedema ('bat's wings')
Kerley B lines (interstitial oedema)
Pleural effusion
Cardiomegaly

Figure 14.2 Peak flow meter and how to measure PEFR

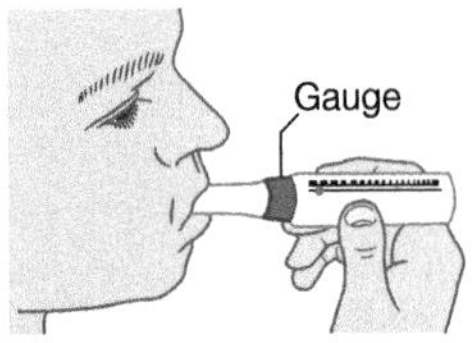

Gauge

Taking an accurate PEFR reading
- Ensure patient in upright position
- Connect a clean mouthpiece to the meter
- Ensure the marker on the flow meter is set at zero
- Check the finger is not obstructing the cursor

Ask the patient to:
- Take as deep a breath as possible and hold.
- Ensure a tight seal on the mouthpiece with the lips
- Breathe out as fast as possible with a quick sharp blow
- Reading in L/min recorded from cursor placement

Return the cursor to the zero position and repeat twice. Record the best reading of three.

Table 14.1 Using a spirometer, tests and simple analysis. Source: NICE, 2010.

Test	Explanation	Normal	Obstructive lung disease such as COPD or asthma
FVC (forced vital capacity)	The total volume of air that the patient can forcibly exhale in one slow steady breath until exhalation complete (measured in litres)	Above 80% of predicted volume	Below 80% of predicted volume
FEV_1 (forced expiratory volume in one second)	The volume of air that the patient is able to exhale in the first second of forced expiration (measured in litres)	Above 80% of predicted volume	Normal or reduced
FEV_1/FVC	The ratio of FEV_1 to FVC, indicating degree of airways obstruction	> 0.7	< 0.7

Figure 14.5 Problem identification using arterial blood gas analysis

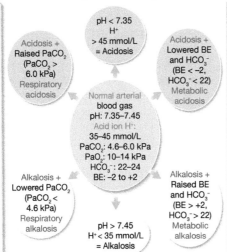

ABG analysis: respiratory problems
Respiratory acidosis:
Decreased ventilation (increased H⁺)
- Depressed respiratory centre due to opiates, sedatives or head injury
- Neuromuscular disorders
- Acute respiratory infection, when patient is nearing exhaustion
- COPD
Respiratory alkalosis:
Increased ventilation (decreased H⁺)
- Hyperventilation e.g. through stress or panic

pH < 7.35
H⁺ > 45 mmol/L
= Acidosis

Acidosis + Raised PaCO₂ (PaCO₂ > 6.0 kPa) Respiratory acidosis

Acidosis + Lowered BE and HCO₃⁻ (BE < –2, HCO₃⁻ < 22) Metabolic acidosis

Normal arterial blood gas
pH: 7.35–7.45
Acid ion H⁺:
35–45 mmol/L
PaCO₂: 4.6–6.0 kPa
PaO₂: 10–14 kPa
HCO₃⁻: 22–24
BE: –2 to +2

Alkalosis + Lowered PaCO₂ (PaCO₂ < 4.6 kPa) Respiratory alkalosis

Alkalosis + Raised BE and HCO₃⁻ (BE > +2, HCO₃⁻ > 22) Metabolic alkalosis

pH > 7.45
H⁺ < 35 mmol/L
= Alkalosis

ABG analysis: metabolic problems
Metabolic acidosis:
(increased H⁺ or decreased HCO₃⁻)
- Shock (anaerobic metabolism due to tissue hypoxia)
- Ketoacidosis (excess H⁺ ions released from ketone bodies)
- Diarrhoea (loss of HCO₃⁻)
- Renal failure (inability to excrete H⁺ as waste)
Metabolic alkalosis:
(Decreased H⁺ (acid) or increased HCO₃⁻)
- Vomiting (loss of H⁺ from stomach)
- Gastric aspiration from NG tube
- Excessive bicarbonate intake, e.g. indigestion remedies

Figure 14.3 Spirometry. Source: NICE, 2010.

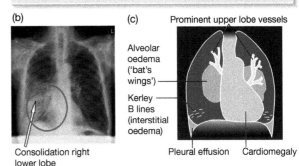

The patient takes a deep breath in, then breathes out completely into the spirometer.

Measurements of air expired in litres, are taken at 1 second (FEV1), and at the end of expiration (FVC)

Figure 14.4 Normal venous blood gas (VBG) ranges

pH: 7.31–7.41
PvO₂: 4.6–5.8kPa
PvCO₂: 5.5–6.8kPa
HCO₃⁻: 22–26 mmol/L
BE: –2+2
O₂ sats: 70–75%

Acute and Critical Care Nursing at a Glance, First Edition. Edited by Helen Dutton and Jacqui Finch
© 2018 John Wiley & Sons, Ltd. Published 2018 by John Wiley & Sons, Ltd.
Companion website: www.ataglanceseries.com/nursing/acutecare

A comprehensive respiratory assessment of the patient presenting with symptoms such as cough, breathlessness or wheeze, is essential if appropriate, timely interventions are to be commenced. Clinical assessment alone, however, does not always give sufficient information to ascertain the underlying reasons for the symptoms presented. Additional investigations may be required to determine the disordered physiology giving rise to respiratory distress. This chapter discusses the investigations which inform diagnosis and management of patients with a range of respiratory symptoms.

Chest X-ray

The chest X-ray (CXR) is a non-invasive painless investigation that gives images of the heart, lungs, airways, blood vessels and the bones of the spine and chest (Figure 14.1). X-ray radiation penetrates soft tissue easily but does not penetrate hard tissue. Areas where radiation cannot penetrate such as bones appear white on the film, with air-filled cavities appearing black. Organs and fat have a darker grey appearance, whilst water appears a lighter grey. Problems such as pneumonia, heart failure (Figure 14.1), pneumothorax and lung cancer can be identified. The sharpest films are obtained in the X-ray department using the standard PA (posterior–anterior) and lateral view. For those who are acutely unwell a portable CXR is required, with the machine brought to the bedside. A portable CXR takes an anterior–posterior (AP) view (or from front to back).

Peak expiratory flow rate

Peak expiratory flow rate measures the rate that air is forcibly expelled from the lungs in litres per minute. This test is used to evaluate the degree of bronchoconstriction occurring in patients who suffer from asthma, COPD, or who have an audible wheeze on auscultation.[1] Charts are to enable comparison with normal values[1] but most importantly the PEFR obtained should be compared with the patient's own 'best' value. Many patients with COPD will have reduced normal values. Peak flow meters are simple devices to use, but the patient needs clear instructions on how to carry out the procedure (Figure 14.2). Measurements are taken before and after bronchodilator therapy to evaluate response. Acutely unwell patients may be too breathless for PEFR, so clinical indicators such as changes in respiratory rate and SpO_2 are used to indicate and/or evaluate therapy.

Spirometry

Spirometry is a non-invasive method of assessing lung function by measuring the volume of air that the patient can expel from the lungs after maximal inspiration. It is often used to aid diagnosis and to assess progression of obstructive lung disorders such as COPD.[2]

Prior to the test patients are asked to refrain from taking:
- Short-acting bronchodilators such as salbutamol for 4 h.
- Long-acting bronchodilators such as Serevent for 12 h.
- Anticholinergic such as Atrovent for 6 h.

Clear explanations are required regarding the different exhalation techniques for measuring FVC and FEV_1 (see Figure 14.3 and Table 14.1):
- Each should be measured at least twice, but no more than eight times, to obtain two values within 150 mL of each other.
- FEV_1/FVC should be measured before, and 15–20 minutes after bronchodilator is given.

COPD is diagnosed by clinical history and the presence of airflow obstruction in postbronchodilator spirometry. Asthma is diagnosed if a marked improvement in FEV_1/FVC in postbronchodilator spirometry is seen, as airways constriction is reversible. Healthcare professionals caring for people with COPD should be competent in spirometry and result interpretation, to monitor patient progress.

Blood tests

Some routine blood tests performed on venous samples can contribute to the assessment of the patient with respiratory symptoms such as: haemoglobin to check for anaemia; white cell count, C-reactive protein and blood cultures to evaluate infection; and alpha-1 antitrypsin deficiency, a major cause of emphysema. Venous blood gas (VBG) samples give insight into respiratory problems (Figure 14.4), but should be interpreted with caution. A series of VBG measurements are required to track patient progress, and should not replace **arterial samples** in the patient who is acutely unwell.

Arterial blood gas analysis

Arterial blood gas (ABG) specimens can be obtained from the radial or femoral artery using a needle and heparinised syringe, by an appropriately competent healthcare professional. This is an invasive procedure that can be uncomfortable, so if multiple samples are required in a critical care setting, an arterial line may be placed using local anaesthetic.

The **pH** scale (1–14) is used to describe serum acidity or alkalinity with a narrow **serum range of 7.35–7.45** required for optimum functioning of the numerous chemical reactions necessary for life. **Hydrogen ions (H^+)** determine acidity. H^+ is generated from the respiratory gas CO_2, which dissolves to form carbonic acid. Adequate ventilation is required to excrete CO_2, to maintain pH range. H^+ generated from metabolic processes are excreted via the kidneys, after initially being buffered by substances including **bicarbonate (HCO_3^-)** to prevent large changes in pH occurring. Figure 14.5 illustrates some common problems identified by ABG interpretation.

A five-step approach can be used to analyse ABGs:

1 Assess the PaO_2 and SaO_2: is this sufficient? Do these values correlate with the patients monitored SpO_2?

PaO_2 <8.0 kPa and /or SaO_2 <90% indicates respiratory failure.

2 Assess the pH: pH <7.35 and $H^+\uparrow$, the patient is acidotic. pH >7.45 and $H^+\downarrow$ the patient is alkalotic.

3 Assess the $PaCO_2$: if $PaCO_2\uparrow$ with pH$\downarrow$ a respiratory acidosis is present. If $PaCO_2\downarrow$ with pH$\uparrow$ then a respiratory alkalosis is present.

4 Assess the HCO_3^- and BE: changes in these values are usually consistent with a metabolic problem. If lowered and pH$\downarrow$, HCO_3^- has been used to buffer excess metabolic H^+, and a metabolic acidosis is present. If raised and pH$\uparrow$, a metabolic alkalosis is present.

5 Determine the imbalance: this is done by finding the value that gives the best explanation for the altered pH.

Compensation occurs when pH or H^+ ions remain within normal limits, despite abnormal CO_2 or HCO_3^- values. A patient with COPD who has a chronically high $PaCO_2$, an elevated HCO_3^- (>26 mmol/L), with a normal pH, has a compensated respiratory acidosis.

Respiratory investigations should always be interpreted within the context of the patient's health history, symptoms and clinical presentation, to aid diagnosis and guide treatment effectively.

15 Oxygen therapy

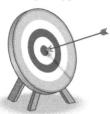

Figure 15.1 Target oxygen saturations

Target saturations are prescribed for all patients who require oxygen therapy, at either 94–98% or 88–92%. Saturations should remain within the prescribed range at all times. On some occasions different target ranges may be set for individual patients by medical staff.

Table 15.1 Patients who may not benefit from oxygen therapy

Oxygen therapy NOT required unless hypoxaemic $SaO_2 < 94\%$
Patient who are breathless but not hypoxaemic require close monitoring

Myocardial infarction and acute coronary syndromes or stroke	• Oxygen should not be given unless hypoxaemic
Pregnancy and obstetric emergencies	• Oxygen therapy may be harmful to foetus if mother not hypoxaemic
Hyperventilation	• Exclude organic illness • Anxiety or panic attacks unlikely to require oxygen therapy • Avoid rebreathing from paper bag as this may cause hypoxaemia
Metabolic and renal disorders	• Most do not need oxygen unless hypoxaemic. Breathlessness caused by metabolic acidosis

Figure 15.3 Venturi masks for controlled oxygen therapy

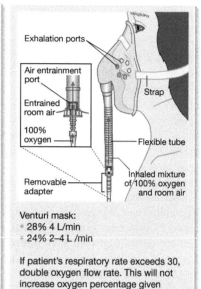

Venturi mask:
• 28% 4 L/min
• 24% 2–4 L /min

If patient's respiratory rate exceeds 30, double oxygen flow rate. This will not increase oxygen percentage given

Table 15.2 Groups of patients requiring oxygen therapy. Source: O'Driscoll B., et al., 2017.

Target saturations 94–98%		Target saturations 88–92%
Critical illness	**Serious illness, requiring moderate supplemental oxygen, if hypoxaemic**	**COPD (and other conditions) requiring low-dose oxygen therapy**
Critical illness: Initial therapy 15 L/min via reservoir mask Then titrate down if target sats met **Cardiac arrest:** Bag valve mask 15 L/min oxygen **COPD or risk of hypercapnia?** Initial 15 L/min via reservoir mask, pending ABG results	**Serious illness:** 2–6 L/min nasal specs OR 5–10 L/min face mask If $SpO_2 < 85\%$ use reservoir mask and seek senior advice **Co-existing COPD?** Target SpO_2 88–92% pending ABG results. If not hypercapnic, target may be revised upwards to 94–98%	**COPD/controlled oxygen therapy:** 24% Venturi mask 2–3 L/min 28% Venturi mask 4 L/min Or nasal cannulae 2 L/min when stable Reduce oxygen (but do not stop) if SpO_2 > 92% **Hypercapnic with an arterial pH < 7.35?** Non-invasive ventilation should be considered
Examples: • Acute hypoxaemia, unknown cause • Major trauma, major head injury • Sepsis, anaphylaxis, shock (BP < 90mmHg), drowning • Status epilepticus • Carbon monoxide poisoning (SpO_2 measurement unreliable, check carboxyhaemoglobin levels)	**Examples:** • Acute asthma, pneumonia • Acute heart failure (consider CPAP or NIV) • Pleural effusion, pneumothorax (drain/aspirate as indicated) • Lung cancer • Pulmonary embolism • Severe anaemia (correct anaemia)	**Examples:** • COPD (may need a lower target SpO_2 range set) • Exacerbation of COPD • Chronic neuromuscular disorders • Chest wall disorders • Morbid obesity, cystic fibrosis

Figure 15.4 Nebulisers in COPD

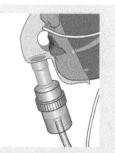

Patients with COPD, with target sats of 88–92%, should have nebulisers driven with 6 L/min of compressed air; oxygen can be given at the same time by nasal cannula if necessary to maintain target saturations. If air is not available limit oxygen-driven nebuliser to 6 minutes

Figure 15.2 Non-rebreathe (reservoir) and simple face masks, nasal specs

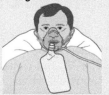

Critical illness: high flow oxygen Target sats 94–98%

Non-rebreathe mask (reservoir bag), 60–80% oxygen flow rate 15 L/min. Reservoir bag must be inflated prior to use. Valve prevents exhaled air entering reservoir bag

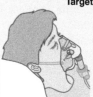

Serious illness: medium flow oxygen Target sats 94–98%

Simple face mask, oxygen flow rate 5–10 L/min. At least 5 L/min required to prevent CO_2 rebreathing

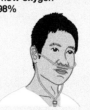

Nasal specs most comfortable for the patient, and therefore tolerated well. Suitable for patients who are stable. Oxygen flow rate 2–6 L/min

Figure 15.5 Oxygen Alert cards

OXYGEN ALERT CARD
Name: _____
I am at risk of type II respiratory failure with a raised CO_2 level.
Please use my _____% Venturi mask to achieve an oxygen saturation of _____% to _____% during exacerbations.
Use compressed air to drive nebulisers (with nasal oxygen at 2 L/min).
If compressed air not available, limit oxygen-driven nebulisers to 6 minutes.

COPD patients should carry an Oxygen Alert card to inform paramedic/healthcare practitioners of agreed target oxygen saturations. Patients may have their own Venturi mask with them

Acute and Critical Care Nursing at a Glance, First Edition. Edited by Helen Dutton and Jacqui Finch
© 2018 John Wiley & Sons, Ltd. Published 2018 by John Wiley & Sons, Ltd.
Companion website: www.ataglanceseries.com/nursing/acutecare

Oxygen is probably the most common drug to be used in the care of patients who present with medical emergencies.[1] **Hypoxaemia** (low level of oxygen in arterial blood), needs to be corrected when identified, as there is good evidence that severe hypoxaemia is harmful, adversely affecting patient outcome. Patients who are breathless, or exhibiting signs of respiratory distress, should be assessed for hypoxaemia as soon as possible using pulse oximetry (SpO_2). Oxygen saturation, considered the fifth vital sign, is recorded at least 12 hourly in all patients in the acute care setting. **Target saturations** are set by medical staff[2] and should be maintained at all times (Figure 15.1) with immediate action required to restore values to within normal, or near normal, range with prescribed supplemental oxygen. Currently there is no evidence of benefit in giving supplemental oxygen to patients who are not hypoxaemic even if they are 'out of breath' (Table 15.1). This group may be at risk of harm from inappropriate supplemental oxygen so caution is required.[2]

Positioning

Hypoxaemic patients benefit from being in an upright position, supported by pillows, maximising FRC (see Chapter 12 & Figure 12.5), thus increasing the surface area available for gaseous exchange to occur. The pressure of the abdomen on the diaphragm is decreased, helping to increase chest expansion and lung volumes.

Oxygen therapy

The British Thoracic Society have published guidelines,[2] for oxygen use in adult patients, that are widely endorsed and adopted.

Patients requiring oxygen therapy are divided into three groups. For each group oxygen is prescribed on the drug chart, with a target range of oxygen saturations clearly identified. Nurses administering oxygen therapy must be competent, understanding the range of appropriate devices and oxygen flow rates likely to achieve the target saturation prescribed. SpO_2, delivery device and oxygen flow rates are recorded on observation charts and signed for on the prescription chart. In emergencies nurses give oxygen first, as per local guidance, then ensure that this is prescribed and documented at the earliest possible opportunity.

Critical illness

In **critical illness** (Table 15.2) hypoxaemic patients require high flow oxygen therapy to prevent tissue hypoxia and organ damage. **Urgent medical review** with **ABG analysis** helps determine the nature of the problem and direct therapy. Further support such as **continuous positive airway pressure** (CPAP) may be indicated. If ABGs reveal hypercapnia and respiratory acidosis, controlled oxygen therapy (with target saturations of 88–92%) and/or non-invasive ventilation may be required.

Serious illness

Serious illness (Table 15.2) requires moderate amounts of supplemental oxygen to treat hypoxaemia, via a simple face mask at flow rates between 5 and 10 L/min or via nasal cannula (NC) at 2–6 L/min, maintaining target saturations between 94 and 98% (Figure 15.2). Nasal cannulae are tolerated well, do not interfere with talking and drinking, and are suitable for stable patients. Drying of the nasal mucosa is sometimes experienced with high flows of 4–6 L/min. If the target range is not met using oxygen via face mask or NC, a reservoir mask with 15 L/min of oxygen is required, with urgent medical review.

Patients at risk of hypercapnia

For patients with COPD or other known risk factors for **hypercapnic respiratory failure** (e.g. neuromuscular disorders or morbid obesity) a target saturation of 88–92% is at least initially recommended, pending the results of ABG analysis. It is possible that target saturations may be adjusted later, if the $PaCO_2$ remains within normal limits. Venturi masks are useful in this group, as known concentrations of oxygen are administered and can be delivered at higher flow rates[2] (Figure 15.3). If required, **nebulisers are air driven**, with supplemental oxygen given via nasal specs to maintain target saturations (Figure 15.4). Oxygen alert cards highlight individual oxygen requirements (Figure 15.5). In those who develop acute hypercapnic failure ($PaCO_2$ >6.5 kPa, and pH <7.35)[3] despite initial medical therapy, non-invasive ventilation in the form of **BiPAP** will be considered as a matter of urgency.

High flow nasal cannula therapy

High flow nasal cannula (HFNC) therapy is an innovative treatment for hypoxaemia, delivering heated humidified medical gas at up to 60 L/min. It is tolerated well by most patients, and its use in adult critical care is increasing. The high flow of gas creates a positive pressure environment, and 'washes out' gases in the nasopharynx, helping CO_2 clearance.[4,5]

Caring for the patient on oxygen therapy

Close monitoring is required, with the frequency of observations influenced by the NEWS. Nurses titrate oxygen therapy upwards or downwards to maintain target saturations. After any change in oxygen flow rate or device, SpO_2 should be monitored for at least 5 min and recorded on the observation chart. Patients who require increased amounts of oxygen need medical review, with ABGs checked within 30 min to 1 h. It is not necessary to remove the oxygen mask prior to ABG analysis; this action increases the risk of tissue hypoxia. The target saturations for the patient should be maintained at all times.

Humidification

Whilst oxygen is a gas which can cause dryness, humidification is not necessary for low flow oxygen (<4 L), or for the short-term use of high flow oxygen (<24 h). In an emergency, humidification can be restricted to those patients with a tracheostomy tube, or who are intubated. Patients with tenacious secretions who are having problems expectorating may benefit from saline nebulisers to loosen secretions.

Discontinuing oxygen therapy

Oxygen therapy can be discontinued when the patient is clinically stable and their oxygen saturations remain within their target range on room air. Monitor SpO_2 for at least 5 min after low flow oxygen has been withdrawn, then again at 1 h, checking and recording observations and NEWS on the chart.

16 Respiratory failure

Figure 16.1 Respiratory failure can be due to failure of gaseous exchange in the lung, or failure to ventilate the lung

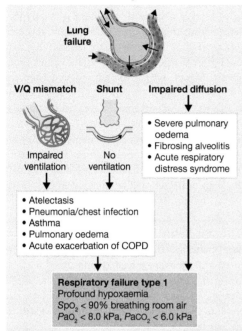

Lung failure

V/Q mismatch	Shunt	Impaired diffusion
Impaired ventilation	No ventilation	• Severe pulmonary oedema • Fibrosing alveolitis • Acute respiratory distress syndrome

• Atelectasis
• Pneumonia/chest infection
• Asthma
• Pulmonary oedema
• Acute exacerbation of COPD

Respiratory failure type 1
Profound hypoxaemia
SpO_2 < 90% breathing room air
PaO_2 < 8.0 kPa, $PaCO_2$ < 6.0 kPa

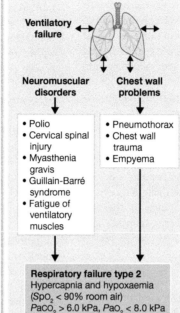

Ventilatory failure

Neuromuscular disorders	Chest wall problems
• Polio • Cervical spinal injury • Myasthenia gravis • Guillain-Barré syndrome • Fatigue of ventilatory muscles	• Pneumothorax • Chest wall trauma • Empyema

Respiratory failure type 2
Hypercapnia and hypoxaemia
(SpO_2 < 90% room air)
$PaCO_2$ > 6.0 kPa, PaO_2 < 8.0 kPa

Table 16.1 Respiratory information from ABG analysis (no metabolic problems included)

PaO_2: 10–13.5 kPa	Normal range
PaO_2: 8.0–10 kPa	Hypoxaemia probably due to VQ mismatch. Supplemental oxygen may be required. Check target oxygen saturations
PaO_2 < 8.0 kPa	Respiratory failure (profound hypoxaemia)
$PaCO_2$ = 4.6–6.0 kPa	Normal range
$PaCO_2$ < 4.6 kPa	Hyperventilation (maybe due to hypoxemia). Increased minute ventilation has reduced partial pressure of CO_2 in arterial blood
$PaCO_2$ > 6.0 kPa	Hypoventilation: failure to maintain adequate minute ventilation
pH 7.35–7.45	Normal range
pH < 7.35	May be caused by increased CO_2 levels. Hypoventilation (respiratory acidosis)
pH > 7.45	May be caused by reduced level of CO_2 Hyperventilation (respiratory alkalosis)
HCO_3^- (bicarbonate) 22–26 mmol/L	Normal range
HCO_3^- > 24	Retention of bicarbonate by the kidneys probably due to chronically raised carbon dioxide in disorders such as COPD. The increased bicarbonate increases buffering, keeping the pH near normal range, despite a raised $PaCO_2$.

Figure 16.2 Oxygen haemoglobin dissociation curve

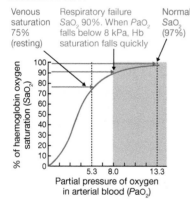

Venous saturation 75% (resting)

Respiratory failure SaO_2 90%. When PaO_2 falls below 8 kPa, Hb saturation falls quickly

Normal SaO_2 (97%)

% of haemoglobin oxygen saturation (SaO_2)
100 90 80 70 60 50 40 30 20 10 0

5.3 8.0 13.3

Partial pressure of oxygen in arterial blood (PaO_2)

Box 16.1 Understanding the oxygen haemoglobin dissociation curve

• The oxygen haemoglobin dissociation curve describes the relationship between PaO_2 and SaO_2
• SaO_2 is measured clinically using pulse oximetry (SpO_2) (normal range 94–98%)
• PaO_2 is measured in arterial blood gas analysis (normal range 10–13.5 kPa)
• Respiratory failure is defined as SaO_2 < 90% or PaO_2 < 8.0 kPa
• It is at this point (SaO_2 90%) that rapid desaturation of Hb occurs, thereby reducing oxygen delivery to the tissues. Further drop in SaO_2 or PaO_2 could cause tissue hypoxia and organ damage
• Further evaluation of $PaCO_2$ and pH and HCO_3^- (bicarbonate) are required to determine type of respiratory failure, so ABG analysis may be required if SpO_2 falls below 93%

Box 16.2 Some useful definitions

• Compliance – the ease with which the lung stretches to accommodate tidal volume
• Resistance – the resistance to air flow through the airways
• Work of breathing – the energy required to breathe. Normally very low!
• Elasticity – the ability of the lung to recoil back to its normal shape on exhalation
• Tidal volume – the amount of air moving into the lung in one breath
• Minute ventilation = tidal volume × respiratory rate

Figure 16.3 Acute respiratory failure: an imbalance of oxygen supply and oxygen demand

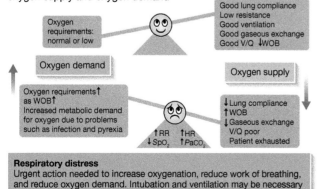

Oxygen requirements: normal or low

Good lung compliance
Low resistance
Good ventilation
Good gaseous exchange
Good V/Q ↓WOB

Oxygen demand

Oxygen supply

Oxygen requirements↑ as WOB↑
Increased metabolic demand for oxygen due to problems such as infection and pyrexia

↑RR ↑HR
↓SpO_2 ↑$PaCO_2$

↓Lung compliance
↑WOB
↓Gaseous exchange
V/Q poor
Patient exhausted

Respiratory distress
Urgent action needed to increase oxygenation, reduce work of breathing, and reduce oxygen demand. Intubation and ventilation may be necessary

Table 16.2 Obstructive and restrictive lung disorders

Obstructive lung disorders	Restrictive lung disorders
Obstruction to air flow such as: • Bronchoconstriction of asthma • Presence of mucus in airways This increases resistance to air flow Work of breathing is increased Mixed pathology: both restrictive and obstructive features	Pathological changes reduce compliance of the lung or chest wall • Pneumonia • Pulmonary oedema • Kyphoscoliosis • Pneumothorax Work of breathing is increased Signs of increased work of breathing: • Mouth or pursed lip breathing • Use of accessory muscles, tripod position • Sensation of breathlessness (dyspnoea) • Smaller breaths, lower tidal volumes • Difficulty in talking in full sentences • Raised respiratory rate and heart rate

Acute and Critical Care Nursing at a Glance, First Edition. Edited by Helen Dutton and Jacqui Finch
© 2018 John Wiley & Sons, Ltd. Published 2018 by John Wiley & Sons, Ltd.
Companion website: www.ataglanceseries.com/nursing/acutecare

Failure to maintain adequate gas exchange across the alveolar capillary membrane gives rise to problems with oxygenation and excretion of carbon dioxide. Acute respiratory failure is one of the most common reasons for deterioration, leading to admission to intensive care. Early identification, with a systematic assessment and the development of an appropriate treatment plan whilst the patient is ward-based, is essential to prevent deterioration. Respiratory failure can be a result of failure of the gaseous exchange mechanism at alveolar level (lung failure), or as failure of ventilation, limiting the flow of gases through the respiratory system (ventilatory failure) (Figure 16.1). The diagnosis of respiratory failure is made on assessment of hypoxaemia (low levels of oxygen in the blood). Hypoxaemia is measured clinically either by SpO_2 monitoring or by evaluation of ABGs as PaO_2. The relationship between oxygen saturations and PaO_2 is demonstrated in Figure 16.2 and Box 16.1. A SpO_2 of <90% is a point at which Hb starts to lose affinity for oxygen and a consequent drop in oxygen content and delivery occurs, a marker for respiratory failure. Obtaining an arterial sample can be uncomfortable for the patient, but extra information obtained regarding PaO_2 pH, $PaCO_2$ and bicarbonate (HCO_3^-) levels, assist in determining the type of failure present and appropriate management strategies (Table 16.1). Failure of the lung can be caused by impedance of airflow through the airways or **obstructive lung disorders**. Changes in the lung that reduce the lung volumes are known as **restrictive lung disorders**; this could be due to damage to the lung tissue itself, or a disease of the chest wall (Table 16.2).

Lung failure

Inadequate **alveolar ventilation**, either reduced (low V/Q) or absent (right-to-left shunt), will result in arterial hypoxaemia. Constriction of the pulmonary capillary blood flow to underventilated alveoli helps in diverting blood to healthy alveoli, but this is not always sufficient to prevent hypoxaemia. Thickening of the alveolar capillary membrane disrupts diffusion of gases and is associated with inflammatory and fibrotic lung disorders. In the early stages of acute respiratory problems, hyperventilation of healthier lung units may result in lower arterial carbon dioxide (CO_2) levels, but do not raise oxygen levels sufficiently. The highly soluble CO_2, is initially excreted even with some areas of hypoventilation.

Work of breathing increases with changes in lung compliance and airways resistance (Box 16.2), observed clinically as a rise in respiratory rate and accessory muscle use. The cardiovascular system responds with an increase in heart rate and blood pressure as part of a sympathetic response. NEWS increases as observations move out of their normal range, alerting the team to deterioration. Arterial blood gas analysis is required, to assist diagnosis and management.

Type 1 respiratory failure or lung failure, is diagnosed when profound hypoxaemia is present, identified by an **SpO_2 <90%**, (or PaO_2 <8.0 kPa), with a **normal or low $PaCO_2$ of <6.0 kPa.**

Ventilatory failure

The physical act of breathing is the cyclical exchange of air during inspiration and expiration known as pulmonary ventilation, and this has been discussed in Chapter 12. It requires coordination of the respiratory centre, nerves, muscles, chest wall and rib cage for effective air movement.

Patients with ventilatory failure may have normal lung tissue, but cannot generate sufficient gas movement or alveolar ventilation for gaseous exchange to occur. As a result, arterial carbon dioxide will rise and arterial oxygen levels will reduce, as indicated by falling SpO_2 measurements. Arterial blood gases are required for diagnosis. **Type 2 respiratory failure** is diagnosed when hypoxaemia is present, identified by an **SpO_2 <90%** (or PaO_2 <8.0 kPa), with an **elevated $PaCO_2$ of >6.0 kPa**.

Mixed respiratory failure

Acute

Whilst identifying whether the primary cause of respiratory failure is lung failure or ventilatory failure is helpful to direct treatment, both aspects may be present. In particular, the patient who presents in type one failure, for example with a chest infection, may struggle to maintain the extra respiratory effort required for sufficient minute ventilation. Eventually the work of breathing (WOB) uses more oxygen to supply respiratory muscles than is gained (Figure 16.3). Inadequate ventilation from exhausted respiratory muscles will cause $PaCO_2$ to rise (as in type 2 failure). In acute hypercapnic respiratory failure the rising CO_2 levels in arterial blood cause the pH to fall below the normal range of 7.35–7.45 and can develop over minutes to hours. If not recognised and treated promptly, respiratory and/or cardiac arrest may ensue. Signs of profound fatigue include reduction in the ability to speak, confusion and/or a deteriorating level of consciousness and a falling SpO_2.

Chronic

Chronic respiratory failure (CRF) develops over days to weeks, thus the symptoms are less dramatic and can be more difficult to identify. Patients with disorders such as COPD may have deranged ABGs that are normal for them. In response to slowly rising CO_2 levels, the kidneys retain bicarbonate as an alkaline buffer, increasing its concentration, and therefore minimising the drop in serum pH. In response to the chronic hypoxaemia, red blood cell production is increased giving rise to polycythaemia, a clinical marker of CRF. In the winter months, additional problems such as chest infection can cause acute deterioration (with acute hypercapnic failure) in addition to the underlying chronic failure. This requires skilled management, careful oxygen titration and the use of additional support such as non-invasive ventilation.[1]

Supporting respiratory function

In respiratory failure, interventions are aimed at treating the problems that cause changes in lung compliance and airways resistance, thereby reducing the work of breathing. Supplemental oxygen is used to restore SpO_2 to within prescribed target oxygen saturations, and in conjunction with positioning, physiotherapy, hydration and appropriate medication such as bronchodilators, steroids or antibiotics, the patient's clinical condition often improves. Specific respiratory problems with their management are discussed in following chapters.

17 Breathing problems: obstructive disorders

Figure 17.1 Asthma and COPD, summary of characteristics

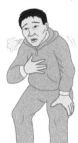

Asthma

- Rarely smokes
- Symptoms evident usually < 35 years, often from childhood
- Variable breathlessness and PEFR from day to day
- Dry cough and wheeze, typically at night time

COPD

- Smoker or ex-smoker
- Symptoms usually evident > 50 years of age
- Persistent and progressive breathlessness
- Chronic productive cough, often worse in the morning

Spirometry
FEV_1/FVC ratio < 0.7 but a good response to bronchodilators returns this to normal

Spirometry
FEV_1/FVC ratio < 0.7 but does not respond to bronchodilators and remains at < 0.7

Spirometry: airflow obstruction is defined as reduced FEV_1/FVC ratio (< 0.7)

FEV_1 is the maximum amount of air forcibly exhaled in 1 second

FVC is the maximum amount of air that can be forcibly exhaled from maximal inspiration to expiration

Box 17.1 Factors that act as asthma triggers.
Source: RCP, 2014.

- Viral infections
- Medicines: aspirin, NSAIDS (i.e. ibuprofen, naproxen)
- Aero allergens: house dust mite, pollens, spores, animal dander
- Exercise
- Oral allergens: eggs, fish, milk, nuts
- Environmental factors: tobacco smoke, fumes, air pollutants, climatic variation

Box 17.2 Risk factors/causes of COPD

- Tobacco smoke
- Occupational pollutants, such as dust and chemicals
- Low socioeconomic status: factors, such as poor nutrition, and overcrowding
- Genetic factors: alpha-1 antitrypsin deficiency

Figure 17.2 Airway changes in acute asthma

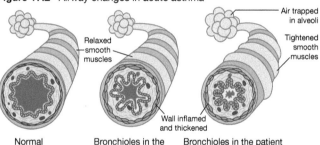

Relaxed smooth muscles

Air trapped in alveoli

Tightened smooth muscles

Wall inflamed and thickened

Normal bronchioles

Bronchioles in the patient with asthma

Bronchioles in the patient having an asthma attack

Figure 17.3 Airway changes in COPD

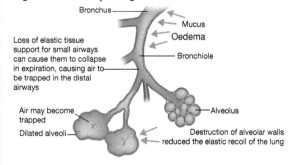

Bronchus

Mucus

Oedema

Bronchiole

Loss of elastic tissue support for small airways can cause them to collapse in expiration, causing air to be trapped in the distal airways

Air may become trapped

Dilated alveoli

Alveolus

Destruction of alveolar walls reduced the elastic recoil of the lung

Table 17.1 Levels of severity of asthma in adults. Source: BTS, 2014.

Moderate asthma	Increasing symptoms PEF > 50–75% of best or predicted No features of acute severe asthma
Acute severe asthma	Any one of: PEF 33–55% of best or predicted Res rate ≥ 25/min Heart rate ≥ 110/min Inability to complete sentence in one breath
Life-threatening asthma	Any one of the following in a patient with severe asthma: SpO_2 < 92% Altered level of consciousness PaO_2 < 8.0 kPa Normal $PaCO_2$ (4.6–6.0 kPa) Hypotension Exhaustion Cyanosis PEF < 33% of best Silent chest Poor respiratory effort
Near-fatal asthma	Raised $PaCO_2$ (> 6.0 kPa)

Table 17.3 Some ABG examples of patients with COPD

COPD patient who normally retains CO_2		COPD patient with acute exacerbation who normally retains CO_2	
pH 7.37	Normal range	pH 7.32	Lower than normal range: acidotic
$PaCO_2$ 6.8 kPa	Raised due to hypoventilation	$PaCO_2$ 7.8 kPa	Raised above patient's normal with deterioration in lung function due to acute exacerbation
PaO_2 8.0 kPa	Hypoxaemic	PaO_2 7.5 kPa	Hypoxaemic
HCO_3^- 31 mmol/L	Raised Kidneys are retaining bicarbonate in an effort to normalise pH	HCO_3^- 31 mmol/L	No further renal compensation for this acute phase
SaO_2 89%	Hypoxaemic	SaO_2 86%	Hypoxaemic

Table 17.2 Arterial blood gas analysis

	Normal ranges	Example of a patient with an acute exacerbation, but without CO_2 retention	
pH	7.35–7.45	7.38	Normal
$PaCO_2$	4–6 kPa	4.5 kPa	Normal
PaO_2	10–14 kPa	7.9 kPa	Hypoxaemic
HCO_3^-	22–24 mmol/L	23 mmol/L	Normal
SaO_2	94–96%	90%	Hypoxaemic

Acute and Critical Care Nursing at a Glance, First Edition. Edited by Helen Dutton and Jacqui Finch
© 2018 John Wiley & Sons, Ltd. Published 2018 by John Wiley & Sons, Ltd.
Companion website: www.ataglanceseries.com/nursing/acutecare

Respiratory problems that increase the resistance to airflow, increasing the work of breathing, are known as **obstructive lung disorders**. Resistance is influenced by the diameter of the lower respiratory airways. The walls of the respiratory tree are supported by cartilage to prevent collapse, smooth involuntary muscle and a mucous membrane inner lining. The narrow lumen of the terminal bronchioles has no cartilage, just smooth muscle. In health, little resistance is offered by these bronchioles as they are so numerous, but the narrow lumens can be easily disrupted by secretions and inflammation, increasing airways resistance and work of breathing. The smooth muscle cells in the respiratory tract lining are supplied by branches of the sympathetic and parasympathetic nervous system, which work together to regulate airways diameter. Asthma and COPD are obstructive lung disorders commonly encountered by nurses working in an acute care environment. Characteristics of each are summarised in Figure 17.1.

Asthma

The UK has one of the the highest number of people in the world affected by asthma.[1] This chronic inflammatory airways disorder is triggered by many factors (Box 17.1). Symptoms include wheeze, breathlessness, chest tightness and cough. Airways swelling, secretion accumulation and airway hyperresponsiveness (twitchiness of the airway muscles) (Figure 17.2) results in airflow obstruction that is variable and reversible. Patients may be symptom free for long periods, punctuated by a few acute episodes. Treatment can be successful with patient education and self-management, but nurses need to be vigilant as acute episodes can be rapid and potentially life threatening.

Assessment of the patient with asthma

Patients with acute severe asthma will be distressed and anxious, presenting with cough, chest tightness and wheeze. The British Thoracic Society (BTS) and Scottish Intercollegiate Guidelines Network (SIGN) (2016) have published guidelines for recognition and management of asthma (brit-thoracic.org.uk).[2] A detailed respiratory assessment, including the PEFR, is necessary to identify the severity of the attack (Table 17.1). Supplementary oxygen to maintain SpO_2 at 94–98% is a priority, often requiring high flow oxygen therapy. Arterial blood gas analysis for those with SpO_2 <92% identifies those at risk from **life-threatening or near fatal asthma** (Table 17.1). Frequent assessment with urgent care escalation is necessary to prevent untimely death.

Nursing management

Positioning is important to maximise chest expansion. Most asthma attacks will respond to nebulised β_2-agonists such as **salbutamol**, with oxygen as the driving gas. Steroid therapy such as **prednisolone 40–50 mg daily**, or intravenous hydrocortisone (400 mg in divided doses) are effective at reducing the inflammatory component of airway lumen reduction and is usually given for at least 5 days. Combining **ipatropium bromide** (Atrovent) with salbutamol may be beneficial if response to salbutamol alone is poor. Patients whose peak expiratory flow (PEF) remains 50% below that expected after bronchodilators should be assessed by senior medical staff, who may prescribe intravenous **magnesium sulphate** (1.2–2 g over 20 min). Frequent assessment of post-treatment PEFR and ABGs for the patient with acute severe or life-threatening asthma is managed best in level 2/3 dependency care, especially if response to ongoing

therapy is poor. Anaesthetic and intensivist support is essential. Transfer to a level 3 unit requires accompanying personnel that are competent in airway management and intubation.

Chronic obstructive pulmonary disease

An estimated 3 million people in the UK have COPD.[3] The airway inflammatory processes of COPD differs from asthma as it is a combination of both airway and lung parenchymal damage, the majority of cases due to the long-term effects of smoking (Box 17.2). COPD is now the preferred term for what has been described as:

- **Chronic bronchitis**: inflammation of the airways and an increase in mucus secretion caused by smoking irritants.
- **Emphysema:** distension and destruction of tissue in the respiratory bronchioles and alveolar sacs, affecting gaseous exchange. Elastic recoil of the airways is reduced (Figure 17.3), with airways collapse and **air trapping** during expiration.

Diagnosis is made from a combination of clinical history and spirometry (Figure 17.1). FEV_1 can vary from mild (<80% predicted) to very severe impairment (<30% predicted)[3] (see Chapter 14). Patients often manage their condition well, but as the disease progresses the irreversible nature of the airways obstruction increases breathlessness. The effective removal of CO_2 often presents no problem, but some, over time, are unable to maintain sufficient minute ventilation. Breathing in this patient group may be reliant on the peripheral chemoreceptors, more sensitive to hypoxemia as the respiratory stimulus, resulting in chronic hypercapnia. The 'hypoxic drive' may be suppressed if oxygen therapy increases the SpO_2 to greater than 92%. Thus the **SpO_2 target range for patients with COPD is 88–92%**. Hypercapnia, causing respiratory depression and possible respiratory arrest, is a risk if SpO_2 rises above this target range.

Assessment of the patient with COPD

During the winter months acute exacerbations (AECOPD), a rapid sustained worsening of symptoms[3] are common, requiring hospital admission. Severe breathlessness, inability to mobilise, impaired level of consciousness, saturations <90% and poor social support suggest admission would be beneficial. Alongside a full respiratory assessment, fluid retention with swollen ankles may be seen, caused by right-sided heart failure (due to the increased work of pumping blood through constricted pulmonary capillaries). Information is gained from: CXR, 12-lead ECG and full blood count to exclude comorbidities. ABG analysis evaluates what may be 'normal' for the patient and those at risk of acute CO_2 retention (examples in Tables 17.2 and 17.3).

Nursing management

Good positioning, physiotherapy, bronchodilators nebulised with air (with supplemental oxygen through nasal specs to maintain target SpO_2 at 88–92%), corticosteroids and possibly antibiotics, will comprise initial management. If despite maximum therapy, hypercapnia is identified on ABG with a lowered pH, this is the threshold for non-invasive ventilation (NIV) (see Chapter 20).[4] Clear plans considering action to be taken in the event of deterioration, considering ceiling of care, should be discussed with patients and their relatives by the senior doctor responsible, as early as possible.[5,6] Regular assessment will identify clinical improvement and assisted discharge schemes can support the transition home, with regular visits by nurses and physiotherapists experienced in managing COPD.

18 Breathing problems: lung (parenchymal) disorders

Figure 18.1 Common symptoms of pneumonia

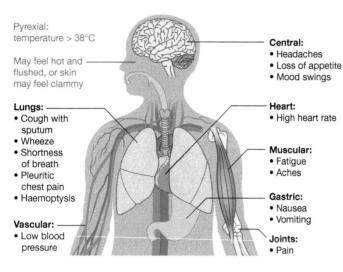

Pyrexial:
temperature > 38°C

May feel hot and flushed, or skin may feel clammy

Lungs:
- Cough with sputum
- Wheeze
- Shortness of breath
- Pleuritic chest pain
- Haemoptysis

Vascular:
- Low blood pressure

Central:
- Headaches
- Loss of appetite
- Mood swings

Heart:
- High heart rate

Muscular:
- Fatigue
- Aches

Gastric:
- Nausea
- Vomiting

Joints:
- Pain

Table 18.1 Features of typical and atypical pneumonia

Typical	Atypical
Presents over 24–46 h	Presents over a few days
Sudden onset of fever with rigours	Non-respiratory symptoms
Cough productive of mucopurulent sputum	Cough may appear after a few days, often non-productive, sputum may be clear
Breathless with pleuritic chest pain	Minimal chest signs or symptoms
CXR shows consolidation, affecting single lobe, a whole lung or both lungs	CXR shows widespread patchy consolidation with interstitial and alveolar infiltrates
WCC raised	WCC may be normal or elevated
Positive sputum sample	Sputum sample often negative

Signs of severe pneumonia
- SpO$_2$ < 90% on 60% supplemental oxygen
- Exhaustion
- Not speaking in full sentences
- Drowsiness
- Not spontaneously talking
- Unconscious
- Does not respond to voice
- Signs of shock
- Tachycardia and lowered BP
- NEWS ≥ 7
- ABG showing severe acidosis with pH < 7.25

Table 18.2 CURB 65 severity assessment

Score 1 for each point presented	Score	Severity assessment
- New confusion - Raised blood urea nitrogen > 7 mmol/L	0–1	**Low risk** (less than 1% mortality risk) Home-based care appropriate
- Raised respiratory rate ≥ 30 breaths/min - Low blood pressure diastolic ≤ 60 mmHg or systolic ≤ 90 mmHg	2	**Intermediate risk** (1–10% mortality risk) Hospital assessment, admission required score
- Age 65 years or more	3–5	**High risk** (more than 10% mortality risk) Hospital admission requiring higher level of care

Figure 18.2 Lobar, bronchial and intersitial pneumonias

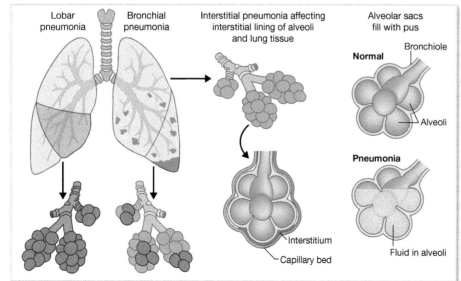

Lobar pneumonia
Bronchial pneumonia
Interstitial pneumonia affecting interstitial lining of alveoli and lung tissue
Alveolar sacs fill with pus

Normal
Bronchiole
Alveoli

Pneumonia
Fluid in alveoli

Interstitium
Capillary bed

Figure 18.3 Chest X-ray showing right-sided lobular pneumonia (see also Figure 14.1). Source: Leach R.M., 2014. Reproduced with permission of John Wiley & Sons.

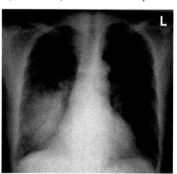

Acute and Critical Care Nursing at a Glance, First Edition. Edited by Helen Dutton and Jacqui Finch
© 2018 John Wiley & Sons, Ltd. Published 2018 by John Wiley & Sons, Ltd.
Companion website: www.ataglanceseries.com/nursing/acutecare

The World Health Organization (WHO) report that 1.4 million people globally each year die as a result of pneumonia.[1] Mortality is high among the most susceptible: the elderly, infants, immunocompromised patients and those taking immunosuppressive drugs, smokers and patients with obstructive lung diseases. Patients admitted to acute care are placed at increased risk, as pneumonia may also occur as a complication in hospital settings secondary to a procedure such as surgery or artificial ventilation.

Acute pneumonia is a respiratory infection which results in inflammation of the interstitial lung tissue. It may be the primary result of an infection or secondary to another disease, e.g. malignancy or AIDS, or it may be due to aspiration of vomit or mucus. The condition is generally classified into two distinct groups classified according to where the infection was acquired:
- **Community-acquired pneumonia** (CAP).
- **Hospital-acquired pneumonia** (HAP) (nosocomial).

Causative agents may be bacterial or viral, and their symptoms are similar (Figure 18.1), but may be more numerous in viral presentations. Untreated pneumonia may cause rapid deterioration, requiring urgent care escalation (see red flag box) and possibly intubation for mechanical ventilation in intensive care.

Community-acquired pneumonia

Community-acquired pneumonia is defined as an infection that is not acquired in hospital, or after recent hospitalisation. It is commonly caused by the pneumococcal bacterium *Staphylococcus pneumonia*, *Staphylococcus aureusi*, or other gram-negative bacteria such as *Klebsiella*, *Pseudomonas*, or *E. coli*. Fungal causes include *Pneumocystis jurovecii* pneumonia. CAP can further be divided into 'typical' and 'atypical' presentations (Table 18.1).

Bacteria that are commonly found in the upper airways enter the lungs causing the alveolar sacs to fill up with pus and fluid (Figure 18.2) reducing the amount of air space in the lungs, leading to hypoxaemia and increased work of breathing. Some bacteria enter the lungs via the bloodstream, for example *Escherichia coli* and *Klebsiella* pneumonia, which normally live in the gut.

Viral pneumonias accounts for 20% of CAP and are seasonal in nature, with the influenza virus often seen in winter months. Touching contaminated surfaces can transfer viruses from the hands to the eyes and nose, other airborne viruses are inhaled, while some, such as measles, are blood borne making their way systemically to the lungs. Inflammatory reactions are localised within the walls of the alveoli. The virus attacks the cell lining causing cell death. As the immune system responds to the invasion, the lungs fill with fluid, fibrin, red blood cells and macrophages. **Cytokines** are released as part of the inflammatory response, causing damage to the alveolar–capillary membrane. Lung compliance is reduced and bronchoconstriction occurs resulting in increased work of breathing and impaired gas exchange.

Diagnosis is made by physical examination, CXR (Figure 18.3) and blood tests including white cell count (WCC), C-reactive protein (CRP) and cultures. Patients with a CRP >100 mg/L, should be commenced on early antibiotic therapy. Pneumococcal and Legionella urinary antigen tests screen for these two organisms, enabling early treatment.

Classification

Pneumonia is classified according to the location of the inflammation (Figure 18.2):
- Lobar – affecting the whole of one lobe.
- Bronchial pneumonia – affecting the lobules and bronchi.
- Interstitial pneumonia – involving the areas between the alveoli (typically viral).

CURB 65 score

Morbidity and mortality are high in the very young and the elderly. In a recent audit, 18% of those affected had an average age of 71 years with death occurring within 24 h in 20% of cases.[2] The CURB 65 (Confusion, Urea, Respiratory rate, systolic Blood pressure) score is used by admitting medical staff to assess severity of CAP and guide the decision to discharge, admit to an acute ward, or to a higher level of care (Table 18.2).

Hospital-acquired pneumonia

Hospital-acquired pneumonia is defined as occurring after the first 48 h of admission excluding an infection that was incubating at the time of admission to hospital. HAP is a common cause of morbidity in the critically ill and has an associated mortality of up to 50%. An episode of pneumonia acquired while mechanically ventilated significantly prolongs critical care and hospital stay, thereby generating considerable additional costs. There is an increased risk for multidrug resistant organisms, e.g. methicillin-resistant *Staphylococcus aureus* (MRSA). Gram-negative bacteria are the most common cause of nosocomial pneumonia in critically ill adults. Diagnosis of HAP is based on clinical examination, CXR, diagnostic blood tests, and sputum and blood cultures.

Aspiration pneumonia is frequently seen in hospitalised patients and those in the community with reduced levels of consciousness. It is associated with high morbidity and mortality as inhalation of gastric or oropharyngeal contents into the lungs cause pneumonitis and extensive damage.

Nursing considerations to reduce risk of pneumonia

Patients who have reduced levels of consciousness, and slow gag and swallowing reflexes such as patients with a stroke, should have their airway protected by careful positioning on their side at a 30° angle if possible. Introducing a mouth care protocol has been demonstrated to reduce HAP, by reducing bacterial load in the oral cavity.[3] Early mobilisation with good nutrition is also beneficial. The use of bundles, e.g. British Thoracic Society Community Acquired Pneumonia Care Bundle[4] may improve outcome.

Care and management

- Administer oxygen therapy as prescribed to maintain SpO_2 within target saturations. Additional support such as CPAP or NIV may be required.
- Encourage mobilisation with nurses and physiotherapists, with high sitting position if too unwell to get out of bed.
- Ensure minimum pain to promote patient comfort, aid mobilisation and deep breathing exercises.
- Ensure frequent monitoring of six key physiological parameters, recording and acting appropriately on NEWS trigger. Early detection may prevent further deterioration.
- Ensure antibiotics, nebulisers and any other medications are safely administered as prescription.
- Ensure good fluid balance management as high fever and tachypnoea will increase insensible fluid loss. Urine output should be monitored hourly in the critically unwell.

19 Breathing problems: pleural disorders

Figure 19.1 The chest wall, visceral and parietal pleura, and pleural space

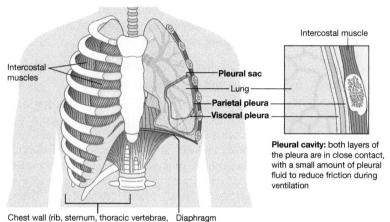

Intercostal muscles

Pleural sac
Lung
Parietal pleura
Visceral pleura

Intercostal muscle

Pleural cavity: both layers of the pleura are in close contact, with a small amount of pleural fluid to reduce friction during ventilation

Chest wall (rib, sternum, thoracic vertebrae, connective tissue, intercostal muscles)   Diaphragm

Table 19.1 Disorders of the pleura

Pleural effusion	Build up of fluid in the pleural space
Pleurisy	Inflammation of the pleura
Pneumothorax	Collection of air in the pleural space
Haemothorax	Collection of blood in the pleural space

Box 19.1   Light's criteria. Source: Hooper C., et al., 2010. Reproduced with permisssion of BMJ Publishing Group Ltd.

Fluid is exudate if it contains any of the following:
- pleural fluid/serum protein ratio > 0.5
- pleural fluid/serum LDH ratio > 0.6
- pleural fluid LDH > two-thirds the normal upper limit for serum

Figure 19.2   Pleural effusion

Pleural effusion symptoms and signs include:
- breathlessness, cough, pain on inspiration and coughing
- a CXR is required for diagnosis

Rib
Parietal pleura (outer layer)
Pleural cavity
Visceral pleura (inner layer)
Pleural effusion

Pleural fluid can be drained, but large effusions > 1.5L will be removed in several stages in 2-hourly intervals

Excess fluid builds up on pleural space, increasing pressure on the lung until part of it collapses

Figure 19.3   Chest drainage of pneumothorax

Pneumothorax:
Air between the pleura tends to rise to apex of lung. Any fluid, e.g. blood, tends to collect at base of the lung

Collapsed lung

Chest drainage tube, normally inserted in 5th or 6th intercostal space, mid axillary line

Air flows down chest tube on expiration as thoracic pressure rises. Air will be prevented from entering the lung in inspiration either by underwater seal or one-way valve

Underwater seal chest drain will bubble as air is drained from the pleural cavity until pneumothorax has resolved OR if the chest drain tube has become blocked. Medical review required if blocked drain suspected

Normal lung

From patient
To atmosphere or suction
Underwater seal bottle

Table 19.2 Transudate and exudate pleural effusion, causes and characteristics

Transudate pleural fluid and characteristics		Exudate pleural fluid and characteristics	
Caused by circulatory problems that increase hydrostatic pressure or reduce colloid osmotic pressure	Clear fluid Protein < 30g/L Specific gravity <1.012	Inflammatory processes in the lung result in fluid formation that is a high protein and white blood cell level	Cloudy fluid Protein > 30g/L Specific gravity >1.020
Collects in both pleural cavities		Collects in one pleural cavity	Meets Light's criteria
Examples		**Examples**	
Left ventricular failure	Hypothyroidism	Malignancy (accounts for about 40% of pleural effusions)	Postmyocardial infarction
Hypoproteinaemia	Mitral stenosis	Pneumonia, increasing capillary permeability	Pulmonary embolism
Constrictive pericarditis	Liver cirrhosis	Tuberculosis	Pancreatitis
Nephrotic syndrome		Postcardiac surgery	

Box 19.2   Removal of pleural chest drains

- Check that chest drain removal has been requested by medical staff
- Explain procedure to patient and gain consent
- Ensure adequate analgesia is given, pleural drain removal can be painful (e.g. morphine)
- Remove suction if applied
- Practice with the patient taking several deep breaths, then performing a Valsalva manoeuvre to increase intrathoracic pressure
- Cut suture. When patient is performing Valsalva manoeuvre remove drain (do not remove on inspiration)
- Cover site immediately with occlusive dressing
- Dispose of clinical waste according to local policy
- Observe patient, noting any signs of respiratory distress
- Take clinical observations and calculate NEWS score at least 4 hourly for the first 24 h postremoval

Acute and Critical Care Nursing at a Glance, First Edition. Edited by Helen Dutton and Jacqui Finch
© 2018 John Wiley & Sons, Ltd. Published 2018 by John Wiley & Sons, Ltd.
Companion website: www.ataglanceseries.com/nursing/acutecare

Problems that affect the integrity of the pleura or movement of the chest wall will impact on the patient's ability to move sufficient air in and out of the lungs, thereby reducing the supply of oxygen to the tissues and carbon dioxide removal. This chapter explores some common pleural diseases.

The pleura

The pleura is a thin double-layered membrane covering the surface of the lungs (visceral layer), and the inside of the chest wall and thoracic surface of the diaphragm (parietal) (Figure 19.1). The pleural cavity is a potential space between the two layers, containing a small amount of fluid to reduce friction. As the parietal pleura is adherent to the chest wall, it moves with the wall during inspiration. The very small amounts of intrapleural fluid are bound by intramolecular forces, so the visceral pleura and lung tissue move with the chest wall, increasing the space within the thorax for air to flow into the lung (inspiration). Pleural fluid is formed, then drained through the lymphatics, with a balance of formation and reabsorption to maintain homeostasis and lung function. Some disorders affecting the pleura are identified in Table 19.1. The British Thoracic Society (2010) have issued guidelines for the management of pleural diseases that can be accessed from https://www.brit-thoracic.org.uk.[1]

Pleural effusion

This consists of an excess of fluid in the pleural space; parts of the lung collapse leading to decreased lung compliance, increased work of breathing and hypoxaemia (Figure 19.2). Common causes are identified in Table 19.2, with pleural fluid classified as **transudate** or **exudate**, according to whether the fluid originates from within the lung tissue, or from circulatory problems.[2] An analysis of a sample of pleural fluid using Light's criteria (Box 19.1) identifies exudate fluid, suggesting possible causes, and guiding treatment. Moderate unilateral effusions may be aspirated by **thoracentesis**, with larger effusions requiring chest drainage and possibly **pleurodesis**. Transudate effusions resolve when circulatory problems have been treated, so removal of fluid may not be indicated. Pleural fluid may become infected (**empyema**), and this may not be detected until the patient becomes unwell. Infected pleural fluid is removed by chest tube drainage to reduce the risk of sepsis. Surgical intervention may be required, but decisions to proceed are made on an individual basis.

Pleurisy

Inflammation of the pleura (pleurisy) causes sharp pain on inspiration. Life-threatening conditions featuring chest pain, such as myocardial infarction, pulmonary embolus and pneumothorax need to be excluded before pleurisy is diagnosed. Common causes include: viral infections, **mesothelioma**, **pericarditis** and pneumonia. Pain relief through positioning, support during breathing and analgesics such as NSAID, are an essential component of nursing management. Treatment focuses on identifying and treating the cause.

Pneumothorax

Pneumothorax is the presence of air between the parietal and visceral pleura. The normal lung has a tendency to collapse, but in health is held open by the two pleural layers. When the pleura are separated, the lung collapses. Large pneumothoraces cause chest pain, shortness of breath, and unequal chest movements. A CXR confirms diagnosis. Pneumothoraces can be categorised as:

- **Primary spontaneous pneumothorax (PSP):** occurs unrelated to any underlying lung disease, and if small may resolve without treatment. Smoking is associated with higher risk, and advice is given to quit. Exercise is not associated with pneumothorax.
- **Secondary pneumothorax (SP):** occurs secondary to existing lung disease, such as tuberculosis, cancer and COPD.
- **Traumatic pneumothorax:** from a penetrating chest trauma such as a stab wound, or blunt trauma causing a fractured rib. **Open:** air enters and leaves pleural space during respiration. **Closed:** air enters, but cannot leave pleural space leading to a tension pneumothorax.
- **Tension pneumothorax: a medical emergency** (see Chapter 36).
- **Iatrogenic pneumothorax:** one that has been induced inadvertently by healthcare interventions, such as after central line insertion, lung biopsy or mechanical ventilation.
- **Haemothorax:** blood collects in the pleural cavity, often results from trauma and may be associated with a pneumothorax, i.e. **haemopneumothorax.**

Management includes supplemental oxygen to maintain SpO_2 within target saturations, sitting the patient upright to maximise lung expansion and close monitoring of physiological signs using NEWS to help detect deterioration. A computed tomography (CT) scan provides the most detailed information regarding size and position, guiding treatment in conjunction with the severity of patient breathlessness.[3] Small pneumothoraces (<15% of lung) where the patient is not breathless resolve spontaneously, with analgesia to control pain. Needle aspiration or chest drain insertion is required for larger symptomatic pneumothoraces (Figure 19.3).

Chest tube drainage

A number of different chest drain devices are available.[4] Nurses must be familiar with the type used for their patients in order to ensure safe, effective care. Types of drainage systems include:

- Underwater seal collecting chambers.
- Dry collecting chambers with one-way valve.
- Drains with low suction applied (10–20 cmH$_2$O or 1–2 kPa).
- For recurrent pleural effusion such as seen with COPD – small pig-tailed drains, with one-way flutter valve and drainage bag.

If no suction is applied, any fluid in the drainage tube should swing with the patient's breathing. The negative pressure of inspiration causes the fluid to move towards the patient, then down again in expiration. If swinging stops, the drain could be blocked risking a tension pneumothorax developing, so medical review is required. Any fluid from the drain should be recorded for amount and appearance. Clamps are available, but only for use if disconnection occurs, if temporarily moving the chamber above the level of the patient's chest, or when draining large pleural effusions. When the pneumothorax or effusion has drained, medical staff will decide when the chest drain can be removed by a competent healthcare professional. Considerations when removing a chest drain are summarised in Box 19.2. A CXR, post removal, checks lung expansion.

20 Respiratory support: non-invasive ventilation

Figure 20.1 Mask options for non-invasive ventilation (CPAP and BIPAP).
Source: Leach R.M., 2014. Reproduced with permission of John Wiley & Sons.

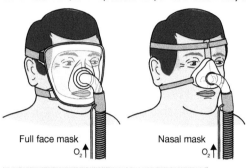

Full face mask $O_2\uparrow$ Nasal mask $O_2\uparrow$ Naso-oral mask $O_2\uparrow$

Figure 20.2 High flow nasal oxygen

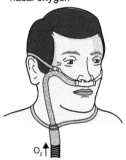

$O_2\uparrow$

Box 20.1 Indications for CPAP

- Acute hypoxaemic respiratory failure
- Cardiogenic pulmonary oedema

Both refractory to conventional medical treatment

Box 20.2 Indications for BIPAP

- Acute hypercapnic respiratory failure in the acute or chronic patient
- $PaCO_2 > 6.5$ kPa
- pH < 7.35
- Increased RR despite optimisation with oxygen therapy OR
- Hypercapnic respiratory failure with chest wall deformity
- Neuromuscular disorder
- Obstructive sleep apnoea
- Type 1 respiratory failure not responding to CPAP, but must be in level 3 environment

Box 20.3 Standard Medical therapy for COPD

- Controlled oxygen therapy to maintain SaO_2 between 88–92%
- Nebulised salbutamol 2.5–5 mg
- Nebulised ipratropium 500 μg
- Prednisolone 30 mg
- Antibiotic agent (if indicated)

Box 20.4 Issues for consideration when starting NIV

- Has the patient consented to NIV? Does patient and their relatives understand the treatment plan?
- If NIV fails, is intubation, ventilation and admission to ITU appropriate?
- If NIV fails is it appropriate to continue as palliation? Is NIV ceiling of care?
- Is it inappropriate to start NIV due to complexity of patient problems and poor prognosis?
- Considering a DNAR? This does not exclude NIV treatment
- pH below 7.25? This is a threshold for considering intubation and full ventilation, with level 3 care

Table 20.1 Inclusion and exclusion criteria.
Source: Davidson A., et al., 2016.

NIV inclusion	NIV exclusion
Primary diagnosis of COPD (neuromuscular disease or obesity) present	Life threatening hypoxaemia pH < 7.15
Able to protect airway	Severe comorbidity
Conscious and co-operative	Glasgow coma score ≤ 8, confusion, agitation Severe cognitive impairment
Potential recovery to quality of life acceptable to the patient	Facial burns/trauma/ recent facial or upper airway surgery
Patient consent gained	Undrained pneumothorax
In level 3 area, NIV may be appropriate if not fully conscious	Upper gastrointestinal surgery Bowel surgery
There is evidence to support the use of NIV in patients who are comatose secondary to COPD-induced hypercapnia	Inability to maintain airway/moribund Is pH < 7.25 with additional adverse features ?

Figure 20.3 Meeting the needs of the patient requiring NIV

Agitation and distress may be relieved by infused sedation, e.g. morphine 2.5–5mg, +/– a benzodiazepine BUT is only appropriate in a level 2 or 3 setting

The pressure from NIV may lead to bloating, nausea and discomfort

Consider inserting nasogastric tube to relieve distension and anti-emetic for nausea as prescribed

Select appropriate type and size of face mask, full mask preferred. Ensure snug fit. Let patient hold mask to face, before securing then gradually commence NIV

Cardiac output can be reduced due to increased intrathoracic pressure

Face mask can be claustrophobic, sore and uncomfortable. Excessive anxiety may be present

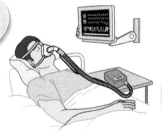

Monitor ECG, HR, RR, BP, SpO_2, AVPU Record fluid balance, check urine output > 0.5 mL/kg/h

Allow plenty of time for questions, and NIV initiation. Stay with patient for at least 5 min after any change in setting

Encourage short 5–10 min breaks for a drink and meals. IV supplements may be required, to replace increased fluid loss through lungs

Explain clearly what NIV involves

Lack of compliance with NIV is a common cause for failure

Box 20.5 Patient safety alert stage one. Source: NHS, 2015.

- A mask for non-invasive ventilation (NIV) was attached to a patient's face but the ventilation machine had not been switched on
- The patient became severely hypoxic and died

Acute and Critical Care Nursing at a Glance, First Edition. Edited by Helen Dutton and Jacqui Finch
© 2018 John Wiley & Sons, Ltd. Published 2018 by John Wiley & Sons, Ltd.
Companion website: www.ataglanceseries.com/nursing/acutecare

An overview has been given of clinical conditions that may require additional respiratory support in the form of **non-invasive ventilation (NIV)** (Chapters 17 and 18) comprising of **CPAP** and **BiPAP**. NIV supports breathing using a variety of snug-fitting face masks (Figure 20.1), enabling pressure to be maintained both in the circuit and the respiratory system. **HFNC** (Figure 20.2) is now being used for adults with **acute hypoxaemic respiratory failure** (Type 1), but as yet has not been incorporated into clinical guidelines. These approaches to respiratory support benefit from the principle of applying positive pressure during expiration thereby increasing oxygenation, but differ in the extent of ventilation support delivered. NIV is now being used frequently in acute care and requires an appropriate environment with appropriately trained staff.[1] Guidance for NIV for patients with acute hypercapnic failure has been published by the British Thoracic Society and Intensive Care Society.[2]

High flow oxygen therapy

Conventional high flow oxygen therapy comprises a flow of around 15 L/min, via a non-rebreathe face mask. A HFNC can generate up to 60 L/min of heated, humidified gas through the nasal cannula. The high flow of gas creates a positive resistance to expiration in the nasopharynx, which whilst small, helps keep alveoli open and improves gaseous exchange.[3] A HFNC is often found more comfortable than the tight-fitting mask of CPAP.

Continuous positive airway pressure

Continuous positive airway pressure can be delivered through a number of devices, using a nasal or nasa/oral or full face mask for patients with **acute respiratory failure, Type 1.** A continuous positive flow of gas is delivered throughout the breathing cycle, with a positive end expired pressure (PEEP) of between 5 and 10 cm H_2O (also referred to as end positive airway pressure, EPAP). Patients breathe spontaneously, benefiting from the continuous flow of gas at above atmospheric pressure which reduces the work of inspiration, and by PEEP holding lung units open during expiration, increasing functional residual capacity and oxygenation. Increased CO_2 clearance may occur with CPAP. Indications for CPAP are given in Box 20.1.

Bi-level positive airways pressure

For those who have difficulty in maintaining sufficient minute volumes to remove carbon dioxide or **type 2 respiratory failure**, extra inspiratory support is required (Box 20.2). BiPAP (preferably delivered by full face mask), reduces both rate of intubation and mortality for COPD patients with respiratory acidosis. It is indicated for those with an arterial **pH <7.35** and a $PaCO_2$ **>6.5 kPa** who have not responded to maximal therapy (Box 20.3). Early ABG analysis and NIV commencement is beneficial.[4] BiPAP should not be commenced if the pH is within normal range. Indications and contraindications for BiPAP are shown in Table 20.1.

The BiPAP machine

Bi-level positive airways pressure is delivered using two levels of pressure: IPAP (inspiratory) and EPAP (expiratory). **Pressure support** (PS) is the difference between IPAP and EPAP. PS determines how much help is given to inspiratory effort: as pressure support increases, the tidal volume increases. Initially an IPAP of 15 cmH$_2$O is selected (or 20 if pH <7.25) and titrated upwards over 10–30 minutes, to a maximum pressure target of 20–30 cmH$_2$O. EPAP settings are commenced at 3 cmH$_2$O and should not exceed 8 cmH$_2$O without expert review.[2] A therapeutic level is reached when the respiratory rate falls below 30, with good tidal volumes, a reducing $PaCO_2$ with SpO_2 within the target range of 88–92%.

Additional BiPAP settings include:

- **Oxygen**: oxygen percentage is set according to target saturations. Oxygen enrichment is best delivered close to the face mask.
- **Back-up rate:** patients on BiPAP can breathe spontaneously – each breath triggers the machine to deliver the IPAP. A back-up rate (usually 16–20 breaths/min) will deliver a breath, even if not triggered.
- **Ti: inspiratory time**, usually about a third of the breath cycle.
- **Rise time**: the time for the pressure to rise from EPAP to IPAP.
- **Ramp time**: the amount of time taken to achieve the pre-set IPAP pressure. A gradual change in pressure over about 10–30 min is often better tolerated by the patient.

Monitoring the patient receiving bi-level positive airways pressure

Patients commencing BiPAP require **close/continuous monitoring** for changes in their condition including: **pulse oximetry**, ECG monitoring, respiratory rate, blood pressure, heart rate and AVPU assessment, for the first 12 h. The intervals between observations are reduced to hourly as clinical status stabilises, then to 4-hourly after 24 h if improvement continues. Nurses must be competent in caring for patients on BiPAP to prevent **adverse incidents**[5] (Box 20.5). Patient care issues are summarised in Figure 20.3.

In additional to clinical evaluation, ABG analysis is integral to determining effectiveness of BiPAP. After initiation, ABGs are checked regularly at 1, 4 and 12 h. ABGs assist in both titrating machine settings and informing the treatment plan. A senior doctor or other competent designated healthcare professional will assess the patient within the first 4 h of NIV to ensure that the treatment plan is appropriate and further escalation is not required.

Escalation

Prior to the initiation of BiPAP a ceiling of treatment should be discussed (Box 20.4) within the multidisciplinary team and be documented in the patient's notes. Patients and their relatives are included in decision making where possible. Escalation if appropriate should take place with the critical care team at an early stage. The patient remains on BiPAP as much as possible for 24 h. Treatment continues until maximum therapeutic interventions have had time to be effective and the acute cause of respiratory failure has resolved. If NIV has failed and it is not appropriate to escalate care, a proactive approach to palliation should be implemented.

Weaning

When the patient parameters have returned to normal (pH >7.35, respiratory rate normalised and underlying cause/symptoms resolved) a weaning plan should be put in place, documented and commenced. Weaning must only be instigated during the day and preferable at the start of the day. Patients often require night time NIV for the first 48 h of weaning from daytime NIV.

21 Principles of thoracic surgery

Table 21.1 Common thoracic procedures

Procedure	Definition	Condition
Lung resection	Removal of part or the entire lung	Tumours (mainly primary lung cancer or metastasis)
Lung volume reduction	Resection of the severely emphysematous lung tissue allowing the remaining, relatively good lung to expand and work better	Advanced emphysema
Bullectomy	Removal of dilated air space in the lung parenchyma (bullae)	Pneumothorax caused by rupture of bullae
Lung decortication	Removal of restricting lung inelastic fibrous peel from the lung parenchyma and pleura to allow the lung to re-expand	Fibrothorax Mesothelioma
Pleurectomy	Resection of pleura	Recurrent pneumothorax Malignant pleural effusion Mesothelioma
Pleuradesis	Mechanical (surgical abrasion) or chemical irritation (by talc instillation) of the visceral and parietal pleura to cause permanent adhesion obliterating the pleural space and attach the lung to the chest wall	Recurrent pneumothorax Recurrent pleural effusion

Figure 21.1 Types of lung resection

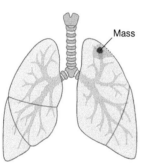

Wedge resection removes a small portion of a lobe

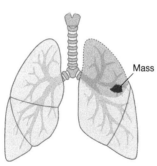

Segment resection removes a larger portion of a lobe

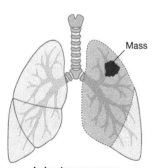

Lobectomy removes an entire lobe

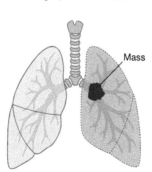

Pneumonectomy removes the entire lung

Figure 21.2 Different approaches for surgical access

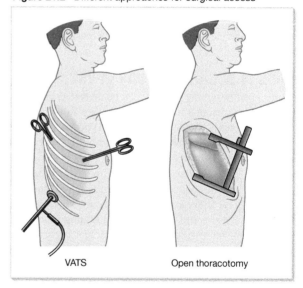

VATS   Open thoracotomy

Figure 21.3 Open thoracotomy wound, with pleural drainage

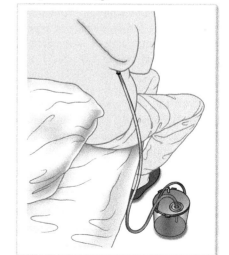

Table 21.2 Complications after thoracic surgery

Respiratory complications	Cardiovascular complications	Others
• Pneumonia • Atelectasis • Respiratory failure • Prolonged air leak • Empyema • Bronchopleural fistula	• Haemorrhage • Pulmonary oedema • Arrhythmias • Myocardial ischaemia/ infarction • Deep vein thrombosis and pulmonary emboli	• Acute and/or chronic pain • Wound infection • Chylothorax • Surgical emphysema

Acute and Critical Care Nursing at a Glance, First Edition. Edited by Helen Dutton and Jacqui Finch
© 2018 John Wiley & Sons, Ltd. Published 2018 by John Wiley & Sons, Ltd.
Companion website: www.ataglanceseries.com/nursing/acutecare

The purpose of thoracic surgery is to treat diseased or injured organs in the chest, including trachea, lungs, mediastinum, pleura and chest wall. Lung cancer is the most common reason for surgical intervention. Different parts of the lung can be removed depending on localisation, type and the extent of tumour (Figure 21.1). Common thoracic surgical procedures and their indications are summarised in Table 21.1.

Types of thoracic surgery

Minimally invasive surgery

Video-assisted thoracoscopic surgery (**VATS**) is performed using a video camera and endoscopic instruments that are inserted into the chest through usually two or three small incisions (ports) made between ribs (Figure 21.2). The notable benefits of VATS to patients include less trauma and pain, lower risk of postoperative complications, less stress on the immune system and faster recovery time. The majority of thoracic procedures can be performed using a minimally invasive approach. However, VATS is contraindicated in markedly unstable patients and those with extensive adhesions obliterating pleural space.

Open surgery

Posterolateral thoracotomy remains the standard approach in patients not suitable for VATS and those requiring major lung resections. It involves opening the chest by making a 10–15 cm incision below the scapula that extends along the fifth or sixth intercostal space to the anterior axillary line. It allows direct visualisation of the thoracic cavity and optimal access to the pulmonary hilum (pulmonary artery and pulmonary veins) (Figure 21.2). A thoracotomy incision involves rib retraction or excision, large muscle cutting and intercostal nerve injury. There is, therefore, a very high level of post operative pain associated with this approach.

Nursing management

Monitoring

The majority of thoracic surgical patients can be transferred from recovery to a high-dependency unit or directly to a surgical ward. The level of care depends on the extent of surgical intervention and the patient's condition before and after surgery. Patients post lobectomy or pneumonectomy and those with impaired respiratory function prior to surgery usually require close observation of cardiac and respiratory status, with continuous ECG and oxygen saturation monitoring for the first 1–2 days. ABG analysis is often performed to determine gas exchange and to guide oxygen therapy. The frequency of observation will be determined by the patient's recovery. The six vital signs are monitored closely. Additional observations should include respiration pattern and depth, chest movements, with assessment of pain and effort associated with breathing and coughing.

Optimising respiratory function

In the early post operative period most patients require oxygen therapy that is titrated according to the oxygen saturation and ABG results. Respiratory failure due to atelectasis and pneumonia is the most common complication after thoracic surgery caused by ineffective airway clearance, increased secretions and diminished cough secondary to pain and fatigue. Therefore, effective pain control is essential to facilitate deep breathing and coughing. Early mobilisation significantly reduces the risk of respiratory complications and promotes lung re-expansion, and it should be initiated on the day of surgery. Nurses should encourage expectoration, effective coughing and deep breathing exercises to avoid retention of secretion. Nebulisers are often administered to aid secretion clearance and treat any bronchospasm.

Postoperative pain management

Pain after thoracic surgery, especially open thoracotomy, is severe and if not treated may have major implications, including respiratory failure and development of chronic pain syndrome. A high level of pain results from surgical incision, irritation of pleura by chest drains, and respiratory effort (breathing, coughing and clearing secretion). Large numbers of patients also experience shoulder pain caused by arm positioning during surgery and phrenic nerve irritation. Different analgesic strategies can be used. However, thoracic epidural analgesia and paravertebral nerve block have been found to be most effective. Other pain relief options include oral and intravenous opioids, PCA, NSAID and paracetamol (see Chapter 5).

An analgesic regimen should be implemented under the guidance of the anaesthetist or pain nurse specialist. Nurses are responsible for regular pain assessment and maintaining adequate pain relief. Pain scores should be measured at rest and during physical activity, documented, acted upon and re-evaluated. Other non-pharmacological strategies, such as positioning, relaxation and distraction can be used to support pain relief.

Chest drain care

Pleural chest drains are usually inserted at the end of surgery to facilitate fluid drainage and re-expansion of the lung that has been deflated during surgery (Figure 21.3). Recording the amount of drainage, observing for air leak (bubbling) and swing, and presence of fresh blood or chyle is necessary to guide therapeutic decisions and detect the possible complications outlined (Table 21.2). Any changes in the drain activity, character and amount of fluid should be reported to medical staff. Chest drains can be connected to suction (usually between 2.5 and 5 kPa) to aid lung re-expansion. Nursing staff need to ensure the suction pressure is correct to prevent lung injury. The chest drain site should be inspected for oozing, presence of surgical emphysema and signs of infection.

Psychological and emotional support

Thoracic surgery is performed mainly in patients with malignant and chronic conditions. In many cases information about cancer and poor prognosis is given following the surgery. In some patients, surgery is performed only as a palliative measure to relieve distressing symptoms. Nurses should ensure that patients' and carers' psychological and emotional needs are identified and addressed to enable them to cope with the stress and impact of the disease on their life. Referral to appropriate specialist teams (palliative care/lung cancer specialist nurses, psychologists) should be made promptly. The patients and their families should be provided with information and advice on available support and resources in the community (patients support groups, charities, smoking cessation services, etc.).

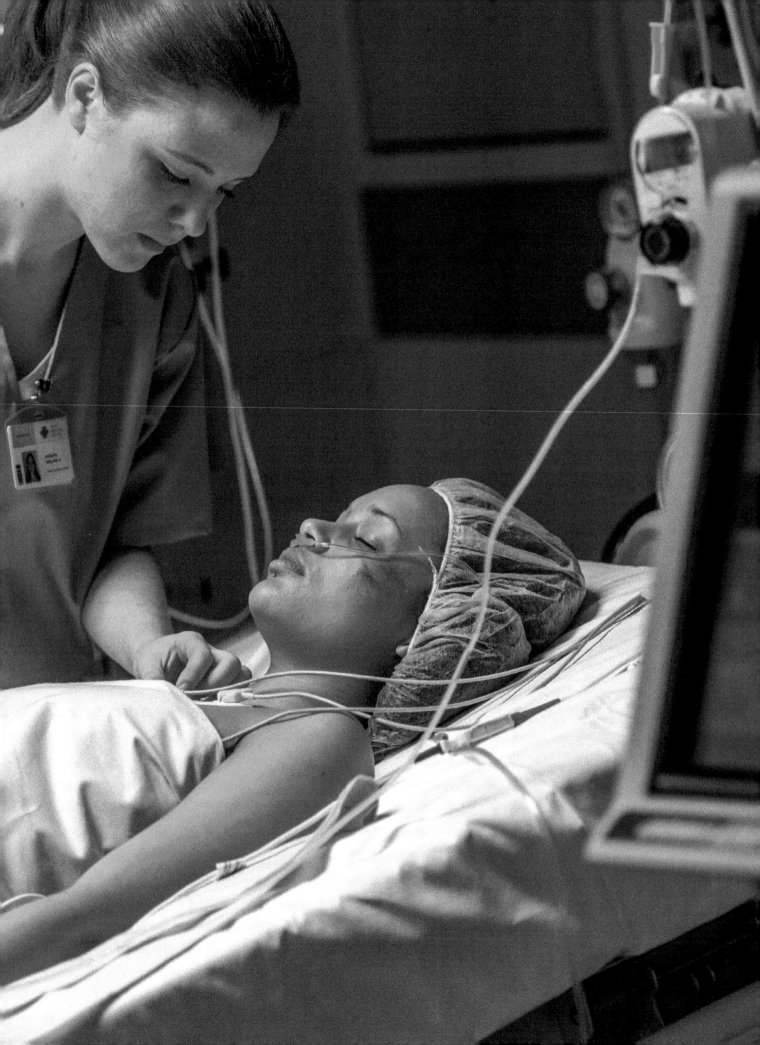

Circulation: patients with circulatory problems

Part 4

Chapters

22 Circulatory physiology 1: circulation   50
23 Circulatory physiology 2: the heart and cardiac cycle   52
24 Circulatory physiology 3: control of circulation   54
25 Assessment of circulation   56
26 Cardiac investigations   58
27 Fluid, electrolytes and intravenous fluids   60
28 Haemodynamic monitoring   62
29 Acute chest pain   64
30 The 12-lead electrocardiogram   66
31 Altered heart rhythm   68
32 Physiology of the immune system   70
33 Acute circulatory failure 1: distributive (sepsis)   72
34 Acute circulatory failure 2: distributive (anaphylaxis and neurogenic)   74
35 Acute circulatory failure 3: hypovolaemia   76
36 Acute circulatory failure 4: obstructive   78
37 Acute circulatory failure 5: heart failure   80
38 Principles of cardiac surgery   82
39 Physiology of the gastrointestinal system   84
40 Acute medical and surgical gastrointestinal problems   86
41 Physiology of the renal system   88
42 Acute kidney injury   90
43 Burns: immediate care   92
44 Major trauma   94
45 Resuscitation   96

22 Circulatory physiology 1: circulation

Figure 22.1 The heart, major structures and blood flow.
Source: Peate I., *et al*., 2014. Reproduced with permission of John Wiley & Sons.

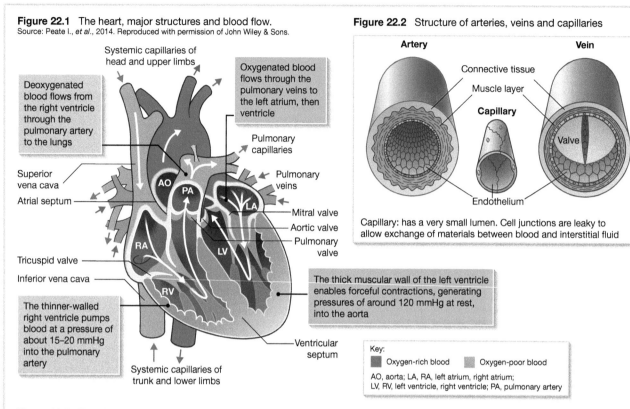

Systemic capillaries of head and upper limbs

Deoxygenated blood flows from the right ventricle through the pulmonary artery to the lungs

Oxygenated blood flows through the pulmonary veins to the left atrium, then ventricle

Superior vena cava

Atrial septum

Pulmonary capillaries

Pulmonary veins

AO

PA

LA

Mitral valve
Aortic valve
Pulmonary valve

RA

LV

Tricuspid valve

Inferior vena cava

RV

The thinner-walled right ventricle pumps blood at a pressure of about 15–20 mmHg into the pulmonary artery

The thick muscular wall of the left ventricle enables forceful contractions, generating pressures of around 120 mmHg at rest, into the aorta

Ventricular septum

Systemic capillaries of trunk and lower limbs

Key:
■ Oxygen-rich blood   ■ Oxygen-poor blood
AO, aorta; LA, RA, left atrium, right atrium;
LV, RV, left ventricle, right ventricle; PA, pulmonary artery

Figure 22.2 Structure of arteries, veins and capillaries

Artery

Vein

Connective tissue

Muscle layer

Capillary

Valve

Endothelium

Capillary: has a very small lumen. Cell junctions are leaky to allow exchange of materials between blood and interstitial fluid

Figure 22.3 The circulatory system

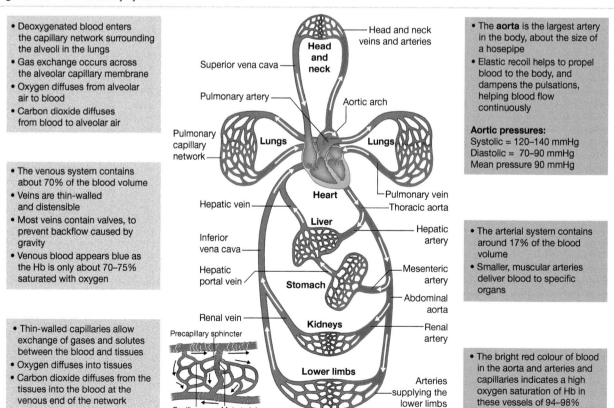

- Deoxygenated blood enters the capillary network surrounding the alveoli in the lungs
- Gas exchange occurs across the alveolar capillary membrane
- Oxygen diffuses from alveolar air to blood
- Carbon dioxide diffuses from blood to alveolar air

- The venous system contains about 70% of the blood volume
- Veins are thin-walled and distensible
- Most veins contain valves, to prevent backflow caused by gravity
- Venous blood appears blue as the Hb is only about 70–75% saturated with oxygen

- Thin-walled capillaries allow exchange of gases and solutes between the blood and tissues
- Oxygen diffuses into tissues
- Carbon dioxide diffuses from the tissues into the blood at the venous end of the network

Head and neck veins and arteries

Superior vena cava

Head and neck

Pulmonary artery

Aortic arch

Pulmonary capillary network

Lungs

Lungs

Heart

Hepatic vein

Pulmonary vein
Thoracic aorta

Liver

Inferior vena cava

Hepatic artery

Hepatic portal vein

Mesenteric artery

Stomach

Abdominal aorta

Renal vein

Kidneys

Renal artery

Precapillary sphincter

Lower limbs

Arteries supplying the lower limbs

Capillary   Metarteriole

- The **aorta** is the largest artery in the body, about the size of a hosepipe
- Elastic recoil helps to propel blood to the body, and dampens the pulsations, helping blood flow continuously

Aortic pressures:
Systolic = 120–140 mmHg
Diastolic = 70–90 mmHg
Mean pressure 90 mmHg

- The arterial system contains around 17% of the blood volume
- Smaller, muscular arteries deliver blood to specific organs

- The bright red colour of blood in the aorta and arteries and capillaries indicates a high oxygen saturation of Hb in these vessels of 94–98%

Acute and Critical Care Nursing at a Glance, First Edition. Edited by Helen Dutton and Jacqui Finch
© 2018 John Wiley & Sons, Ltd. Published 2018 by John Wiley & Sons, Ltd.
Companion website: www.ataglanceseries.com/nursing/acutecare

A continuous supply of oxygen and nutrients is required by the cells in order for them to function. The cardiovascular system consists of the heart as a pump, arteries that transport blood away from the heart, the thin-walled capillaries allowing diffusion of gases to, and metabolites from, the tissues and veins returning blood back to the heart. The system is constantly working to ensure each cell, tissue and organ has an adequate blood supply to carry out their functions.

The heart

The heart's modest size, that of a human fist with a weight of around 250–300 g, seems inconsistent with its strength and endurance. This four-chamber muscular pump is enclosed in the mediastinum of the thorax, with about two-thirds lying left of the mid sternal line (Figure 22.1). The atria act as the receiving chambers for blood flowing into the heart assisting ventricular filling, whilst the ventricles perform the work of pumping the blood round **the pulmonary and systemic circulations**. It is largely self-regulating, its beating initiated by its own pacemaker, but it is also responsive to the changing needs of the body, influenced by the autonomic nervous system (Chapter 24). The heart pumps blood simultaneously around both the pulmonary and systemic circulations. Valves, placed between the atria and ventricles (atrioventricular valves) and in the outflow tracts (pulmonary artery and aorta) are essential to ensure blood continues to flow in the right direction. They open and close in response to pressure changes generated by the heart muscle contracting (systole) and then relaxing (diastole) whilst the chambers refill with blood.

Blood flow through the heart (Figure 22.1)

The right side of the heart receives venous blood from the superior and inferior vena cava draining from the body into the right atrium. Blood then flows through the **tricuspid (right atrioventricular) valve** in to the right ventricle. Ventricular contraction conveys the blood through the **pulmonary valve** into the pulmonary artery and pulmonary capillaries. Most arteries carry oxygenated blood, the pulmonary artery being an exception, carrying deoxygenated blood away from the heart to the lungs. The pulmonary circulation is comparatively short having close proximity to the heart, and offers only a low resistance to blood flow. The right ventricle therefore does not have to generate a very high pressure (15–20 mmHg), and so its muscular wall is not as thick as its harder working counterpart, the left ventricle. It does, however, have to move exactly the same volume of blood, about 70 mL in each heartbeat (known as **stroke volume**, SV), in order to deliver sufficient volume through the pulmonary circulation to the left ventricle. Oxygen diffuses from the air-filled alveoli to the blood in the pulmonary capillaries and carbon dioxide moves in the opposite direction from the blood to be expelled through pulmonary ventilation. Pulmonary venous blood, now enriched with oxygen, flows through the pulmonary veins into the left atrium.

Blood returns to the left atrium from the lungs via the pulmonary veins (note these veins are transporting oxygenated blood), through the **mitral (left atrioventricular) valve** into the left ventricle. The systemic circulation is a large system, requiring the blood to be transported some distance through vessels which offer a high resistance to flow. The left ventricle needs to generate a systolic pressure of 100–140 mmHg, and the thick ventricular

cardiac muscle (**myocardium**) helps generate this higher pressure. The left ventricle has to work considerably harder than the right to move the same amount of blood. The left side of the heart is more prone to problems, both with the heart valves (pulmonary and aortic) and damage from ischaemic events such as a myocardial infarction. The strong left ventricular contraction ejects blood through the **aortic valve**, into the **aorta**, where the large rise in pressure during ventricular systole stretches the elastic walls of this major artery. Elastic recoil propels the blood through the vessels of the vascular system during the resting or diastolic phase of the cardiac cycle.

The vascular system

The vascular system provides the conduit for blood to reach the cells, and then returns it back to the central pump.

Arteries and **veins** (Figure 22.2) both consist of three layers:
- The innermost layer, the **endothelium** (also tunica intima), provides a smooth surface allowing uninterrupted blood flow, discouraging clot formation.
- The middle, smooth muscle and elastic tissue of the **tunica media**, is thicker in arteries than in the thinner walled veins. This enables arteries to stretch and recoil in response to pressure changes in the left ventricle. Arteries which supply muscles and specific body organs have more smooth muscle and less elastic tissue and this facilitates active vasoconstriction and vasodilation, regulating blood flow to these areas.
- The **tunica externa** is made of fibrous/connective tissue and provides support and protection to the vessels.

The circulatory system (Figure 22.3) conveys blood around the body. The haemoglobin in aortic blood is almost fully saturated with oxygen (about 94–98%), giving this arterial blood a bright red appearance. Major arteries branch off from the aorta, then divide to become progressively smaller arteries. Smaller muscular arterioles, with lumen diameters ranging from 30 to 10 μm, regulate blood flow into the capillary beds. Microscopic capillaries with lumen diameters of 8–10 μm, just large enough for a red blood cell to squeeze through, are thin walled and porous, enabling oxygen and nutrients to diffuse into the adjacent cells. Cells are only able to gain nutrients from their immediate environment so an extensive capillary network is essential for nutrient delivery and waste product removal. The higher oxygen content in the capillary blood relative to the cell creates a concentration gradient, so oxygen diffuses into the interstitial space, then through the cell wall. Waste products of metabolism, including carbon dioxide, move from the cell by diffusion into venules at the venous end of the capillary bed.

Venules converge into veins where blood now has a low oxygen saturation of around 70–75%, with increased amounts of carbon dioxide and waste products. Veins, particularly in the legs, contain valves to resist the effect of gravity which causes backflow. Leg muscles massage the deep veins in the leg encouraging venous return. Venous return continues with abdominal pressure driving the blood upwards through the inferior vena cava, with the negative intrathoracic pressure of inspiration drawing blood back to the right atrium. The pressure of blood as it enters the right atrium, known as the central venous pressure, is around 2–6 mmHg, much lower than high aortic pressure at the beginning of the systemic circulation. The circuit is now complete, but continues as the blood drains into the ventricles ready for the next contraction.

23 Circulatory physiology 2: the heart and cardiac cycle

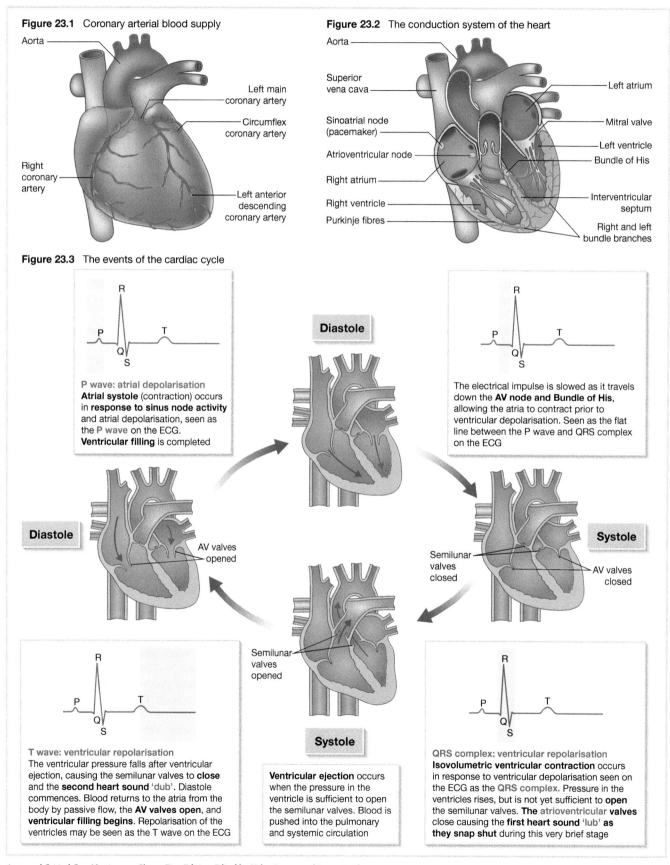

Figure 23.1 Coronary arterial blood supply

Aorta
Left main coronary artery
Circumflex coronary artery
Right coronary artery
Left anterior descending coronary artery

Figure 23.2 The conduction system of the heart

Aorta
Superior vena cava
Sinoatrial node (pacemaker)
Atrioventricular node
Right atrium
Right ventricle
Purkinje fibres
Left atrium
Mitral valve
Left ventricle
Bundle of His
Interventricular septum
Right and left bundle branches

Figure 23.3 The events of the cardiac cycle

Diastole

Systole

Diastole

Systole

AV valves opened

Semilunar valves closed

AV valves closed

Semilunar valves opened

P wave: atrial depolarisation
Atrial systole (contraction) occurs in **response to sinus node activity** and atrial depolarisation, seen as the **P wave** on the ECG.
Ventricular filling is completed

The electrical impulse is slowed as it travels down the **AV node and Bundle of His**, allowing the atria to contract prior to ventricular depolarisation. Seen as the flat line between the P wave and QRS complex on the ECG

T wave: ventricular repolarisation
The ventricular pressure falls after ventricular ejection, causing the semilunar valves to **close** and the **second heart sound** 'dub'. Diastole commences. Blood returns to the atria from the body by passive flow, the **AV valves open**, and **ventricular filling begins**. Repolarisation of the ventricles may be seen as the T wave on the ECG

Ventricular ejection occurs when the pressure in the ventricle is sufficient to open the semilunar valves. Blood is pushed into the pulmonary and systemic circulation

QRS complex: ventricular repolarisation
Isovolumetric ventricular contraction occurs in response to ventricular depolarisation seen on the ECG as the **QRS complex**. Pressure in the ventricles rises, but is not yet sufficient to **open** the semilunar valves. **The atrioventricular valves** close causing the **first heart sound** 'lub' as **they snap shut** during this very brief stage

Acute and Critical Care Nursing at a Glance, First Edition. Edited by Helen Dutton and Jacqui Finch
© 2018 John Wiley & Sons, Ltd. Published 2018 by John Wiley & Sons, Ltd.
Companion website: www.ataglanceseries.com/nursing/acutecare

Chapter 22 introduced the structures that make up the cardiovascular system. This system is relatively simple but the mechanisms that ensure a healthy myocardium, a regular heartbeat with matched output for both right and left ventricles, are more complex.

The coronary arteries

The **myocardium** (or heart muscle) is continuously beating and requires a reliable supply of blood delivering oxygen to fuel the muscle contractions. The left and right coronary arteries arise from just above the leaflets of the aortic valve. The **left coronary artery** quickly branches into two and is the main supply for the left ventricle (Figure 23.1). During systole, when the ventricle is contracting, the pressure in the left ventricular myocardium is so great that coronary artery flow is squeezed, almost halting it. The majority of **myocardial perfusion** (about 85%) occurs during **diastole**, the resting stage of the **cardiac cycle**. An increase in heart rate (HR) can be bad news for myocardial perfusion, as diastole shortens progressively as HR rises. The HR should normally be below 100 beats/min. The myocardium is able to extract 70–80% of the oxygen delivered to it, compared with only 25% extracted by tissues in the rest of the body. The **right coronary artery** supplies the right ventricle and as this does not generate such high pressure, flow is present throughout the cardiac cycle. The myocardium is damaged if the blood supply is interrupted, reduced or even stopped. This causes the chest pain of acute coronary syndrome (ACS, Chapter 29), possible altered heart rhythms (Chapter 31), or even cardiac arrest and death.

The conduction system

The cardiac conduction system (Figure 23.2) comprises **autorhythmic cells**, able to generate their own impulses and transmit electrical waves across the heart, stimulating the myocardium to contract. The **sinoatrial node (SAN)**, the pacemaker of the heart, consists of a region of specialised cells spontaneously depolarising at around 100 beats/min. The SAN is under the influence of the vagal branch of the autonomic nervous system and at rest it normally is slowed down to around 70 beats/min. Atrial depolarisation causes a sweeping wave of atrial muscle contraction. The electrical stimulus arrives at the **atrioventricular node (AVN)** where it moves down to the bundle of His. This slight pause allows atrial contraction to complete before the impulse travels through the **bundle branches** to the apex of the heart, closely followed by a coordinated contraction of the ventricular muscle.

The electrical activity of the heart causes voltage changes that can be recorded and visualised on a cardiac monitor as an ECG complex. The **P wave** reflects atrial depolarisation, the **PR interval** includes the time taken to move through AV node and bundle of His, the **QRS** complex reflects ventricular depolarisation, and finally the **T wave** ventricular repolarisation (see also Chapter 30 and Figure 30.3).

The cardiac cycle

The electrical conduction system initiates a chain of mechanical events that enables the heart to cycle between systole and diastole, maintaining blood flow through the systemic and pulmonary circulation (Figure 23.3). The cardiac cycle is based on a number of simple principles:
- An electrical stimulus (wave of depolarisation) causes the myocardium to contract.
- Myocardial contraction causes the pressure to rise in the atria and/or ventricle.
- Blood will always move from an area of high pressure to lower pressure, unless prevented by a cardiac valve.
- One-way valves direct the blood to the appropriate chamber/vessel: atrioventricular valves from atria to ventricle and the pulmonary and aortic valves from ventricles to the pulmonary artery and aorta respectively.

Cardiac output and blood pressure

Measuring blood pressure is an essential nursing observation used to assess cardiovascular status, but what is it actually telling us? **Blood pressure (BP)** is the force the blood exerts on the walls of the arteries of the cardiovascular system and is determined by **cardiac output** and the resistance to flow offered by the **systemic vascular system**:

$$BP = CO \times SVR$$

where SVR is systemic vascular resistance. Blood pressure is recorded clinically as systolic and diastolic pressures. In addition, **mean arterial pressure (MAP)** is often calculated when assessing critically ill patients and is normally >70 mmHg. MAP gives information regarding organ perfusion throughout the cardiac cycle, and is calculated by:

$$MAP = diastole + one\text{-}third\ pulse\ pressure$$

where pulse pressure is the difference between systolic and diastolic pressure.

Both cardiac output and perfusion pressure are necessary for effective transport and delivery of oxygen to the tissue beds. The amount of blood that is pumped into the systemic and pulmonary circulation in one minute is the **cardiac output**, and this is a product of **stroke volume** and **HR**, normally around 5 L per minute. It is defined by the equation

$$CO = SV \times HR$$

Preload, afterload and contractility

Stroke volume, an essential component of CO and BP, is determined by preload, afterload and contractility.
- **Preload** is related to the blood volume in the ventricle at the very end of the diastolic, or filling stage of the cardiac cycle. This volume distends the ventricular myocardium, immediately before systole. The **Frank–Starling Law** defines the relationship between preload and stroke volume. Increased preload increases myocardial stretch, causing a stronger contraction and therefore greater stroke volume.
- **Afterload** can be viewed as the work the ventricle has to do in order to overcome the resistance of the semilunar valves in the **isovolumetric systolic** stage of the cardiac cycle (the muscle is contracting, the pressure rising, but the valve is not yet open). If the pressure opposing the opening of these valves is increased by factors such as a raised diastolic pressure, increased SVR, or valve disease, the ventricle has to work much harder to eject its volume. An increased afterload may result in a reduced stroke volume and reduced cardiac output.
- **Contractility** refers to the ability of the myocardium to shorten and contract. A healthy heart will contract effectively in response to the amount of volume or stretch (preload) at the end of diastole. A damaged or failing heart has reduced contractility however, and will not pump so well for the same preload.

In order for the cardiovascular system to be successful, all the elements discussed are required to work together; failure of any element reduces oxygen delivery causing organ dysfunction, failure and eventually death.

24 Circulatory physiology 3: control of circulation

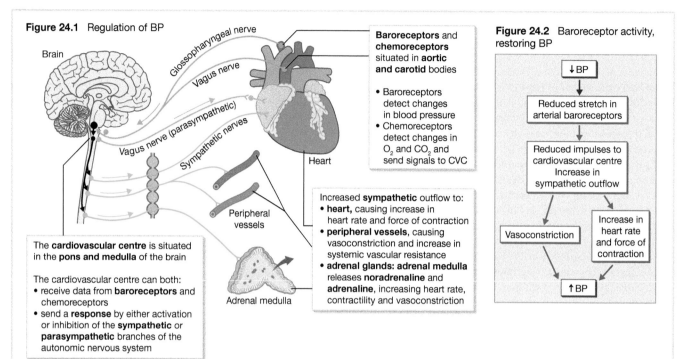

Figure 24.1 Regulation of BP

Brain

Glossopharyngeal nerve

Vagus nerve

Vagus nerve (parasympathetic)

Sympathetic nerves

Heart

Peripheral vessels

Adrenal medulla

The **cardiovascular centre** is situated in the **pons and medulla** of the brain

The cardiovascular centre can both:
- receive data from **baroreceptors** and chemoreceptors
- send a **response** by either activation or inhibition of the **sympathetic** or **parasympathetic** branches of the autonomic nervous system

Baroreceptors and **chemoreceptors** situated in **aortic and carotid** bodies

- Baroreceptors detect changes in blood pressure
- Chemoreceptors detect changes in O_2 and CO_2 and send signals to CVC

Increased **sympathetic** outflow to:
- **heart,** causing increase in heart rate and force of contraction
- **peripheral vessels,** causing vasoconstriction and increase in systemic vascular resistance
- **adrenal glands: adrenal medulla** releases **noradrenaline** and **adrenaline**, increasing heart rate, contractility and vasoconstriction

Figure 24.2 Baroreceptor activity, restoring BP

↓BP
↓
Reduced stretch in arterial baroreceptors
↓
Reduced impulses to cardiovascular centre Increase in sympathetic outflow
↓
Vasoconstriction | Increase in heart rate and force of contraction
↓
↑BP

Box 24.1 BP control by hormones

- Adrenaline – increases blood pressure by vasoconstriction, increasing HR and SV
- Noradrenaline – increased BP by vasoconstriction
- Aldosterone – increases Na^+ and H_2O reabsorption in kidneys, increasing volume and CO
- Angiotensin II – increases BP by vasoconstriction. Also increases aldosterone production
- Aldosterone – increases Na^+ and H_2O reabsorption in kidneys, increasing volume and CO

Table 24.1 ANS influence via adrenergic and cholinergic receptor type

Target organ	Sympathetic adrenergic receptor subtype ($\alpha_1\beta_1\beta_2$) and response	Parasympathetic cholinergic receptor type, muscarinic (mAChR) and response
Heart muscle	β_1: ↑in HR and contractility	mAChR: ↓HR and contractility
Coronary arterioles	β_2: vasodilation	mAChR: vasoconstriction
Bronchiole smooth muscle	β_2: bronchodilation	mAChR: bronchoconstriction
Skeletal muscle	β_2: vasodilation	None
Liver	β_2: gluconeogenesis, glycogenolysis	Glycogen synthesis
GI tract	$\alpha_1\beta_2$: reduced motility	Increased motility
Skin arterioles	α_1: vasoconstriction	None
Sweat glands	α_1: increased sweating	None

Figure 24.3 Effects of the sympathetic and parasympathetic nervous system

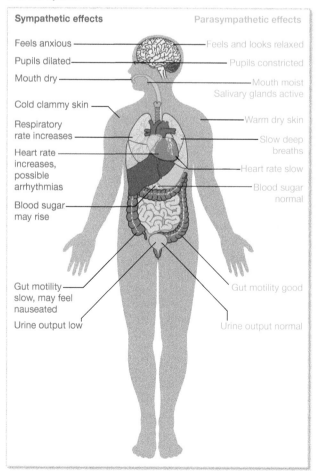

Sympathetic effects

Feels anxious
Pupils dilated
Mouth dry
Cold clammy skin
Respiratory rate increases
Heart rate increases, possible arrhythmias
Blood sugar may rise
Gut motility slow, may feel nauseated
Urine output low

Parasympathetic effects

Feels and looks relaxed
Pupils constricted
Mouth moist Salivary glands active
Warm dry skin
Slow deep breaths
Heart rate slow
Blood sugar normal
Gut motility good
Urine output normal

Acute and Critical Care Nursing at a Glance, First Edition. Edited by Helen Dutton and Jacqui Finch
© 2018 John Wiley & Sons, Ltd. Published 2018 by John Wiley & Sons, Ltd.
Companion website: www.ataglanceseries.com/nursing/acutecare

Cardiac output needs to vary greatly in order to meet the varying physiological demands for oxygen at cellular level. It is necessary, however, for BP to be maintained at a level that does not cause organ damage; such as a stroke through hypertension, or acute kidney injury through hypotension. Patients at risk of deterioration often display subtle changes clinically as a result of alterations in cardiac output and blood flow. Understanding the normal regulation of BP and cardiac output is helpful as it enables the nurse to interpret clinical assessment findings, relating them to the regulatory systems attempting to restore homeostasis.

Neurohormonal mechanisms of blood pressure control

Regulation of BP occurs automatically via a number of control mechanisms, predominantly the **autonomic nervous system** and **hormonal regulation**.

Autonomic nervous system

The autonomic nervous system is a branch of the central nervous system, which contributes to maintaining homeostasis. This autoregulatory system is controlled by centres within the brain stem and hypothalamus and works independently of conscious thought. It is subdivided into the **sympathetic nervous system (SNS)** and **parasympathetic nervous system (PNS)**.

Neural mechanisms lie within the medulla of the brain (Figure 24.1) in the **cardiovascular centre (CVC)**. The CVC receives information from sensors, such as the **baroreceptors** situated in the common carotid arteries and aortic arch. These receptors are sensitive to changes in stretch caused by an increase or decrease in mean arterial pressure. This information is conveyed to the CVC, which responds by altering the balance of parasympathetic and sympathetic outflow to restore homeostasis (Figures 24.1 and 24.2). The autonomic nervous system has specific receptor sites which respond to neurotransmitters. The receptors of the SNS respond to the neurotransmitter **noradrenaline**, and are known as **adrenergic receptors**. The PNS **cholinergic receptors** respond to the neurotransmitter **acetylcholine**. A summary of receptors and responses is found in Table 24.1.

Adrenergic and cholinergic receptors respond to autonomic activity, to ensure that BP is kept constant throughout the range of everyday activities, such as getting up in the morning, or running to catch a bus. During exercise CO can increase from 5 to 30 L to give the active muscles enough oxygen, but if the BP was to vary by this amount (times six), the pressure achieved would not be compatible with life! Vasodilation to decrease vascular resistance is one of the autonomic responses to reduce the rise in pressure and maintain BP within normal range. When the BP drops precipitously, however, the resultant sympathetic mediated activity causes peripheral vasoconstriction, cooling the skin and causing the heart rate to increase, giving rise to the symptoms of shock.

Information from the higher centres of the brain will also precipitate an autonomic response. Perceived fear, pain and stress is communicated to the CVC, giving rise to an increasing heart rate and BP, common physical manifestations of stress. Relaxing music or a quiet, calm environment may reduce SNS activity and reduce BP. The nurse has an active role in recognising signs of anxiety and sympathetic stimulation (Figure 24.3), and can employ stress-reducing interventions, to try and reduce the sympathetic response, allowing the PNS to dominate.

Hormonal response

Hormonal responses by the **adrenal glands**, **posterior pituitary** and **renin-angiotensin-aldosterone-system** (RAAS), contribute to BP regulation, but take longer to respond than the autonomic nervous system.

The **adrenal glands** release **adrenaline** and **noradrenaline** directly into the bloodstream in response to sympathetic activity. Adrenaline will cause an increase in blood flow to cardiac and skeletal muscles and increase heart rate, contractility and, vascular tone of the vessels supplying the skin and gut, increasing BP. Blood flow to the vital organs of the brain, heart and lungs will increase. Some hormonal influences on BP are shown (Box 24.1).

The RAAS is central to BP regulation. This more complex system consists of a chain of events, activated by low mean arterial BP, detected as low renal blood flow. As the kidneys receive approximately 25% of the cardiac output, this system is well placed to detect a reduction in BP. **Juxtaglomerular cells** are situated in the **nephron** of the kidney, where the **glomerular afferent arteriole** and **distal convoluted tubule** combine to form the juxtaglomerular apparatus. Low BP is sensed, and **renin** is released into the blood stream. A series of reactions result in the formation of the hormone **angiotensin 2**, a powerful vasoconstrictor, which restores pressure to the central organs. **Aldosterone** release is triggered, increasing renal sodium and water reabsorption. **Antidiuretic hormone**, released from the **posterior pituitary**, also increases water reabsorption in the nephron, increasing blood volume.

Common medications

An understanding of the neurohormonal mechanisms of BP control is essential if the actions of some common medications used to control and treat high BP and/or heart failure, or to support the circulation in those patients who have become critically ill, are to be understood.

In brief:

• **Beta blockers** block the beta-adrenergic receptors of the SNS, reducing heart rate, force of contraction and the work done by the heart. Beta blockers are used in heart failure and acute myocardial infarction (AMI) to reduce heart work, and in some arrhythmias to reduce heart rate.

• **Angiotensin-converting enzyme inhibitors (ACEI)** and **angiotensin receptor blockers (ARB)**, block angiotensin 2 production, causing vasodilation, and increasing urine output. ACEIs and ARBs reduce afterload, BP and heart work, so are used to treat heart failure and AMI. They are also used in the treatment of hypertension, to lower BP.

• **Dopamine, adrenaline**, and **noradrenaline** are examples of drugs sometimes used in the treatment of the critically ill patient with a low cardiac output, and/or low BP. These are **adrenergic receptor agonists**; that is, they enhance the effect of the adrenergic receptors of the sympathetic nervous system. They result in increased heart rate, contractility and peripheral vasoconstriction, which have the combined effect of increasing BP and cardiac output. These drugs are given in higher levels of care (level 2 or 3) as they have to be given through a central line, via a volumetric infusion pump. Continuous cardiovascular monitoring (Chapter 28) is required, as small doses cause changes in HR and BP that need careful evaluation.

25 Assessment of circulation

Figure 25.1 Assessment using the look, listen, feel, measure, investigate, approach

Patient history

- Hypertension
- Heart failure
- Stroke
- Thromboembolic disease
- Ischaemic heart disease
- Cardiac valve disease
- Peripheral vascular disease
- Myocardial infarction
- Unstable angina

Medication
- beta blockers ↓HR
- amiodarone, digoxin ↓HR ?existing AF
- diuretics
- anticoagulants
- antihypertensives
  - ACE, ARB calcium channel blockers
  - nitrates (GTN)
- statins

Look: any signs of acute respiratory distress? Note position and use of accessory muscles
Listen: dry or productive cough, pink frothy sputum
Measure: respiratory rate, oxygen saturations

Measure: blood pressure. Know normal range for patient. Calculate pulse pressure and mean arterial pressure

Look: fingers for peripheral cyanosis (blue tinge). Check capillary refill time
Feel: are they warm (?sepsis) or cold (reduced cardiac output)
Feel: dry to touch or cold and clammy?

Look: for swelling and tenderness in calves associated with DVT
Feel: assess for pitting oedema

Any signs of new confusion can indicate alterations in cerebral perfusion or the development of cerebral hypoxia

What is going on? Where am I?

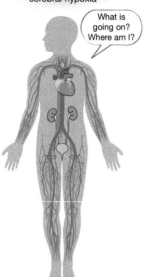

Look: are they flushed or pale?
Listen: complains of being too hot or too cold
Feel: temperature along limbs
Measure: central temperature

Pain: chest pain?
Evaluate: PQRST

Feel: peripheral pulse Is it regular? Is it thready or bounding?
Measure: rate, fast or slow?
Investigate: think ECG

Urine output
Look: colour
Measure: assess in mL/kg/h if possible Calculate fluid balance

Feel: for skin turgor

Investigate

- **Respiratory distress:** SaO_2, ABG, CXR
- **Pyrexia:** sample of sputum, urine, swabs from all invasive sites for MSC&S blood cultures (septic screen) Bloods: check WCC and CRP
- **Irregular pulse, tachycardia/bradycardia:** 12 lead ECG, cardiac monitor, bloods K^+ and Mg^{2+}
- **Chest pain:** 12 lead ECG, bloods for cardiac markers (Troponin)
- **Pale, cool, clammy, ↑CRT, ↑HR:** Hb, urea and electrolytes Find source of fluid loss/ bleeding
- **Warm, dilated, ↑HR↓BP:** septic screen, possible allergic reaction?

Box 25.1 Assessing CRT

- Hold hand at heart level
- Press firmly on nail bed for 5 s until blanched
- Release pressure, observe reperfusion
- Pink colour should return in < 2 s
- Prolonged refill time suggests reduced cardiac output

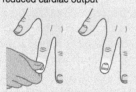

Box 25.2 Manual palpation of radial pulse

- Palpate pulse manually
- What is the rate?
- Is it regular?
- Does it feel strong or weak?

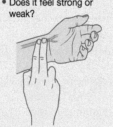

Cardiovascular clinical red flags. Source: RCP, 2013.
- Cardiac chest pain lasting longer than 20 minutes
- Palpations associated with syncope
- Painful swollen calf

Box 25.3 To calculate minimum urine output in mL/kg/h

- Patient weight × 0.5 = minimum in mL/h
- For a patient who weighs 80 kg, minimum urine output expected is 80 × 0.5 = 40 mL/h

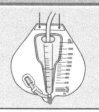

Box 25.4 BP monitoring – example 120/70 mmHg

Sphygmomanometer
- Cuff is placed around limb to compress artery
- Cuff inflated to stop arterial flow
- Cuff slowly deflated (3 mmHg/s)
- As blood resumes flowing through the artery, pulsation can be heard (Korotkoff sounds) with a stethoscope, placed over brachial artery
- Systolic pressure identified with 1st sound, diastolic on sound cessation.

DINAMAP device (device for indirect non-invasive automatic mean arterial pressure), senses pressure oscillations via a transducer. Takes blood pressure as a one-off, or at regular preset intervals if required. Systolic, diastolic and mean arterial pressure measurements available

Figure 25.2 Non-invasive BP measurement

Pressure in cuff greater than 120 mmHg
Artery closed
120
Rubber cuff inflated with air

Pressure in cuff drops below 120 mmHg
120
Sounds audible in stethoscope

Pressure in cuff below 70 mmHg
70
Sounds stop

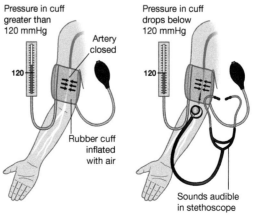
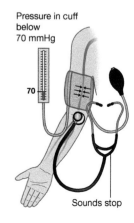

Acute and Critical Care Nursing at a Glance, First Edition. Edited by Helen Dutton and Jacqui Finch
© 2018 John Wiley & Sons, Ltd. Published 2018 by John Wiley & Sons, Ltd.
Companion website: www.ataglanceseries.com/nursing/acutecare

Assessment of circulation is the third step of the ABCDE approach. The nurse needs not only a sound knowledge of normal circulatory physiology (Chapters 22, 23 and 24) but must be cognisant of normal clinical parameters and be able to interpret even subtle changes. A systemic approach to data collection, using the 'look, listen, feel, measure, investigate' approach contributes to a comprehensive assessment (Figure 25.1).

Cardiovascular assessment: look

Focused observation of the patient can almost immediately yield clues as to their circulatory status. A relaxed, comfortable patient, readily engaging in conversation, has adequate perfusion of the brain and vital organs. Restlessness, with the unsettled patient fiddling with sheets or constantly moving to get comfortable, suggests that a more detailed assessment is required.

Noting the position of the patient, the possible use of accessory muscles signifies the extent to which the work of breathing and therefore the potential for respiratory compromise has increased. The respiratory and cardiovascular systems are interdependent; respiratory symptoms may be the presenting feature of cardiac problems. Severe dyspnoea (sensation of breathlessness) is a common feature of acute heart failure[1] and often the patient may not be able to talk in complete sentences. Orthopnoea (difficulty in breathing when lying flat), may be noticed at night, with the patient waking due to extreme breathlessness. Paroxysmal nocturnal orthopnoea, often a feature of heart failure, is relieved when sitting upright. Extreme anxiety, accompanied by a cough and pink frothy sputum, suggests pulmonary oedema, caused by acute left ventricular failure. The nurse, alongside immediate interventions such as positioning the patient upright and commencing oxygen therapy to meet the prescribed target oxygen saturation, should seek urgent medical assistance. Raised respiratory rate, reduced oxygen saturations and oxygen therapy will all score on NEWS.

Good lighting is essential so the patient's colour can be observed. Excessive pallor and peripheral cyanosis is associated with circulatory problems. Bluish-tinged fingers and toes (peripheral cyanosis) are the result of increased oxygen extraction due to vasoconstriction, with sluggish peripheral blood flow. A reduced cardiac output results in increased sympathetic nervous system activity; the arterioles supplying the capillary beds constrict, diverting the blood to the central circulation. Capillary refill time will change as perfusion reduces (Box 25.1). The nurse, however, should also consider other possibilities, such as the ambient temperature, as cold can also reduce peripheral perfusion and capillary refill time!

Cardiovascular assessment: listen

Reports of unpleasant symptoms such as breathlessness, palpations causing dizziness and/or chest pain require detailed assessment to help ascertain the origin and risk of a life-threatening event, such as arrhythmia, acute myocardial infarction or dissecting aortic aneurysm. A 12-lead ECG recording and urgent referral is required.

The experienced nurse may be competent in lung auscultation. Pulmonary oedema caused by acute left ventricular failure causes fluid to accumulate in the alveolar sacs, with movement of air through the fluid giving rise to crackles (a discontinuous popping sound heard through the stethoscope when placed over the lung fields). Specialist cardiac nurses may listen for added cardiac sounds, checking that the heart valves are not leaky or stenotic.

Cardiovascular assessment: feel

Manual palpation of the pulse is increasingly advocated as automated blood pressure measuring devices do not detect a range of essential information (Box 25.2). Pulses may feel bounding (full and strong) or thready (weak). Normally rates will vary from 60 to 100 beats/min. An irregular pulse that differs in strength from beat to beat, making the rate difficult to count, or an abnormally slow or fast rate, prompts a 12-lead ECG recording for review by staff appropriately skilled in ECG interpretation.

Pitting oedema in ankles, legs or sacrum suggests right-sided heart failure. A warm, swollen tender calf is associated with deep vein thrombosis. Progressive cooling along the limbs is evidence of reduced cardiac output possibly due to dehydration, haemorrhage or cardiac failure. Excessive sweating or clammy skin, a sign of very poor cardiac output, requires urgent review.

Cardiovascular assessment: measure

The six key physiological indicators are measured, recorded and the NEW score calculated (Chapter 3). In addition, clinical red flags identify where increased risk is present, but do not score on NEWS[2] (see red flag box). Pyrexia or a raised temperature occur as part of a systemic inflammatory response to trauma or infection. Blood pressure (BP) is taken manually by sphygmomanometer, or an automated system such as the DINAMAP (Box 25.4 and Figure 25.2). A difference in BP of >10–20 mmHg in each arm is associated with increased cardiovascular risk[3] and problems such as aortic aneurysm. Lying and standing differences in BP, or postural hypotension, requires further investigation. Hypertension (BP >140/70 mmHg) is associated with many causes of premature ill health and must be managed long term to avoid preventable deaths.[4] Severe hypertension (systolic blood pressure [SBP] >180 mmHg and/or diastolic BP >120 mmHg) is associated with acute complications and needs prompt attention.[4] Hypotension with systolic pressures below 110 mmHg has the potential to result in inadequate organ perfusion, but for many younger adults this could be a normal BP. The average pressure throughout the cardiac cycle, or MAP, needs to be above 70 mmHg and is calculated by automatic BP devices. Normally the SBP is higher than the HR, a falling SBP and rising HR is a cause for concern. The sympathetic nervous system is triggered by poor cardiac output, it increases HR and respiratory rate and causes peripheral cooling by vasoconstriction.

Whilst most patients do not have urinary catheters, urinary output and fluid balance needs to be assessed. A reduced urine output of <0.5 mL/kg/h (Box 25.3) indicates poor renal perfusion. This early sign of organ damage requires urgent medical review.

Cardiovascular assessment: investigate

Following assessment of circulation, additional information gathered from investigations (Chapter 26) is necessary to guide treatment.

26 Cardiac investigations

Figure 26.1 Exercise tolerance test

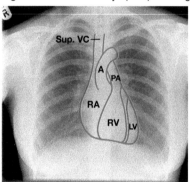

- Blood pressure cuff
- Nurse checks blood pressure
- Electrodes attached to chest
- Electrocardiogram (ECG) recorded on a machine
- Electrodes connected to a machine
- Patient walking on treadmill

Table 26.1 Reference values for venous blood samples in SI units

Venous blood sample	SI unit
Hb male	130–180 g/L
Hb female	115–165 g/L
K+	3.6–5.1 mmol/L
Mg2+	0.75–1.0 mmol/L
Urea	2.5–6.6 mmol/L
Creatinine	55–120 µm/L
Clotting tests	
Activated partial thromboplastin time	26–37 s
Prothrombin time	8.0–10.5 s
Bleeding time	< 8 min

Figure 26.3 Echocardiography

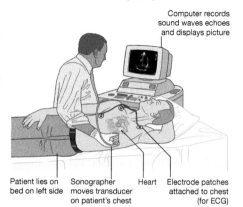

- Computer records sound waves echoes and displays picture
- Patient lies on bed on left side
- Sonographer moves transducer on patient's chest
- Heart
- Electrode patches attached to chest (for ECG)

Figure 26.2 Chest X-rays (CXR) showing cardiac borders and size

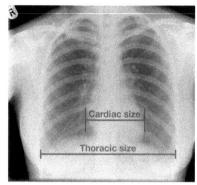

(a) Normal chest X-ray showing cardiac borders

Sup. VC, A, PA, RA, RV, LV

(b) Normal CXR heart size < 50% of thorax

Cardiac size
Thoracic size

(c) CXR showing enlarged heart (heart size > 50% of thorax) consistent with heart failure

Cardiac size
Thoracic size

A, aorta; PA, pulmonary artery; Sup. VC, superior vena cava; RA, right atrium; RV, right ventricle; LV, left ventricle.

Figure 26.4 Carotid Doppler

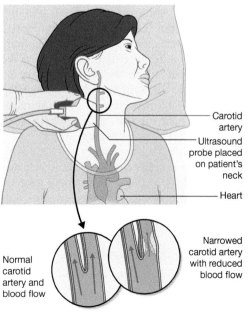

- Carotid artery
- Ultrasound probe placed on patient's neck
- Heart
- Normal carotid artery and blood flow
- Narrowed carotid artery with reduced blood flow

Figure 26.5 Coronary angiography

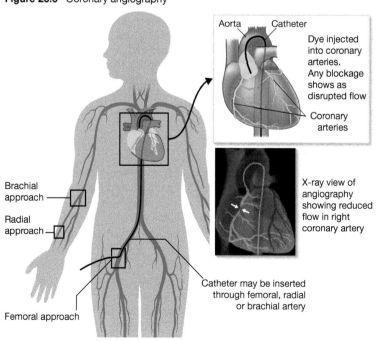

- Aorta
- Catheter
- Dye injected into coronary arteries. Any blockage shows as disrupted flow
- Coronary arteries
- Brachial approach
- Radial approach
- Femoral approach
- Catheter may be inserted through femoral, radial or brachial artery
- X-ray view of angiography showing reduced flow in right coronary artery

Acute and Critical Care Nursing at a Glance, First Edition. Edited by Helen Dutton and Jacqui Finch
© 2018 John Wiley & Sons, Ltd. Published 2018 by John Wiley & Sons, Ltd.
Companion website: www.ataglanceseries.com/nursing/acutecare

Assessment of the cardiovascular system for patients presenting with chest pain, palpations, breathlessness or dizziness is essential for evaluating the problems associated with cardiovascular disease. This chapter discusses additional investigations used to inform the diagnosis and management of patients with a range of cardiovascular problems. Tests should not be interpreted in isolation but in conjunction with clinical findings.

The 12-lead ECG

A 12-lead ECG is a routine non-invasive investigation regularly performed by healthcare professionals on adults in both hospital and community settings. The patient's chest is exposed during this procedure, so after an explanation is given, consent gained and equipment prepared, privacy and dignity must be maintained. A supine position is preferred. To ensure good electrode contact, skin may need to be washed and dried or excess hair removed by shaving. Ensure the patient is relaxed whilst the recording is taken; the name of the patient, hospital number, date and time is recorded on the ECG printout. The ECG then requires interpretation by a competent member of the healthcare team. Cardiac arrhythmias, evidence of heart failure, myocardial ischaemia or infarction may be diagnosed with the aid of the 12-lead ECG. Chapter 30 discusses lead placement and ECG interpretation in more detail.

Exercise tolerance testing

Exercise tolerance testing is a non-invasive test which is used to help determine the presence of significant coronary heart disease. It is mostly carried out using the Bruce protocol, which has seven stages, each lasting 3 min. The procedure involves exercising on a treadmill for 21 min (Figure 26.1), beginning with a gentle walk, then a gradual increase in speed and incline during each stage. Heart rhythm and blood pressure is monitored throughout. The development of chest pain or ECG changes would be considered a positive test. The accuracy of exercise tolerance testing is only about 70%, so some people with coronary heart disease may be missed, but some false positives may lead to inaccurate diagnosis. For this reason, exercise tolerance testing is being progressively superseded by cardiac imaging techniques, such as myocardial perfusion scans.

Chest X-ray

This simple non-invasive investigation (Figure 26.2) provides information regarding the size, shape, and anatomical location of the heart, and also changes in the structure of major vessels. Lung abnormalities are often present with cardiac problems; these are also evident in the CXR (Chapter 14).

Blood tests to investigate cardiac status

Routine blood tests performed on venous samples contribute to the assessment information of the patient with cardiovascular problems (for normal ranges see Table 26.1). Tests may include:
- **Haemoglobin (Hb)** to check for anaemia.
- Serum electrolytes: **potassium (K^+)** and **magnesium (Mg^{++})**: low levels of either of these can contribute to arrhythmias such as ectopic beats or atrial/ventricular fibrillation.

- Renal function tests such as **serum urea** and **creatinine**. Elevation of these could be an indication of poor cardiac output causing renal dysfunction or failure.
- Clotting times.

Additional blood tests would be requested for specific problems, such as heart failure, acute coronary syndrome (ACS) or myocardial infarction (MI):

- **B-type natriuretic peptide (BNP)** or **N-terminal pro-B-type natriuretic peptide [NT-proBNP]** is an important blood test for patients with suspected **heart failure**.[1,2] BNP is secreted from cardiac myocytes in response to the stretch that occurs when intravascular volume is raised. A raised serum BNP of >100 pg/mL, NT-proBNP >300 pg/mL (acute) or NT-proBNP >400 pg/mL (chronic) in an untreated patient, is diagnostic of heart failure.
- Cardiac biomarkers are checked in patients with acute chest pain or suspected acute coronary syndrome. Troponin (I and T), creatinine kinase-MB, and myoglobin are all released when heart muscle cells are damaged. Troponin I or T are the preferred biochemical markers to diagnose AMI, measured on initial assessment on admission. Traditional troponin tests may not detect raised levels for 6–12 hours following myocardial necrosis, so are checked again at 10–12 hours after onset of symptoms[3]. Recently the use of high-sensitivity troponin I or T assays, can rule out AMI within 3 hours[4] and are often used in emergency care. Serial ECG recordings are an important aid to diagnosis (see Chapter 29 and 30).

Echocardiography

An echocardiogram is a non-invasive procedure involving an ultrasound scan of the heart (Figure 26.3) providing information on the amount of blood ejected in each heartbeat, how well the heart valves are working, and wall-motion abnormalities. Doppler echocardiography technology allows determination of the speed and direction of blood flow by utilising the Doppler effect. Patients with raised BNPs require Doppler echocardiography to determine the extent and type of heart failure (Chapter 37).

Doppler ultrasound

This is also used to visualise the passage of blood through arteries and veins, such as observing flow through narrowed carotid arteries (Figure 26.4). Reduced cerebral blood flow increases the risk of stroke and brain injury. Doppler ultrasound can also detect clots that reduce flow in the veins of the legs, as with a DVT. Sections of blood clot in the veins of the leg can break loose and travel to the lungs, causing a pulmonary embolus.

Coronary angiogram

Patients with suspected or confirmed coronary artery disease may undergo cardiac angiography. A catheter is inserted into the femoral or brachial artery; this is threaded up the aorta into the coronary arteries (Figure 26.5). Contrast medium is injected and X-ray imagery used to view the coronary arteries. Visualising blood flow in the beating heart enables evaluation of the extent and location of any coronary artery narrowing or disease.

27 Fluid, electrolytes and intravenous fluids

Figure 27.1 The composition and movement of fluids and electrolytes through cells, interstitial space, interstitial and intravascular compartments

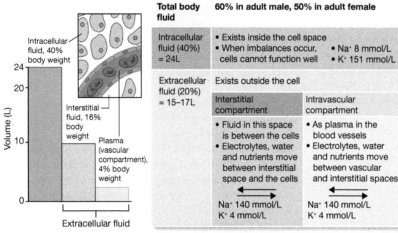

	Total body fluid	60% in adult male, 50% in adult female	
	Intracellular fluid (40%) = 24L	• Exists inside the cell space • When imbalances occur, cells cannot function well	• Na⁺ 8 mmol/L • K⁺ 151 mmol/L
	Extracellular fluid (20%) = 15–17L	Exists outside the cell	
		Interstitial compartment	**Intravascular compartment**
		• Fluid in this space is between the cells • Electrolytes, water and nutrients move between interstitial space and the cells Na⁺ 140 mmol/L K⁺ 4 mmol/L	• As plasma in the blood vessels • Electrolytes, water and nutrients move between vascular and interstitial spaces Na⁺ 140 mmol/L K⁺ 4 mmol/L

Intracellular fluid, 40% body weight

Interstitial fluid, 16% body weight

Plasma (vascular compartment), 4% body weight

Volume (L)

Extracellular fluid

Table 27.1 Examples of constituents of IV fluids

Crystalloid solution	Na⁺ content	Colloid solutions	Na⁺ content
0.9% saline	154 mmol/L	Voluven	154 mmol/L
Hartman's or Ringer's Lactate	131 mmol/L	Gelofusin	154 mmol/L
Plasmalyte	140 mmol/L	Albumin 4%	148 mmol/L
Cheap, safe		More expensive, no evidence of clinical benefit over crystalloids	

• These are solutions of small water-soluble molecules
• The fluid is clear and close to the concentration of the blood (isotonic)
• IV crystalloids move into the circulation, and freely into the interstitial and intracellular space

• Colloids contain large non-soluble molecules
• These attract water to stay in the circulation as they maintain the colloid osmotic pressure of the blood
• Stays in the systemic circulation for longer

Figure 27.2 Movement of water and solutes across the capillary membrane (Starling's law of capillaries)

Hydrostatic pressure forces water and dissolved substances out of the vessel and into the interstitial space, where it surrounds the cells

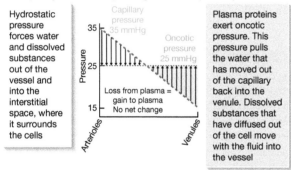

Capillary pressure 35 mmHg

Oncotic pressure 25 mmHg

Pressure

Loss from plasma = gain to plasma
No net change

Arterioles

Venules

Plasma proteins exert oncotic pressure. This pressure pulls the water that has moved out of the capillary back into the venule. Dissolved substances that have diffused out of the cell move with the fluid into the vessel

Figure 27.4 Assessing the need for IV fluids. Source: NICE, 2013.

Ensure nutritional and fluid needs are assessed and met

NEWS ≤ 4
Is there a need for fluid replacement?

ABCDE assessment
Look for clinical signs of fluid depletion

Yes → Can patient eat and drink normally? ← Yes

No

Seek medical review
Complex fluid requirements?
Ensure IV fluid regime of **'replacement and redistribution'** is given as prescribed
No special problems?
Ensure IV fluid regime **'routine maintenance'**, IV fluids are prescribed and given

Is there a risk of deterioration?
For example: NEWS ≥ 5
Does passive leg raise suggest there would be a good response to IV fluids?

↓ Yes

Escalate for medical review
Fluid resuscitation required
See Chapter 35

Figure 27.3 Problems leading to fluid and electrolyte imbalance

Gastric losses
Through vomiting/nasogastric drainage/aspiration
• Sodium
• Potassium
• Chloride

Severe sepsis, burns
Leaky epithelium allows plasma proteins to seep through
• Loss of albumin from circulation
• Water moves from vascular to interstitial space
• Oedema

Hypo/hyperglycaemia
Requires close monitoring of
• Blood sugars
• Hydration status
• Potassium
• Sodium
• Bicarbonate

Diarrhoea, or excessive loss from colostomy
• Sodium loss (Na⁺)
• Chloride loss (Cl⁻)
• Bicarbonate loss (HCO₃⁻)
• Water loss

Water loss through sweat, fever, respiratory rate↑
• Water loss
• Sodium loss (Na⁺)

Pancreatic drain or fistula
• Sodium loss (Na⁺)
• Chloride loss (Cl⁻)
• Bicarbonate loss (HCO₃⁻)

Loss through ileostomy or fistulae
• Sodium and chloride loss

Renal failure, excessive urine loss (polyuria)
• Potassium and sodium disturbances
• Requires close monitoring of electrolytes and fluid status

Blood loss, malaena, haematemesis, wounds/trauma
• Requires close monitoring of Hb electrolytes
• Fluid resuscitation/blood replacement
• Check clotting factors

Table 27.2 Consequences of electrolyte imbalances

Ion (normal range SI units)	Abnormality	Consequences
Sodium (132–144 mmol/L)	Hypernatraemia Na⁺ ↑ Dehydration, excessive IV NaCl	Thirst, confusion, lethargy. If severe, coma, twitching and convulsions
	Hyponatraemia Na⁺ ↓ Excessive loss Burns, diuretics, excess H₂O ingestion	If due to excessive water: brain swelling, mental confusion, giddiness, coma. If due to water and Na⁺ loss, then circulatory shock
Potassium (3.6–5.1 mmol/L)	Hyperkalaemia K⁺ ↑ Renal failure IV KCL	Bradycardia, peaked T waves on ECG, arrhythmias, cardiac arrest Nausea, muscle weakness
	Hypokalaemia K⁺ ↓ GI disturbance Diuretic therapy	Cardiac arrhythmias, muscle weakness, confusion
Calcium (2.12–2.62 mmol/L)	Hypercalcaemia Ca²⁺ ↑ Hyperparathyroidism	Cardiac arrhythmias, muscle weakness, confusion, nausea
	Hypocalcaemia Ca²⁺ ↓ Renal failure diarrhoea	Tingling fingers, cramps, tetany, convulsions
Magnesium (0.75–1.00 mmol/L)	Hypermagnesaemia Mg²⁺↑ Rare	Lethargy, respiratory depression, cardiac arrest
	Hypomagnesaemia Mg²⁺ ↓ Alcoholism, chronic diarrhoea, diuretic therapy	Tremors, tetany convulsions

Acute and Critical Care Nursing at a Glance, First Edition. Edited by Helen Dutton and Jacqui Finch
© 2018 John Wiley & Sons, Ltd. Published 2018 by John Wiley & Sons, Ltd.
Companion website: www.ataglanceseries.com/nursing/acutecare

Intravenous (IV) fluid therapy is one of the most common interventions in patients who are acutely unwell. Inappropriate IV fluid therapy has been associated with patient harm and an increased risk of death in postsurgical patients.[1] Guidelines issued by NICE (2013) emphasise the importance of healthcare professionals who are involved in delivering IV fluid therapy, having a good understanding of patients' fluid and electrolyte requirements.[2] There is a need for nurses to be trained and competent in the administration and monitoring of IV fluid therapy.

Fluid and electrolyte balance

The movement of fluids and electrolytes through the fluid body compartments (Figure 27.1) ensures that adequate supplies of oxygen, nutrients and electrolytes, essential for cellular function, are delivered. Electrolytes are solutions in which compounds have dissociated to form charged particles called ions. Examples are: Na^+ (sodium), K^+ (potassium), Cl^- (chloride), Mg^{++} (magnesium), Ca^+ (calcium) and HCO_3^- (bicarbonate). These are essential for regulating acid base balance, neuromuscular excitability, neural function and enzyme reactions. Ions move through **passive transport mechanisms**, down a **concentration gradient**, often through a **semipermeable membrane** such as the cell wall, or the endothelial lining of the blood vessel. Movement of ions or particles occurs by:

• **Diffusion**: the movement of **particles** (or **solute**) from a higher concentration of the particle to a lower concentration. Smaller particles move freely down a gradient, but some larger molecules such as glucose, are transported across cell membranes via a **carrier protein**.
• **Osmosis**: the movement of **water** (or **solvent**) from an area of higher concentration of water, to a lower concentration of water.
• **Active transport** mechanisms use energy to move ions (small charged particles of an electrolyte) against a concentration gradient, such as the Na^+/K^+ pump in the cell. Different concentrations of electrolytes (for example Na^+ and K^+) can therefore be maintained in different compartments (Figure 27.1).

Plasma proteins

Larger, more complex molecules such as **plasma proteins** (e.g. **albumin**) are normally unable to move between the intravascular and interstitial space. Whilst the **hydrostatic pressure** (pressure of the fluid against the vessel wall) within the circulation tends to drive fluid out at the arterial end of the capillary bed, plasma proteins exert an **oncotic pressure** that draws fluid back in from the interstitial spaces at the venous end of the capillary bed (Figure 27.2). Patients with low albumin levels, higher venous pressures (as in right-sided heart failure, or liver failure), or leaky capillaries allowing proteins to escape into the interstitial space (possibly due to sepsis), will have fluid accumulate in the interstitial space, seen clinically as oedema.

Fluid and electrolyte imbalance

Maintaining fluid and electrolyte balance in the acutely unwell patient is complex. Physiological stressors trigger inflammatory responses, increasing vascular permeability, allowing plasma proteins, water and electrolytes to leak into the interstitial space. The vascular compartment becomes depleted causing a relative hypovolemia, with reduced cardiac output. Antidiuretic hormone (ADH), aldosterone and activation of the RAAS, can trigger the retention of sodium, via a number of pathways. IV fluid resuscitation with sodium-containing fluids can contribute to electrolyte imbalance.[2] Figure 27.3 identifies possible patient problems leading to fluid and electrolyte disturbances. Symptoms and possible consequences of some of these losses are considered in Table 27.2.

Intravenous therapy

Patients who are unable to eat or drink require replacement of normal water and electrolyte losses. Maintenance IV fluids are prescribed, indicating type of fluid, volume given and rate of administration. They are regulated by a volumetric pump to ensure accuracy of the infusion amount. Initially a 24h plan is devised, but should be regularly reviewed by the ward team, stopping IV fluids when possible. Prescription fluids should include each of the following:

• 25–30 mL/kg/day of water.
• 1 mmol/kg/day of K^+, Na^+ and Cl^-.
• 50–100 g/kg/day of glucose.

An IV infusion of sodium chloride 0.18%, in 4% glucose, with 27 mmol of potassium, at 25–30 mL/kg daily, is an example of a fluid that would meet maintenance requirements. Further prescriptions are guided by suitably skilled and competent staff. At least daily monitoring of fluid balance, laboratory electrolytes (including urea and creatinine), in conjunction with measuring weight twice weekly is recommended. Caution is required in those who are obese, older and frail, or have risk of renal impairment or heart failure.[2]

Fluid and electrolyte replacement

Figure 27.4 summarises assessment and evaluation of ongoing IV fluid needs. See https://www.nice.org.uk/guidance/cg174 for full algorithm.[2] A five Rs approach is recommended:
• **Resuscitation** (Algorithm 2) (also Chapter 35).
• **Routine maintenance** (Algorithm 3).
• **Replacement and redistribution** (Algorithm 4).
• **Reassessment.**

IV fluid therapy is integral to the care required by the acutely ill patient. **Crystalloid** solutions have been associated with better clinical outcomes than **colloids**, and are usually the initial choice, unless individual requirements are complex[3,4] (Table 27.1). Acute care nurses must be trained, competent and confident with IV fluids, being alert to the consequences of mismanaged therapy, such as:
• Pulmonary oedema.
• Peripheral oedema.
• Volume depletion and inadequate cardiac output.
• Electrolyte imbalance.

Prescriptions must be checked for accuracy and timeframe. A fluid balance chart, recording fluid input and output, needs to be accurately completed by the nurse, with at least daily assessment of balance status. However, greater frequency is often required. Clinical observations are recorded as the patient's condition (and NEWS) dictates, and this will aid early detection of impending problems. Swift escalation is required for problems such as reducing oxygen saturations and a rising respiratory rate (causing a NEWS trigger), to prevent complications of IV fluid therapy.

28 Haemodynamic monitoring

Box 28.1 Indications for arterial monitoring

- Hypotension
- Complex fluid management, for example post major surgery, burns, or trauma
- Requirements for vasoactive support infusions, so rapid feedback on patient's response to medication can be evaluated
- Requirement for frequent arterial blood gas measurement

Box 28.2 Hazards of arterial monitoring

- Air emboli
- Distal limb ischaemia
- Haemorrhage
- Inadvertent injection of drugs into artery
- Thrombus formation and limb ischaemia

Figure 28.1 Arterial pressure wave form

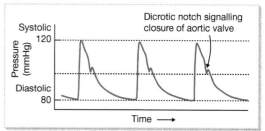

Figure 28.2 Elements of an arterial monitoring system

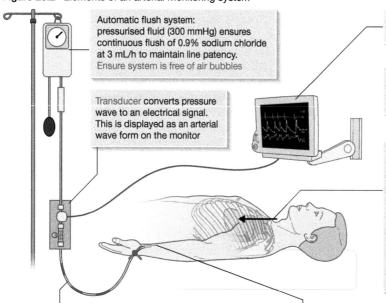

Automatic flush system: pressurised fluid (300 mmHg) ensures continuous flush of 0.9% sodium chloride at 3 mL/h to maintain line patency. Ensure system is free of air bubbles

Transducer converts pressure wave to an electrical signal. This is displayed as an arterial wave form on the monitor

Bedside monitor displays ECG and monitored pressure waves (arterial and CVP)

Patient should be on their back for accurate measurements, but may be raised through to 45°. Transducer will need to be repositioned

Transducer should always be at same level as right atrium (fourth intercostal space, mid-axillary line). Transducer needs to be calibrated to atmospheric pressure or zero regularly

- Mute alarm briefly (automatic 2 min).
- Close three-way tap to patient and open tranducer to air
- Press button on monitor to calibrate to zero
- Check 'zero' on arterial trace
- Return tap to original position, flush, and check arterial trace and pressure

Non-compliant pressure tubing, fluid-filled, will transmit pressure wave to transducer. Fluid line 'red flashed' and/or labelled to identify that it is part of arterial circuit

Radial artery cannulation. Three-way tap (red) allows arterial blood sampling. Arterial line should be clearly labelled

Box 28.3 Arterial sites

- Radial (preferred) (shown in picture)
- Femoral
- Brachial
- Dorsalis pedis

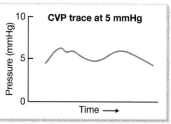

Box 28.4 Care of CVC site. Source: Loveday H.P., et al., 2013. Reproduced with permission from Elsevier.

- Cover site with single transparent dressing, change at least every 7 days
- Cleanse with 2% chlorhexidine gluconate in 70% isopropyl alcohol, allow to dry when changing dressing
- Consider use of chlorhexidine impregnate sponge dressing
- Consider daily cleansing with chlorhexidine

Figure 28.3 Central venous pressure wave form

Box 28.5 Indications for central venous monitoring

- Patients who have complex fluid requirements
- Requirements for drugs, such as vasoactive support and inotropes, that require continuous infusion via central lines rather than a peripheral line
- Requirements for long-term medication such as parenteral nutrition
- Require extra monitoring such as mixed venous oxygen saturations

Box 28.6 Hazards of central venous monitoring

- Arrhythmias
- Infection
- Pneumothorax/haemothorax
- Air embolus (air entering central vein)
- Thrombus formation, and potential pulmonary emboli

Box 28.7 Location for central venous sites

- Internal jugular (preferred) (shown in picture)
- Subclavian
- Femoral (rarely)

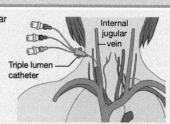

Internal jugular vein

Triple lumen catheter

Haemodynamic monitoring

Haemodynamic monitoring is used to assess and evaluate the effectiveness of the circulatory system in conveying blood and oxygen to body organs. Non-invasive monitoring is usually sufficient for patients who are unwell whose NEWS remains ≤6. Deteriorating patients with NEWS ≥7, who do not respond to initial interventions, require more detailed monitoring in level 2 care/HDU.

Non-invasive approach

A non-invasive assessment approach has been discussed (Chapter 25). Measurements such as non-invasive blood pressure are taken intermittently, at a frequency determined by the patient's clinical condition and NEWS. If deterioration is evident such that continuous non-invasive blood pressure measurement is required, then these can be taken at 5 min intervals whilst intra-arterial blood pressure monitoring is commenced.

Invasive approaches

Invasive monitoring is indicated for use in acutely unwell patients (Boxes 28.1 and 28.5). Arterial and central venous catheter (CVC) insertion sites are chosen for their accessibility and reduced risk of complications (Boxes 28.3 and 28.7). In order to ensure harm-free care, only healthcare professionals who have been assessed as competent should care for patients who require invasive haemodynamic monitoring.

Arterial blood pressure monitoring

Arterial pressure monitoring is an accurate, direct, invasive method which allows a beat-to-beat continuous display of blood pressure, via a catheter directly inserted into an artery. The pressure and flow, changing with each heart contraction, is detected and displayed on a monitor. The arterial waveform (Figure 28.1) gives real time information to enable the nurse to titrate specific treatments, such as intravenous fluids and/or vasoactive medication, safely and effectively. Figure 28.2 illustrates the components of a monitoring system for a patient with an arterial line *in situ* and some essential steps for reliable, consistent and accurate measurements.

Hazards associated with arterial monitoring

Box 28.2 summarises potential hazards with arterial pressure monitoring. Any air entering the arterial flush system is at risk of entering the artery; small amounts of air can cause localised tissue ischaemia. The correct flush fluid, normal saline, must be checked, as alternative fluids such a 5% dextrose give rise to sample error when measuring blood glucose.[1] The system is completely flushed through before connection to the patient, checking for small bubbles. The hand (distal limb) should be checked for colour, warmth, sensation and capillary refill, to confirm adequate perfusion. The arterial insertion site and distal limb need to be visible, to enable early identification of ischaemia. The lumen of the arterial line is small, but the pressure of blood in the artery will cause significant blood loss if disconnection occurs. Connections are secured and **alarms set** appropriately to detect any drop in blood pressure.

No drugs should be given through the arterial lines. The high concentration of injectate will cause tissue damage and necrosis, often requiring the distal limb to be amputated. For this reason, all lines are **clearly labelled** to prevent drug administration error.

Central venous pressure monitoring

The CVC is a wide-bore catheter inserted into a major vein that directly measures pressure in the superior vena cava, enabling a continuous central venous pressure (CVP) waveform display (Figure 28.3). CVP gives a good indication of fluid status, right ventricular preload or filling pressure, with normal values ranging from 2 to 8 mmHg. Patients who are acutely unwell often have complex fluid requirements. NICE (2013) have formulated a fluid resuscitation algorithm (Chapter 35, Table 35.2) which directs therapy for hypovolaemic patients.[2] For those who require ongoing fluid resuscitation, CVP measurements help guide management. The most valuable information is gained from the response of CVP to a fluid bolus (of 250–500 mL) rather than single measurements. CVP values that quickly return to baseline after a fluid bolus suggest that more fluid is required. A sustained, increased CVP indicates normovolaemia has been reached. A rapidly rising CVP, in conjunction with deteriorating circulatory and respiratory status, requires urgent attention. Vasopressors and/or inotropes may be required to improve the patient's clinical status. Transfer to ICU may be necessary.

Hazards associated with central venous pressure monitoring

Box 28.6 identifies potential hazards with CVP monitoring. Arrhythmias can occur on CVC insertion as the floor of the atrium is irritated. Pneumo/haemothorax can occur if, on cannula insertion, the needle penetrates though the vessel wall and punctures the lung. Signs of respiratory distress (chest pain, asymmetrical chest wall movement, rising heart and respiratory rates) are indicative of pneumothorax and a chest X-ray is always required post CVC insertion to exclude this. Air embolism can cause cardiac arrest if sufficiently large, so connections need to be tightly secured. The patient should also be positioned in a head downwards position on line insertion and removal, increasing pressure in the central veins, preventing air from being drawn into the catheter during inspiration. Symptoms of air emboli may be seen if 10–20 mL of air enters the right ventricle, lungs or brain. Positioning the patients on their left side, with legs raised, allows air to rise and remain in the right ventricle for absorption, preventing it travelling to the vessels supplying the lungs or brain.[3]

Hazards: arterial and central lines

A continuous flush system is required to ensure patency (Figure 28.2). Thrombus formation may occur if the pressure bag in the flush system has deflated below 300 mmHg, or the flush fluid runs out, occluding the lumen and causing a reduction in blood flow. The pressure trace will be dampened, or flat, and blood cannot be withdrawn from the catheter. The thrombus may move, giving rise to pulmonary embolism (CVC) or vessel occlusion and limb ischaemia (arterial line), so line replacement may be required.

Catheter-related bloodstream infections (CRBSI) occur when a systemic infection is present and the same organism is isolated from both blood cultures and the intravascular catheter. Organisms are often transferred from the hub and surrounding skin. Meticulous hand decontamination (Chapter 4) is essential, with trained and competent healthcare workers adhering to Epic 3 guidelines,[4] if mortality from CRBSI is to be reduced. A summary of recommendations for insertion site care is given in Box 28.4.

29 Acute chest pain

Figure 29.1 Chest pain: potentially life-threatening and non-life-threatening causes

Potentially life-threatening causes of chest pain:
- acute coronary syndrome
- aortic aneurysm rupture
- aortic dissection
- tension pneumothorax
- pulmonary embolism
- pericarditis

Crushing

Had it for about 20 mins

I feel sick and sweaty

I am really scared

Like a hippo sitting on my chest

Non-life-threatening causes of chest pain:
- angina
- chest infection
- fractured rib
- gallstones
- gastro-oesophageal reflux, or indigestion
- panic attack
- pleurisy
- pneumothorax
- shingles

Box 29.1 Psychological support
- Psychological support is a vital part of patient recovery
- Standardised screening tools such as the 'Hospital Anxiety and Depression Scale', are useful to assess for depression soon after acute cardiac event
- Information should be tailored to patient needs, and attendance at cardiac rehabilitation encouraged

Box 29.2 Nursing priorities for a patient with suspected ACS
- Pain assessment and management with morphine as prescribed. Reassurance that pain can be controlled
- Assess need for antiemetics for nausea
- Oxygen therapy to keep within 94–98% target range as prescribed
- Serial ECGs as requested. IV access established
- Recognising the importance of blood tests such as troponin T and I
- Ensuring prescribed medication to inhibit clotting, or to reduce heart work is given promptly
- Explaining to patient and relatives each element of planned care

Table 29.1 PQRST: mnemonic tool to aid symptom assessment

P	Provocation or palliation	What makes the pain better? / What makes the pain worse?
Q	Quality and/or quantity	What does it feel like? / Is it stabbing, piercing, dull, crushing? / How does it affect what you can do?
R	Severity	How would you rate it on a scale of 1–10, with 10 being the most severe? / Is it getting better, or worse?
T	Timing	When did the pain start? / Was it gradual or sudden? / What were you doing when the symptoms started?
U	Understanding	Have you any thoughts on what could be causing this pain?

Figure 29.3 Aortic dissection and Type A and B aortic aneurysm

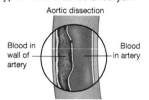

Aortic dissection

Blood in wall of artery — Blood in artery

Blood seeps and collects via tear in aortic intima. High risk of rupture and internal bleeding. Blood pressure should be taken in both arms. A difference of ≥ 20 mmHg may indicate aortic dissection

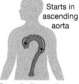 Starts in ascending aorta

 Starts in descending aorta

Type A dissection:
- Involves ascending aorta
- Requires urgent surgical intervention or stent insertion

Type B dissection:
- Does not involve ascending aorta
- May be managed conservatively with blood pressure control

Figure 29.2 Non-modifiable and modifiable risk factors for atherosclerosis and ACS

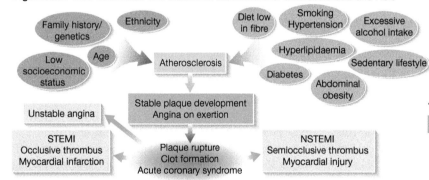

Family history/genetics · Ethnicity · Low socioeconomic status · Age → Atherosclerosis · Diet low in fibre · Smoking · Hypertension · Excessive alcohol intake · Hyperlipidaemia · Sedentary lifestyle · Diabetes · Abdominal obesity

Unstable angina · Stable plaque development Angina on exertion · STEMI Occlusive thrombus Myocardial infarction · Plaque rupture Clot formation Acute coronary syndrome · NSTEMI Semiocclusive thrombus Myocardial injury

Table 29.3 Risk stratification: TMI risk score

Risk factor	Points
Age > 65	1
≥ Three coronary artery disease risk factors: family history, hypertension, diabetes mellitus, smoker, peripheral vascular disease	1
Known coronary artery disease (stenosis 50%)	1
Aspirin use in past seven days	1
Severe angina (≥ two episodes in last 24 h)	1
↑ raised cardiac markers	
ST deviation ≥ 0.5 mm	1

RISK score = total points 1–7
High risk: 5–7 – early invasive strategy, e.g. PCI in 72 h
Intermediate risk: 1–4 – inpatient or outpatient, investigations, e.g. angiography

Table 29.2 ACS by troponin T concentration and ECG changes. Source: adapted from SIGN, 2013; Roffi et al., 2016.

ACS category	Unstable angina	NSTEMI with myocardial cell death	STEMI clinical myocardial infarction
Serum troponin concentration	Normal, or very slightly raised (0 – +)	Mildly raised (+)	Significantly raised (++)
Common ECG findings	No new changes	ST segment depression	ST segment elevation
Coronary artery thrombus occlusion	Partial occlusion	Partial occlusion	Full occlusion

Acute and Critical Care Nursing at a Glance, First Edition. Edited by Helen Dutton and Jacqui Finch
© 2018 John Wiley & Sons, Ltd. Published 2018 by John Wiley & Sons, Ltd.
Companion website: www.ataglanceseries.com/nursing/acutecare

The patient presenting with chest pain

Chest pain is a distressing symptom associated with a 'heart attack' and death. The priority is to establish whether the pain indicates a life-threatening problem (Figure 29.1). The PQRST mnemonic assists in gathering information from the patient regarding the nature of the chest pain, and aids in selecting the most likely cause from a range of diagnosis[1] (Table 29.1). Psychological support is essential during both the acute phase and recovery (Box 29.1). Acute myocardial infarction and sudden cardiac death are leading causes of death, so must be considered as a diagnosis.[2]

Atherosclerosis and stable angina

Atherosclerosis, the underlying pathology, develops and progresses decades before symptoms occur. The inner lining of the arteries (intima) becomes inflamed due to a range of risk factors; some of which cannot be avoided (non-modifiable) and some reducible with lifestyle changes and medication (modifiable) (Figure 29.2). As the disease progresses, plaques consisting of inflammatory cells, smooth muscle cells, and cholesterol form, reducing the artery lumen size. Fibrous caps develop over the plaque and if stable, blood flow may only be insufficient in times of increased physical activity or stress, giving rise to the symptoms of angina, which disappear on rest. Sublingual glyceryl trinitrate (GTN), helps relieve angina symptoms. Medication reducing heart work may be prescribed (Chapter 24).

Acute coronary syndromes

Acute coronary syndrome (ACS) is an umbrella term for:
- Unstable angina.
- Non-ST-segment elevated myocardial infarction (**NSTEMI**).
- ST-segment elevated myocardial infarction (**STEMI**).

Clot formation, triggered by plaque erosion or plaque rupture, reduces blood flow down the coronary arteries, causing myocardial injury and/or death due to lack of oxygen supply.

Unstable angina

Blood clots forming on top of the plaque partially block the coronary artery, causing chest pain even at rest. The clot partially dissolves and reforms, causing variable, prolonged chest pain. Unstable angina is not relieved by medication such as GTN spray. ECG changes are not evident. The blood cardiac markers, troponin T and troponin I, are normal or very slightly elevated (Table 29.2).[3]

Non-ST-segment elevated myocardial infarction

This involves the rupture of the fibrous cap with a partially occlusive thrombus forming. The damage to the heart muscle is **not** sufficient to cause the characteristic ST segment elevation ECG changes seen in myocardial necrosis, but ST depression and T wave inversion may be evident. Raised serum Troponin T or I, indicate myocardial injury and damage (Table 29.2). Perfusion of blood to the heart muscle needs to be re-established to prevent further injury.

ST-segment elevated myocardial infarction

This is total occlusion of the coronary artery by the thrombus. STEMI is diagnosed by noting ST elevation on the 12-lead ECG and specific changes indicating the location of the infarct can also be seen (Chapter 30). Cardiac markers will be significantly elevated too (Table 29.2). Time is of the essence if myocardial damage is to be avoided, so prompt reperfusion treatment is required.

Management of acute coronary syndrome

Patients with suspected ACS require urgent nursing assessment, with a 12-lead ECG review, troponin levels preferable using a high sensitivity troponin assay, are taken on arrival and repeated, serial ECGs are taken.[4,5] Plasma glucose and cholesterol tests assess risk factors for coronary heart disease. Patients diagnosed with acute myocardial infarction, with blood glucose levels of over 11 mmol/L, are commenced on a sliding scale insulin regime for at least 24 h. Continuous cardiac monitoring can detect arrhythmias early, enabling prompt treatment. Patients with NSTEMI ACS should be assessed for risk using scores such as thombolysis in myocardial infarction (TIMI) (Table 29.3). High-risk NSTEMI patients may benefit from early **primary percutaneous coronary interventions (PPCI)**. Nursing priorities (Box 29.2) include pain relief, with intravenous **morphine** 2.5–5 mg titrated against pain. **Opiates** relieve anxiety, reducing sympathetic drive, HR and BP. **Nitrates** also relieve heart work (by vasodilation reducing afterload), as do **beta blockers** reducing HR, BP and myocardial oxygen demand. Antiemetics relieve nausea and vomiting. Hypoxaemic patients require oxygen therapy as per prescription, but there is no evidence of benefit in patients with ACS in increasing SpO_2 beyond 94–98%.

Reducing thrombus size is a key element of trying to restore blood flow through the coronary artery. Aspirin (300 mg) is given immediately, reducing thromboxane A2 production and platelet activation, limiting clot growth. Adding one of clopidogrel, prasugrel or more recently ticagrelor, enhances this antiplatelet effect, improving outcomes. For those with ischaemic changes, additional anticoagulation with low molecular weight heparin or fondaparinux is also given.

Urgent PPCI is also recommended to restore perfusion for patients with STEMI. Further anticoagulation with a glycoprotein 11a/11b receptor antagonists (e.g. abciximab, tirofabin) is given. At PCI a catheter is inserted through either the femoral or radial artery and manoeuvred into the blocked coronary artery. A balloon is inserted to dilate the artery and compress the thrombus, often with a metal cage (stent) inserted to keep the artery open.

Patients with ACS may develop added complications such as pulmonary oedema, hypotension, heart failure or cardiogenic shock and transfer to level 3 care may be required.

Other life-threatening causes

A severe tearing pain in the chest and back radiating to the scapula describes the pain felt by patients with dissecting aortic aneurysm. A defect in the wall of the aorta allows blood to flow in-between the layers (Figure 29.3). Systolic BP needs to kept <120 mmHg, whilst interventions are planned. Pericardial tamponade, tension pneumothorax and pulmonary embolism are life-threatening events also presenting with chest pain. (see Chapter 36)

The 12-lead electrocardiogram

Figure 30.1 Lead ECG electrodes placement.
Source: Aaronson P.I., et al., 2013. Reproduced with permission of John Wiley & Sons.

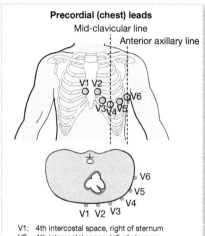

Precordial (chest) leads

Mid-clavicular line
Anterior axillary line

V1: 4th intercostal space, right of sternum
V2: 4th intercostal space, left of sternum
V3: Midway between V2 and V4
V4: 5th intercostal space, mid-clavicular line
V5: Same horizontal line as V4, anterior axillary line
V6: Same horizontal line as V4, mid-axillary line

Limb leads

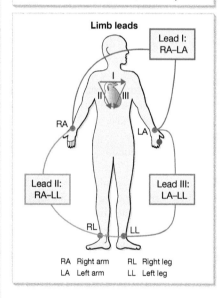

Lead I:
RA–LA

Lead II:
RA–LL

Lead III:
LA–LL

RA Right arm   RL Right leg
LA Left arm   LL Left leg

Figure 30.3 ECG waveform components.
Source: Aaronson P.I., et al., 2013. Reproduced with permission of John Wiley & Sons.

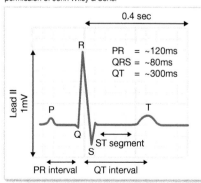

0.4 sec

PR = ~120ms
QRS = ~80ms
QT = ~300ms

Lead II
1mV

ST segment

PR interval   QT interval

Figure 30.2 Origin of ECG waveform

☐ Depolarisation ■ Repolarisation

SA node

AV node

1 Electrical impulse from SA node causes atrial depolarisation resulting in atrial contraction

2 Impulse enters AV node where it is delayed. Atrial depolarisation is complete

3 Impulse is conducted down to the ventricles, causing ventricular depolarisation and contraction

4 No further electrical current passed through myocardium. Ventricular depolarisation is complete

5 Ventricular repolarisation begins causing ventricular relaxation

6 Ventricular repolarisation is complete

Figure 30.5 Normal 12-lead ECG with rhythm strip

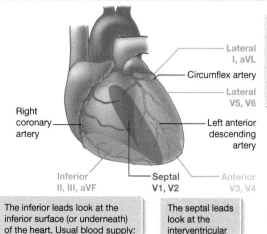

Figure 30.4 Contiguous ECG leads (looking at the same anatomical area)

Any precordial leads that are next to each other, e.g. V2 and V3

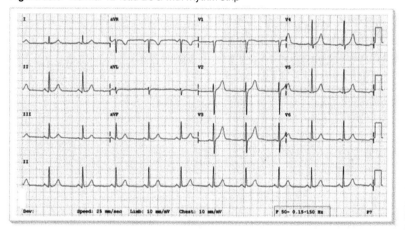

The lateral leads look at the lateral (or side) walls of the left ventricle. Usual blood supply: circumflex branch of left coronary artery

Lateral
I, aVL

Circumflex artery

Lateral
V5, V6

Right coronary artery

Left anterior descending artery

Inferior
II, III, aVF

Septal
V1, V2

Anterior
V3, V4

The inferior leads look at the inferior surface (or underneath) of the heart. Usual blood supply: right coronary artery

The septal leads look at the interventricular septum (LAD)

The anterior leads look at the anterior surface (or front wall) of the right and left ventricle Usual blood supply: left anterior descending (LAD) branch of left coronary artery

Acute and Critical Care Nursing at a Glance, First Edition. Edited by Helen Dutton and Jacqui Finch
© 2018 John Wiley & Sons, Ltd. Published 2018 by John Wiley & Sons, Ltd.
Companion website: www.ataglanceseries.com/nursing/acutecare

A 12-lead ECG records changes in electrical activity of the heart during each part of the cardiac cycle that is observed from 12 different views (leads). The conduction of the heart's electrical impulses is detected through the skin by 10 electrodes, six placed on the chest and four on the limbs (Figure 30.1). The trace is displayed on a cardiac monitor or recorded by the ECG machine.

Electrocardiogram waveform

The heart muscle contracts and relaxes in response to the electrical impulse that arises in the sinoatrial node and spreads through the conduction system across the atria and ventricles. This electrical activity is recorded as the ECG waveform on graph paper. The paper is divided into small squares of 1 mm each. Standard ECG paper speed is 25 mm/s per one square (1 mm) which equals 0.04 s horizontally or 0.1 mV vertically. Each waveform deflection is related to the electrical events of **depolarisation** and **repolarisation** occurring in the cardiac tissue. A normal ECG waveform (Figures 30.2 and 30.3) consists of:

• **P wave:** should be symmetrically rounded and, except for the lead aVR, it should be positive (upright).
• **PR interval:** starts from the beginning of the P wave and ends at the beginning of the QRS complex.
• **QRS complex:** it is made up of three waves. If the first deflection of the QRS complex is downward, it is called Q wave and it represents septal depolarisation. The normal Q wave should not be wider than 1 mm and deeper than a quarter of the height of the R wave. Small Q waves may be seen in leads I, II, aVL, V5 and V6. The first upward deflection is called the R wave and it is generated by the depolarisation of the bulk of the ventricles. The R wave in the **precordial leads** must progress in height from V1 to V6. A downward deflection after an R wave is called an S wave and it represents depolarisation of ventricular muscle around major valves. The QRS complexes can be 'positive' (above **isoelectric line**) or 'negative' (below isoelectric line), depending on whether the R or S wave is bigger; this depends on the lead from which it is recorded.
• **ST segment:** should not deviate below or above the isoelectric line.
• **T wave:** should follow the direction of the QRS. Therefore, it is normally upright in leads I, II and V3–V6.
• **QT interval:** represents total time taken by ventricular depolarisation and repolarisation (Figure 30.3).

Electrocardiogram leads

Information from the four limb electrodes is transformed by the ECG machine to create six limb leads (I, II, III, aVR, aVL and aVF) which represent six views of the heart along a **vertical plane**. The six chest electrodes are placed in a **horizontal plane** along the chest wall and provide information of the heart's electrical activity for six precordial (chest) leads V1–V6. Each lead records the electrical activity from a specific anatomical area of the heart (Figure 30.4). The leads that look at the same general anatomical area are called **contiguous leads**. The knowledge of contiguous leads is necessary in identifying ischaemia or myocardial infarction. Lead AVR offers no specific view of the left ventricle and it is not used in ECG interpretation.

Electrocardiogram interpretation

There are two form of ECG interpretation: rhythm strip and 12-lead ECG analysis. A systematic approach to ECG interpretation should be used to enable identification of abnormal changes and to make a correct diagnosis.

Rhythm strip interpretation

Lead II tends to be the standard lead used for continuous monitoring of patients and it is usually displayed at the bottom of the 12-lead ECG as a strip (Figure 30.5). It provides a good recording of atrial and ventricular activity allowing identification of cardiac arrhythmias. All features in lead II (P wave, QRS complex and T wave) should be positive. The following needs to be answered on rhythm strip interpretation:

• **Are there changes that necessitate resuscitation or urgent medical intervention?** Look for life-threatening arrhythmias (ventricular tachycardia, ventricular fibrillation), or problems such as ST elevation or depression and T-wave changes suggestive of **acute myocardial ischaemia.**
• **What is the rate?** Determine whether the rate is normal, bradycardic or tachycardic.
• **Is this rhythm regular?** Assess whether the rhythm is regular, irregular or regularly irregular.
• **Is the QRS complex narrow or wide?** QRS complex that is wider than 0.12 seconds (three small squares, Figure 30.3) suggest ventricular arrhythmias or ventricular conduction blocks.
• **Is this a sinus rhythm?** Check whether there are positive P waves preceding every QRS complex. Absence of P waves is commonly associated with atrial flutter or fibrillation.
• **Is every P wave followed by the QRS complex?** Calculate P:QRS ratio. Second- or third-degree heart block should be suspected if there are more P waves than QRS complexes.
• **Is the PR interval normal and constant?** Consider presence of atrioventricular block if PR interval is prolonged (>0.2 s or five small squares, Figure 30.3) or its duration changes.

A 12-lead electrocardiogram analysis

A 12-lead ECG can be analysed using the following steps:
• Analyse major shape of QRS complexes: look for life-threatening arrhythmias and signs of infarction (presence of ST elevations in contiguous leads).
• Determine rate.
• Assess rhythm regularity.
• Analyse precordial leads: look for **ST segment elevation** (above the isoelectric line by more than 1 mm in limb leads and 2 mm in precordial leads). **ST depression** (more than 1 mm) and T-wave abnormalities (flattening, inversion) in contiguous leads. Assess QRS complexes for ventricular conduction blocks (broad QRS over 0.12 s). Check R wave progression from lead V1 to V6; abnormally tall R waves (>26 mm) and deep S waves (>30 mm) indicate ventricular hypertrophy.
• Analyse limb leads in a similar way to precordial leads. Limb leads can determine cardiac axis; this is the mean direction of the depolarisation flow through the heart.
• Analyse the P wave and PR interval in a similar way to the rhythm strip. Look at shape of P waves: tall peak P waves (>2.5 mm) or notched P waves suggest atrial enlargement.
• Determine QT interval: a prolonged QT interval may lead to ventricular tachycardia or sudden cardiac death.

31 Altered heart rhythm

Figure 31.1 (a, b, c and d) Supraventricular tachyarrhythmias

(a) Sinus tachycardia: impulses originate at SA node

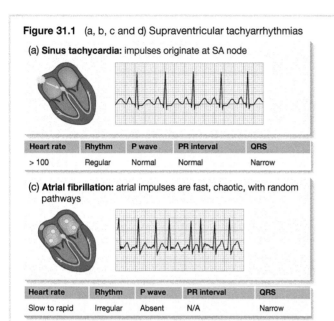

Heart rate	Rhythm	P wave	PR interval	QRS
> 100	Regular	Normal	Normal	Narrow

(b) Atrial flutter: impulses travel in circular course in atria

Variable block

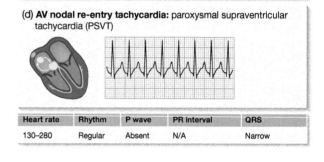

Heart rate	Rhythm	P wave	PR interval	QRS
A 220-430 V <200	Mostly regular	Saw-toothed waves	N/A	Narrow

(c) Atrial fibrillation: atrial impulses are fast, chaotic, with random pathways

Heart rate	Rhythm	P wave	PR interval	QRS
Slow to rapid	Irregular	Absent	N/A	Narrow

(d) AV nodal re-entry tachycardia: paroxysmal supraventricular tachycardia (PSVT)

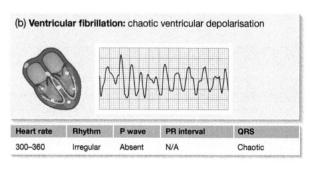

Heart rate	Rhythm	P wave	PR interval	QRS
130–280	Regular	Absent	N/A	Narrow

Figure 31.2 (a, b) Ventricular arrhythmias

(a) Ventricular tachycardia: impulses originate at a ventricular pacemaker

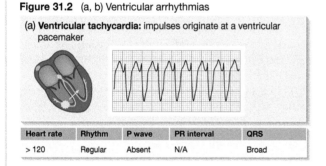

Heart rate	Rhythm	P wave	PR interval	QRS
> 120	Regular	Absent	N/A	Broad

(b) Ventricular fibrillation: chaotic ventricular depolarisation

Heart rate	Rhythm	P wave	PR interval	QRS
300–360	Irregular	Absent	N/A	Chaotic

Figure 31.3 (a, b, c and d) Atrioventricular blocks

(a) First degree AV block

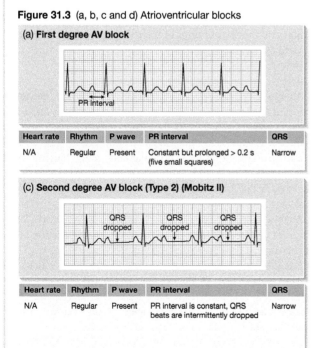

PR interval

Heart rate	Rhythm	P wave	PR interval	QRS
N/A	Regular	Present	Constant but prolonged > 0.2 s (five small squares)	Narrow

(b) Second degree AV block (Type 1) (Mobitz I)

QRS dropped

PR interval   PR interval   PR interval

Heart rate	Rhythm	P wave	PR interval	QRS
N/A	Regular	Present	PR progressively lengthens until QRS is dropped	Narrow

(c) Second degree AV block (Type 2) (Mobitz II)

QRS dropped   QRS dropped   QRS dropped

Heart rate	Rhythm	P wave	PR interval	QRS
N/A	Regular	Present	PR interval is constant, QRS beats are intermittently dropped	Narrow

(d) Third degree AV block (complete heart block)

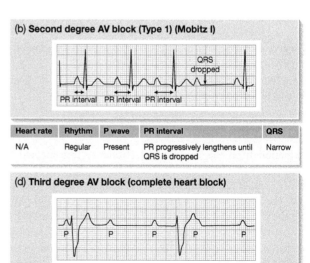

P   P   P   P   P

Heart rate	Rhythm	P wave	PR interval	QRS
N/A	Regular	Present	Dissociation between P waves and QRS complexes; impulses from SA node are blocked; wide QRS generated by impulse in the ventricle	Narrow

Acute and Critical Care Nursing at a Glance, First Edition. Edited by Helen Dutton and Jacqui Finch
© 2018 John Wiley & Sons, Ltd. Published 2018 by John Wiley & Sons, Ltd.
Companion website: www.ataglanceseries.com/nursing/acutecare

In health, the SAN regulates the heart, resulting in a regular rhythm and coordinated muscle contraction. Acutely unwell patients are at risk of developing rhythm problems, so assessment, recognition and timely escalation by the nurse is essential for safe, effective care. Arrhythmias are abnormalities of heart rate or rhythm, caused by:

- **Pacemaker problems**: when the SAN, the heart's natural pacemaker, fails to generate an electrical impulse, or is overcome by the generation of impulses from non-pacemaker cells (i.e. myocardial cells).
- **Conduction problems**: the path of an electrical impulse may be blocked, or the electrical signal circles back to stimulate a second impulse, instead of naturally ending (re-entry circuit).

Common disorders that may lead to arrhythmias include: MI, cardiomyopathy, heart failure, congenital heart disease, cardiac surgery, electrolyte and acid-base imbalance, drugs (e.g. digoxin, beta blockers) and hypoxaemia.

Tachyarrhythmias

These occur when the HR >100 beats/min. They can be **supraventricular** (impulse is generated above the ventricles with narrow QRS complexes), or **ventricular** (impulse is generated in the ventricles producing a wide QRS complex). Common tachyarrythmias are shown in Figure 31.1 (a–d), and are discussed below.

Supraventricular arrhythmias

- **Sinus tachycardia** may be a normal response to stress, pain and exercise. It can also occur as a compensatory mechanism (in shock, anaemia, respiratory distress, heart failure) or it can be related to the use of some drugs such as caffeine and nicotine. Treatment includes managing underlying causes.
- **Atrial flutter** results from circuit re-entry within the right atrium.
- **Atrial fibrillation** (AF) is a chaotic firing of numerous cells in the atria at a rate >300/min causing the atria to quiver instead of contract. AF is the most common arrhythmia in people >65 years. Both atrial flutter and atrial fibrillation with a rapid ventricular response and ↓BP, require immediate treatment. **Rhythm control** involves **cardioversion** with drugs such as **amiodarone** to restore to sinus rhythm. **Rate control** is achieved by drugs such as **digoxin**, or **beta blockers**. Anticoagulation with drugs such as **warfarin,** or **apixabam** is required to prevent stroke, MI or pulmonary embolism from atrial thrombus.[1]
- **AV nodal re-entry tachycardia** (paroxysmal sustained supraventricular tachycardia [SVT]) arises when re-entry circuit forms within or next to the AVN. Impulses travels down the normal AV pathway but return via the abnormal pathway. It circles round the two pathways repeatedly activating the atria and ventricles. Intravenous **adenosine** or **cardioversion** may be used if the patient has a low BP. Radiofrequency catheter ablation may also be used to destroy abnormal pathways.

Ventricular arrhythmias

Ventricular tachycardia (VT) (Figure 31.2, a & b) may occur in a short burst lasting <30 s, causing few or no symptoms (non-sustained VT). Sustained VT (>30 s) usually causes haemodynamic instability and often precedes **ventricular fibrillation** (VF). Treatment of **recurrent VT** includes implantation of cardioverter defibrillator (ICD) to prevent sudden death and/

or antiarrhythmic drugs (amiodarone, beta blockers). VF is a disorganised activity of the heart in which electrical impulses arise from many different foci causing uncoordinated ventricular contraction, with no output. **Pulseless VT and VF** are life-threatening arrhythmias with rapid loss of cardiac output, causing **cardiac arrest**. Immediate defibrillation and other advanced life support interventions must be initiated as per cardiopulmonary resuscitation algorithm (Chapter 45).[2]

Bradyarrythmias

These occur when the HR <60/min. These are usually caused by delayed or blocked conduction. A HR <50/min with pauses between ventricular beats of >2 s often causes symptoms related to reduced cardiac output and poor perfusion.

Sinus bradycardia

Sinus bradycardia contains normal complexes but the rate is <60. It is often well tolerated and left untreated. Occasionally treatment with drugs such as **atropine** or **isoprenaline** is required to increase heart rate if the patient feels dizzy or unwell.

Atrioventricular heart blocks

In **atrioventricular (AV) heart block** the impulse between the atria and ventricles is blocked, partially blocked or delayed. The AV block can occur at the AVN, the Bundle of His, or the bundle branches. ECG features are shown in Figure 31.3 (a–d) and discussed below.

- **First-degree AV block**: the impulse from the atria is consistently delayed as it passes through the AVN. It rarely causes symptoms and generally does not require treatment.
- **Second-degree AV block** (Type 1) (Mobitz I): impulses are delayed increasingly with each heartbeat, until a beat is skipped entirely. No treatment is needed if the patient is asymptomatic.
- **Second-degree AV block** (Type 2) (Mobitz II): some of the electrical impulses from the SAN are unable to reach the ventricles giving dropped beats, and this can progress to complete heart block. **Temporary/ permanent pacing** may be required.
- **Third-degree AV block** (complete heart block): impulses from the atria are completely blocked at the AVN and do not reach the ventricles. With no atrial impulse the ventricles fire on their own but at a very slow rate; it is a life-threatening arrhythmia requiring immediate pacing.

Nursing management

Patients with serious arrhythmias require continuous ECG monitoring on designated wards with nurses appropriately skilled in basic ECG interpretation. Initial management should involve: an ABCDE assessment, 12-lead ECG, intravenous access, supplemental oxygen as required to meet target saturations and early referral for help and expert advice. Regular NEWS calculation is essential to identify deterioration. Symptoms and signs of reduced cardiac output such as hypotension, dizziness, decreased urinary output and chest pain are monitored and used to determine the patient's response to treatment or to escalate as appropriate for medical review. Potential causes of arrhythmia such as infection, hypoxaemia, ischaemia, some medicines, and acid base and electrolyte imbalance (particularly K^+ and Mg^{++}) should be identified and managed appropriately.

32 Physiology of the immune system

Figure 32.1 First lines of defence preventing pathogens entering the body

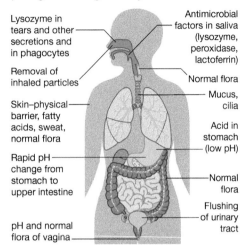

- Lysozyme in tears and other secretions and in phagocytes
- Removal of inhaled particles
- Skin–physical barrier, fatty acids, sweat, normal flora
- Rapid pH change from stomach to upper intestine
- pH and normal flora of vagina
- Antimicrobial factors in saliva (lysozyme, peroxidase, lactoferrin)
- Normal flora
- Mucus, cilia
- Acid in stomach (low pH)
- Normal flora
- Flushing of urinary tract

Figure 32.2 Cells of the immune system.

Source: Peate I. and Nair M., 2011. Reproduced with permission of John Wiley & Sons.

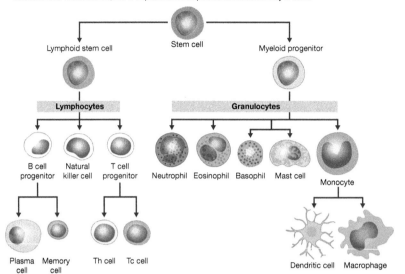

Table 32.1 Reference ranges for white blood cell (leucocyte) count

Total WBC	Adult males Adult females	$3.7–9.5 \times 10^9$/L $3.9–11.1 \times 10^9$/L
Neutrophils	40–75% of total white cells	$2.5–7.5 \times 10^9$/L
Lymphocytes	20–40% of total white cells (of which 70% T cells; 30% B cells)	$1.5–4.0 \times 10^9$/L
Monocytes	2–10% of total white cells	$0.2–0.8 \times 10^9$/L
Eosinophils	1–5% of total white cells	$0.04–0.44 \times 10^9$/L
Basophils	Less than 2% of total white cells	$0.01–0.10 \times 10^9$/L

Figure 32.3 Phagocytic cell and phases of phagocytosis

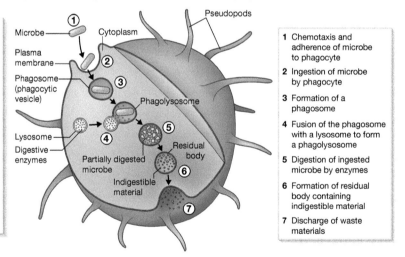

1 Chemotaxis and adherence of microbe to phagocyte
2 Ingestion of microbe by phagocyte
3 Formation of a phagosome
4 Fusion of the phagosome with a lysosome to form a phagolysosome
5 Digestion of ingested microbe by enzymes
6 Formation of residual body containing indigestible material
7 Discharge of waste materials

Table 32.2 Cytokine examples and their role in the immune response

Tumour necrosis factor α (TNFα)	Enhances production of T cells, promotes production and differentiation of B cells in the presence of IL-2
Interleukin 4 (IL-4)	Promotes production and differentiation of activated B cells
Interleukin 5 (IL-5)	Promotes growth and differentiation of eosinophils
Interleukin 13 (IL-13)	Reduces proinflammatory cytokine production. Helps B monocyte and B cell differentiation and proliferation

Figure 32.4 Complement enhances the destruction of pathogens/invaders

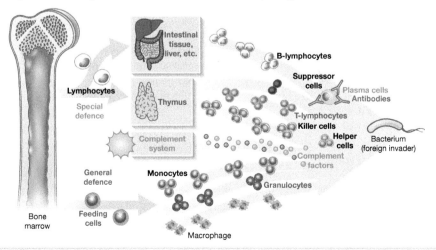

Acute and Critical Care Nursing at a Glance, First Edition. Edited by Helen Dutton and Jacqui Finch
© 2018 John Wiley & Sons, Ltd. Published 2018 by John Wiley & Sons, Ltd.
Companion website: www.ataglanceseries.com/nursing/acutecare

A good understanding of the immune system can help health practitioners identify factors and interventions that will impact on it and explore strategies for minimising harm. Some of these are preventative such as: avoiding the insertion of urinary catheters, encouraging effective coughing to prevent chest infections, ensuring patients receive sufficient fluid and nutrition and early mobilisation. Early detection of an infection that may lead to a sepsis response is an essential skill for nurses, especially those working with acutely unwell patients who are vulnerable to infection.

The immune system, when working efficiently, is able to differentiate 'self' from 'non-self' and mount an immune response, against harmful agents, such as bacteria, viruses or fungi. An **antigen** initiates an immune response, and includes microorganisms such as bacteria, viruses, fungi and protozoa, as well as non-infectious substances such as pollen or transplanted tissue. At times, this system can turn on itself and cause disorders such as allergic diseases and arthritis.

Immunity is divided into two systems, the **non-specific or innate immune system** and the **specific or acquired immune system,** although in reality these two components frequently work together. The immune system is made up of a number of organs, cells, substances and physical barriers that, when working together in a coordinated fashion, provide protective immunity. Communication between all of these is paramount to initiate an effective immune response.

Non-specific or innate immune response

This part of the immune response is innate or inborn to all human beings. It is responsible for the first response to antigens and can be considered in terms of the 'first' and 'second' lines of defence.

The first lines of defence include preventing microorganisms from entering the body (Figure 32.1). Microorganisms can enter through routes such as the skin, nose, mouth, eyes, vagina and rectum. The skin, with its 'waterproof' nature, prevents easy entry of microorganisms. The pH of 4–7 provides an acidic environment that is hostile to many microorganisms. The mucous membranes covering and lining the entry sites are more delicate but still offer protection. Microorganisms entering via the nose and mouth can be trapped in mucous and transported via the cilia before being coughed out, avoiding entry to the lungs. Microorganisms gaining entry into the stomach will often be killed by the acid bath they fall into and if not, they might die due to the alkaline nature of bile as they progress through the digestive system. Peristaltic action of the bowel will keep things on the move and make attachment to the bowel lining difficult (once attached, invasion and multiplication through the tissues is easier). Unwanted microorganisms can be removed by vomiting, or failing that, be rushed through the bowel in diarrhoea, ensuring that they leave the gut as quickly as possible. In addition, anatomical the length of the male urethra, convolution of the outer ear, eye lashes, and the action of blinking make it harder for microorganisms to enter. The shorter nature of the female urethra makes entry easier, but the acid environment of the vagina between puberty and menopause offers some protection during the childbearing years. If however microorganisms do manage to enter the tissues of the host, there are a number of cells and substances, or a second line of defence that can prevent further progression.

Components of the immune system

This second line of defence includes the white blood cells (WBC) (Table 32.1 gives normal ranges). Like red blood cells and platelets, they originate from stem cells in the bone marrow of long bones. From stem cells, WBCs differentiate into myeloid and lymphoid stem cells (Figure 32.2) and from these into **granulocytes** and **lymphocytes** are formed. Granulocytes consist of:
- **Neutrophils** – these are the largest subgroup of the **granulocytes** and are 'phagocytic' cells containing chemicals that 'eat' and break down the microorganisms they ingest (Figure 32.3).
- **Eosinophils** and **basophils** are much smaller in number. **Eosinophils** deal with parasitic infections by spraying their chemicals onto larger microorganisms that are too big to engulf. **Basophils** are active in allergic reactions and work together with mast cells found in the skin and mucous membranes.
- **Monocytes** circulate in the blood but can migrate to the tissues and develop into **macrophages**: 'fixed macrophages' (found in tissues in the brain, liver, lungs, kidneys) and 'wandering macrophages' that are able to respond immediately to signs of infection. They have phagocytic properties and can act as scavengers, destroying old cells and other debris.

Lymphoid cells are more specialised and form part of the acquired immune system. Lymphoid cells give rise to **natural killer cells**: these are special lymphocytes containing granules filled with powerful chemicals that attack many foreign cells lacking the 'self' molecules. They are important in destroying virally infected and neoplastic cells that develop into cancers.

Complement, a series of substances activated by the non-specific and specific immune systems, enhances the destruction of pathogens and makes the immune response more effective (Figure 32.4). **Cytokines** (Table 32.2), chemical messengers that can recruit more immune cells enhance complement. Cytokines, which are active systemically, also instruct the immune system to 'stand down' when the fight is over to avoid self-destruction, but with continuing infection may not do this, with severe clinical consequences for the patient. **C-reactive protein (CRP)** is produced by the liver in response to inflammation, injury or infection, and is a trigger for the complement system. CRP rises within 2 h of injury, so is a useful early marker for infection or injury, rising before any change in WCC.

Specific 'adaptive' immune response

If the innate immune structures, cells and substances are unable to prevent or overcome the infection, 'special' cells of the adaptive (or specific) immune system called **lymphocytes, from the lymphoid stem cells** (Figure 32.2), are activated. Lymphocytes are programmed to become either B or T lymphocytes and although they work together they have specific roles. **B lymphocytes** provide 'humoral' immunity and deal with 'extra cellular' pathogens. Once activated by the presence of an antigen, they develop into large plasma cells that secrete antibodies or immunoglobulins. These either block the entry of a virus, or attack bacteria that could trigger a sepsis response. **T lymphocytes** provide 'cell-mediated immunity' which means they deal with organisms that hide and multiply inside cells, such as viruses, the unusual bacterium tuberculosis and cancer cells. T cells act by either directing and regulating the immune responses, or directly attacking infected or cancerous cells. Once T and B lymphocytes overcome an infection memory cells remain that give long lasting immunity. Knowledge of the immune response assists nurses to interpret blood results, swiftly identifying the presence of infection and the efficacy of its management.

33 Acute circulatory failure 1: distributive (sepsis)

Figure 33.1 Signs and symptoms of infection

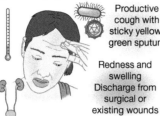

Fever, feeling unwell Sickness and/or diarrhoea

Productive cough with sticky yellow/green sputum

Urinary infection, frequency, pain on micturition, offensive-smelling urine

Redness and swelling Discharge from surgical or existing wounds

Figure 33.2 Three simple bedside tests to identify patients at risk of sepsis. SOFA (quick sequential [sepsis related] organ failure assessment). Source: Singer M., et al., 2016.

Respiratory rate ≥ 22

Score 1

Altered cognition

Score 1

Systolic blood pressure ≤ 100 mmHg

Score 1

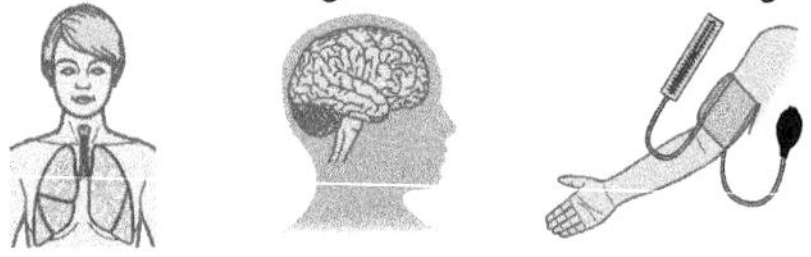

Total score   0 = mortality < 1%
1 = mortality 2–3%
≥ 2 = mortality ≥ 10%

Figure 33.3 Assessment findings in a patient at risk of sepsis

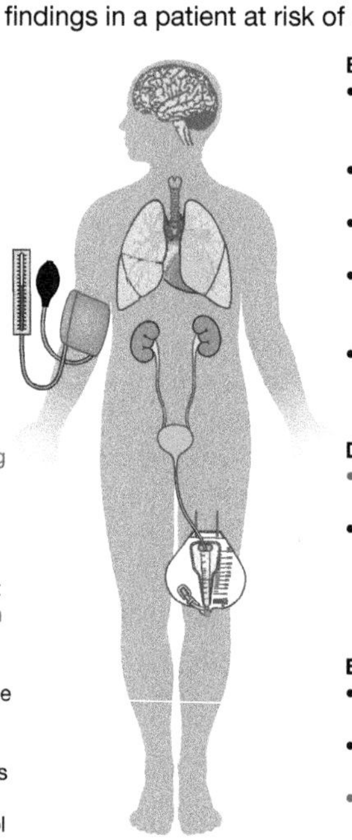

Airway:
- At risk if severely hypoxaemic with reduced consciousness
- Central cyanosis (blue mouth or lips) high risk
- Repeated vomiting risks inhalation

Circulation:
- Tachycardia (91–130 medium to high risk, > 130 high risk)
- New arrhythmia
- Hypotension, medium risk, systolic < 91–100, < 90 mmHg high risk
- Either pyrexia or temp < 36°C
- Warm peripheries caused by dilation of sepsis
- Check urine output and report if below 0.5 mL/kg/h as a high risk for sepsis, due to low perfusion pressure
- Send sample for culture if urine looks cloudy or has offensive smell
- Establish IV access as IV fluids may be required
- Treat pyrexia with paracetamol as prescribed

Breathing:
- Raised RR associated with deterioration. 21–24 medium to high risk, > 24 high risk of sepsis
- SpO₂ falling below target range, increasing oxygen requirements
- Give oxygen as required to maintain target saturations
- Raised RR may be raised due to temperature, increased work of breathing (chest infection)
- Obtain sputum sample and refer to physiotherapist if signs of chest infection are present

Disability:
- Any altered mental state, such as new confusion or drowsiness
- Blood glucose may be elevated due to stress response. Inform medical staff as blood glucose should be kept within normal range

Exposure:
- Look for any signs of infection (Figure 33.1)
- Take swabs or send culture if any infection is suspected
- Examine for any non-blanching rashes, bruises or mottling of skin, a high risk of sepsis

Box 33.1 Lactate

- An elevated lactate is typically abnormal and must be explained; usually it indicates organ dysfunction
- DO remember lactate elevations may be influenced by other conditions, such as a medication, hepatic problems, or due to primarily cardiac causes of hypoperfusion
- A raised lactate > 2 mmol/L, plus hypotension is associated with 42.3% mortality (Shankar-Hari et al., 2016)
- Is an arterial or venous lactate sample required? Either collection is appropriate for evaluating sepsis risk but if lactate raised, an arterial sample will accurately direct therapy

Figure 33.4 Assessment finding with NEWS and actions for those with moderate to high risk of death/severe illness from sepsis.
Source: drawn from NICE, 2016. https://www.nice.org.uk/guidance/ng5/resources.

Moderate to high risk criteria for severe illness and death from sepsis
- RR 21–24 (NEWS 2)
- HR 91–130 (NEWS 1 or 2) or new onset arrhythmia
- Systolic BP 91–100 mmHg (NEWS 2)
- Not passed urine for 12–18 hours, or if catheterised passing between 0.5–1 mL/kg/h
- Temp < 36°C (NEWS 1 [or 3 if < 35°C])
- Signs of infection
- Altered mental state

Two or more of these criteria, suggest organ dysfunction and sepsis

Inform medical team
Bloods will need to be taken for cultures, full blood count, C reactive protein urea and electrolyte, clotting screen, blood gas and lactate

Clinical and blood results reviewed within 1 h

If lactate > 2 mmol/L OR Renal problems (AKI) present
High risk identified, senior clinical review required

Figure 33.5 Assessment finding with NEWS and actions for those with high risk of severe illness/death from sepsis. Source: NICE, 2016.

High risk criteria for severe illness and death from sepsis
- Altered mental state
- RR ≥ 25 (NEWS 3) or new supplemental oxygen requirement of 40% or more to keep SpO₂ > 92% (or 88% if known COPD) (NEWS 2, or more if SpO₂ < 95%)
- HR ≥130 (NEWS 3)
- Systolic BP ≤ 90 mmHg (NEWS 3) or > 40 mmHg below normal
- Not passed urine for 12–18 hours, or if catheterised passing < 0.5 mL/kg/h
- Mottled/ashen cyanosis of skin, lips or tongue
- Non-blanching rash

Any criteria present
Urgent escalation
Senior medical review
Antibiotics within 1 h

If lactate < 2 mmol/L Discuss with consultant Consider fluids

Bloods taken for cultures, full blood count, C reactive protein clotting screen, urea and electrolytes and lactate

If lactate 2–4 mmol/L IV fluid bolus Consultant medical review

If lactate > 4 mmol/L IV fluid bolus Consultant medical review level 3 care

Or two or more of moderate to high risk criteria

Box 33.2 Two clinical criteria to identify patients with septic shock. Source: Singer M., et al., 2016.

- Persisting hypotension requiring vasopressors to maintain mean arterial pressure > 65 mmHg
- Blood lactate > 2 mmol/L despite adequate volume resuscitation

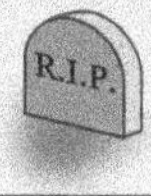

Sepsis 10% mortality
Septic shock 40% mortality

Acute and Critical Care Nursing at a Glance, First Edition. Edited by Helen Dutton and Jacqui Finch
© 2018 John Wiley & Sons, Ltd. Published 2018 by John Wiley & Sons, Ltd.
Companion website: www.ataglanceseries.com/nursing/acutecare

Acute circulatory failure occurs when poor tissue perfusion and oxygenation result in cellular hypoxia. Oxygen is required for ATP production. This essential energy source is required to maintain cellular function. Anaerobic metabolism generates less ATP, altering cellular activities producing lactate as a by-product. Distributive shock describes problems with blood distribution through the vessels, due to profound vasodilation, reduction in BP and reduced organ perfusion. Abnormalities of the peripheral circulation are seen in sepsis, anaphylaxis and some neurogenic disorders (Chapter 34).

Mechanisms and consequences of sepsis

Sepsis involves an inflammatory response to infection, causing damage to organs, which may progress to shock and death.[1] Invading organisms breach defences; an inflammatory response occurs to contain the organism and repair tissue damage. Inflammatory mediators (e.g. histamine, kinins, leukotrienes, prostaglandins and complement) initiate vasodilatation, enhancing blood flow to the affected area. Increased capillary permeability permits defensive proteins, antibodies and clotting agents to trap and remove microbial toxins. The body may be successful in containing the infection or it may be overwhelmed, with the process becoming exaggerated, or dysregulated, failing to respond to inhibitory pathways, leading to organ damage, dysfunction or even death.

Sepsis, a major cause of distributive shock, affects millions worldwide. In developed countries the overall mortality from infection has decreased in the last 10 years, but one in four affected still die from sepsis or septic shock. In the UK an estimated 37 000 patients die from sepsis every year.[1] A further 65 000 people survive but suffer long-term physical and psychological complications.

From 1991 to 2016 the sepsis spectrum has been defined as: SIRS (systemic inflammatory response); sepsis (SIRS plus suspicion of infection); severe sepsis (sepsis with organ dysfunction); septic shock (organ dysfunction non-responsive to fluid resuscitation).[2] Singer et al. (2016) suggest revised definitions to focus on the risk of poor clinical outcome from sepsis-related illness.[3]

Sepsis-3

The European Society of Intensive Care Medicine's and the Society of Critical Care Medicine's Third International Consensus Definitions for Sepsis and Septic Shock (Sepsis-3),[3] offer this changed perspective. Sepsis is defined as a life-threatening organ dysfunction caused by a dysregulated host response to infection, arising when the body's response to infection injures its own tissues and organs. Sepsis replaces the previous 'severe sepsis' category, highlighting that even a small degree of organ dysfunction is associated with an increase in mortality.

Recognising the patient at risk from sepsis

Infection

Infection can be identified by a number of symptoms (Figure 33.1). Many people with an uncomplicated infection will recover with appropriate antibiotics, rest and fluids, demonstrating an appropriate regulated response to infection/injury.

Sepsis

Patients with infection, however, may develop a dysregulated response causing the organ damage of sepsis. A new, quick and easy to use screening tool (qSOFA)[3] consists of three warning signs that, without the need for a blood test, help early identification of sepsis (Figure 33.2). If two or three components of qSOFA are present, blood tests to screen for organ failure, including for example lactate (Box 33.1), increased monitoring, screening for the source of infection, establishing IV access and giving antibiotics are actioned. Clinicians also need to consider additional risk such as; a history of rigors, change in mental alertness, or impaired immunity caused by existing medical treatment, such as chemotherapy or steroids. Nurses require excellent assessment skills (Figure 33.3) to enable early recognition and prompt clinical intervention, optimising patient survival.[4] NICE (2016) identify criteria that place the patient at:[5]

- **Moderate to high risk** of developing severe illness or death from sepsis.
- **High risk** of developing severe illness or death from sepsis.

Actions to be taken for each to move care forward are summarised (Figures 33.4 and 33.5).

Septic shock

A subset of patients with infection will develop sepsis, and a smaller group of these will become very ill with septic shock with its increased mortality of 40%. Lack of response to interventions such as fluid therapy and vasopressors (usually noradrenaline), plus a raised lactate with hypotension, defines septic shock (Figure 33.2).[6] Septic shock's high mortality remains, despite the many organ-supportive therapies available in intensive care.

Management of the patient with sepsis

The healthcare team need to work together to ensure elements of care are completed within the first 3 h of sepsis recognition.

- **Oxygen** is titrated to achieve target saturations.
- Collect samples, and send for microscopy to try and **identify causative organisms**. **Blood cultures** should be drawn percutaneously and through invasive lines present for more than 48 h, by an appropriately trained healthcare professional.
- **Serum lactate:** if >2 mmol/L, organ damage is present. Immediate fluid resuscitation is considered if lactate raised (or other signs of organ dysfunction evident), the patient is hypotensive, tachypnoeic, or has a low urine output. Crystalloid **IV fluid bolus** (500 mL) over 15 min will be given and repeated as required. Consider inserting a **urethral catheter** for accurate urine output assessment.
- Broad spectrum **antibiotics** are prescribed and given as soon as possible (within 1h if '**high risk**' sepsis features are present) (Figure 33.5).
- **HR >130/min, RR >25** and **responding only to voice (V)** have been identified as '**red flags**'.[7] Any feature of **high risk** sepsis identified (Figure 33.5) requires urgent escalation with **senior** medical review, outreach support, and timely interventions.

Frequent monitoring (every 30 min if high risk, or if NEWS ≥7, continuously) is required. Prompt review of blood results by senior clinical staff and the NEWS is used to evaluate the effectiveness of interventions given. If clinical response is poor, with signs of organ failure (e.g. lactate remains >2 mmol/L, not reducing with fluid resuscitation), or red flags remain, urgent review with transfer to a higher level of care is required to optimise treatment and prevent untimely death.

34 Acute circulatory failure 2: distributive (anaphylaxis and neurogenic)

Box 34.1 The patient with anaphylactic shock

- **Airway:** swelling of tongue, laryngeal oedema, stridor, hoarse voice, difficulty in swallowing with drooling
- **Breathing:** bronchospasm wheezing, increased respiratory rate, hypoxaemia. May lead to respiratory arrest
- **Circulation:** cyanosis, tachycardia, severe hypotension, syncope, warm body with cold extremities. May lead to cardiac arrest
- **Disability:** confusion due to hypoxaemia. May lead to loss of consciousness
- **Exposure:** urticarial rash which may be accompanied by pruritis, angio-oedema
- **Other signs and symptoms:** diarrhoea and vomiting with abdominal spasm

Box 34.2 The patient with neurogenic shock

- **Airway:** may be compromised due to hypoxaemia and/or injury
- **Breathing:** bronchoconstriction wheezing, increased respiratory rate, hypoxaemia, cough, retained secretions. May lead to respiratory arrest
- **Circulation:** hypotension and bradycardia due to lack of sympathetic activity (low systemic vascular resistance), cyanosis, increased venous capacitance with blood pooling and risk of thromboembolism
- **Disability:** confusion due to hypoxaemia. Loss of consciousness may occur
- **Exposure:** inability to regulate own temperature (poikilothermia). May be hypothermic (cold) or hyperthermic (warm). Risk of skin breakdown due to poor tissue perfusion
- **Other signs and symptoms:** bowel and bladder dysfunction. Paralytic ileus and gastric distension if due to trauma

Figure 34.1 Management of anaphylaxis. Source: Resuscitation Council (UK) 2008, revalidated 2011.

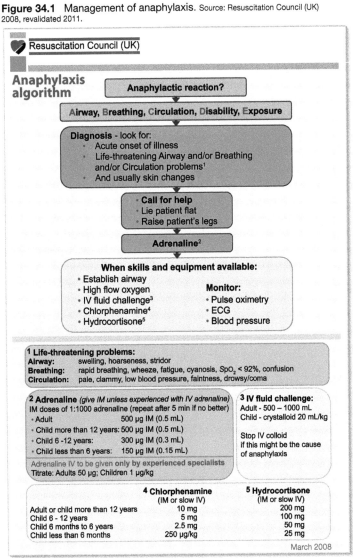

Table 34.1 Management of neurogenic shock

A	• Have all emergency equipment and drugs nearby and ready to use • Maintain airway, use airway adjuncts if required • NB: if spinal injury is the cause of the shock, specialist airway management is required as there is a high risk of vagal stimulation
B	• Monitor respiratory rate • Monitor SpO_2 readings and give oxygen therapy as prescribed to meet target saturations • Auscultate chest to assess for added sounds such as crackles indicating chest infection or wheezing • Observe chest movement for asymmetry • Observe for and record type of sputum produced • Monitor for signs of respiratory distress
C	• Observe colour of skin, mucous membranes and nail beds for signs of cyanosis • Monitor heart rate, blood pressure (and CVP if line *in situ*) for signs of further deterioration • Monitor capillary refill • Check full blood count, urea and electrolyte levels • Administer fluid therapy as prescribed and maintain an accurate fluid balance chart • Insert urinary catheter and monitor urine output, report if less then 0.5 mL/kg/hr • Administer vasopressors and antimuscarinic agents as per prescription and trust drug policies • Observe for venous thromboembolism and administer VTE prophylaxis/anticoagulants as prescribed
D	• Monitor GCS and report any changes • Monitor blood glucose levels, maintain within normal range • Monitor temperature closely, maintain normothermia • Observe for any signs of pain and administer prescribed analgesia • **For spinal injury immobilisation will be required**
E	• Monitor skin for tissue breakdown • Monitor gut function and ensure adequate nutrition • Monitor bowel function and administer laxatives as prescribed

Acute and Critical Care Nursing at a Glance, First Edition. Edited by Helen Dutton and Jacqui Finch
© 2018 John Wiley & Sons, Ltd. Published 2018 by John Wiley & Sons, Ltd.
Companion website: www.ataglanceseries.com/nursing/acutecare

The patient with anaphylactic or neurogenic shock will present with intense peripheral vasodilatation. Both are a distributive form of shock. These disorders, whilst having this common pathophysiological characteristic, vary greatly in their aetiology, clinical presentation and the therapeutic interventions required to successfully manage them.

The immune response, allergy and anaphylaxis

An **antigen** is a substance that provokes immune response and reactivity in the body and in health, the immune system effectively protects against the foreign and infectious antigens that it encounters. Sometimes, however, it reacts inappropriately to them with either a deficient or an exaggerated 'hypersensitive' response. There are four different types of hypersensitivity, three of which are mediated by antibodies and one by T lymphocytes. An **allergen** is defined as an antigen that causes an allergic reaction. Most common allergic reactions are mediated by immunoglobulin E (IgE) (type 1 hypersensitivity). Primary exposure to an allergen leads to the production of IgE and this binds to special receptor sites on the plasma membranes of mast cells, found in connective tissue. Subsequent exposure will cause the allergen to combine with the IgE on the mast cell surface, initiating a degranulation process whereby histamine and a plethora of other inflammatory agents are released. There are many triggers for this type of hypersensitive reaction including food, venom and drugs. Whilst in hospital, certain types of intravenous fluid administration or the use of contrast media can cause reactions. Patients should be assessed for allergies and all findings documented and communicated to colleagues. They should also be closely observed for the emergence of new allergic reactions. By definition, patients are more likely to react to a substance that they have previously been exposed to, so it is important to remember that in the case of a drug, for example, it may *not* be the first dose that causes an allergic response, but later doses.

Many allergic reactions that patients experience will manifest with only mild skin and/or gastrointestinal disturbances. However, some may be more serious. Anaphylaxis is defined as 'a severe, life–threatening, generalised or systemic hypersensitivity reaction' and in England alone it is thought to affect one in 1333 of the population at some point in their lives. A large number of cases are due to either a venom-induced reaction such as a bee sting or as a result of a nut allergy. A serious ongoing problem, there are estimated to be 20 deaths each year in the UK due to anaphylactic shock.[2]

Clinical presentation and management of anaphylaxis

Anaphylaxis can lead to rapid deterioration. The nurse's use of a systematic ABCDE approach, with particular vigilance in airway assessment and management, with timely escalation is essential if safe and effective care is to be delivered. Common assessment findings are outlined in Box 34.1. As a direct result of the inflammatory cascade taking place, respiratory and cardiovascular collapse may occur within minutes. A medical emergency situation should be anticipated with all necessary resuscitation equipment checked and ready to use. The Resuscitation Council UK (2008, revalidated 2011) have published guidelines on the management of anaphylaxis.[1] The aim of treatment (Figure 34.1) is to reverse the ill effects with a combination of: **airway maintenance**, **high flow oxygen therapy** to maintain SpO_2 within target saturations, and **fluid resuscitation** to improve blood pressure. Pharmacological interventions include:

- Hydrocortisone to dampen the inflammatory response.
- Chlorphenamine to directly counteract histamine release.
- Adrenaline (an alpha and beta receptor agonist). This is administered in order to constrict blood vessels, increase myocardial contractility and dilate bronchioles. Intramuscular adrenaline is the preferred route. Pulse, blood pressure, ECG and pulse blood pressure ECG and pulse oximetry should be monitored.

Neurogenic shock: definition and clinical presentation

Neurogenic shock is a much rarer distributive disorder, characterised by overstimulation of the parasympathetic autonomic nervous system or inhibition of sympathetic activity; an example of the latter occurs in spinal cord injury which is a common cause of this type of shock. This disorder is distinct from **spinal shock**, which is the absence of all voluntary and neurological reflexes below the level of an injury.

The spinal cord contributes to homeostasis by conducting sensory and motor nerve impulses (Chapter 46). Sympathetic autonomic nerves arise from the lateral grey column of the spinal cord, beginning at T1 and ending at L2. This pathway is known as the **thoracolumbar outflow** and it regulates sympathetic activity throughout the body. Parasympathetic stimulation, in contrast, is controlled by the **craniosacral outflow** originating from cranial nerves 3, 7, 9 and 10 and portions S2–S4 of the spinal cord, but unlike the sympathetic system, it does not innervate the peripheral vasculature. Neurogenic shock can occur as a result of a partial or full severance of the spinal cord and it is most commonly seen in patients with lesions at T6 or above. Many systemic, physiological problems can occur as a result of disrupted ascending and descending nerve impulses below the level of the transection (Box 34.2) and careful assessment of the patient using an ABCDE approach is required. In particular, the nurse must remember that whilst this is 'shock', the usual physiological stress response will not be seen.

Clinical management

The first goal of management in neurogenic shock is to secure the airway (if compromised) and maintain oxygenation. If the patient has sustained a spinal injury, CT scanning will determine the location and extent of the injury and it may be that strict spinal immobilisation, with specialist airway management will be required. Assisted ventilation may also be necessary. The second goal will be to manage the unopposed parasympathetic outflow that is occurring via the vagus nerve, as this will lead to acute onset haemodynamic instability. A combination of fluid administration, vasopressors (such as noradrenaline or vasopressin) and antimuscarinic agents (such as atropine or glycopyrrolate), blocking parasympathetic activity, may all be necessary to counteract the lack of sympathetic response. Other specific factors to consider include temperature control and the prevention of venous thromboembolism. For the nurse, care delivery is complex (Table 34.1), as the patient may have multiple, physiological disturbances, some of them potentially life threatening.

35 Acute circulatory failure 3: hypovolaemia

Table 35.1 Causes of hypovolaemia

Blood loss (haemorrhage)	• There may be visible bleeding • Bleeding may be concealed, as in abdominal trauma, or internal bleeding postoperatively	• Loss of red blood cells decreases oxygen-carrying ability of blood • Loss of blood volume reduces heart's ability to pump (reduced preload, stroke volume and cardiac output)
Reduced fluid Intake	• Reduced oral intake • Excessive vomiting	• Loss of blood volume as fluid moves from vascular to interstitial to intracellular space • Reduced ability of heart to pump effectively • BP↓
Excessive fluid loss	• Diarrhoea • Excessive perspiration • Excessive urine output (caused by drugs or pituitary problems) • GI problems, fluid may accumulate in gut, but not be absorbed back into circulation, e.g. paralytic ileus	• Loss of blood volume as fluid moves from vascular to interstitial to intracellular space • Reduced ability of heart to pump effectively • BP↓
Plasma loss	• Substantial burns	• Loss of plasma water and blood volume

Box 35.1 Symptoms and signs associated with hypovolemic shock

- RR raised
- Increased effort and depth of breathing
- Reducing SpO_2
- Pale cool peripheries, peripheral cyanosis, reduced capillary refill
- HR increasing
- BP systolic the same or lowering
- Pulse pressure < 35 mmHg
- CVP/JVP reduced
- Patient may be thirsty with a dry mouth
- Decreasing urine output
- Confusion
- NEWS increasing to trigger threshold

Figure 35.1 Automatic, cardiovascular and renal homeostatic responses to low circulating volume

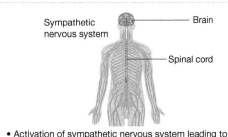

Sympathetic nervous system — Brain — Spinal cord

- Activation of sympathetic nervous system leading to the release of noradrenaline and adrenaline
- Peripheral vasoconstriction occurs and this re-diverts blood to major organs
- Heart rate and myocardial contractility increases:
  SV, CO and BP↑

Remember:
Heart rate × stroke volume = cardiac output
and
Cardiac output × systemic vascular resistance = blood pressure

Low circulating volume detected by baroreceptors in carotid bodies and aortic arch and receptors in the kidney

Baroreceptor response ← **Initiates** → Renal response

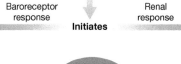
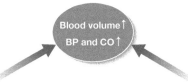

Blood volume↑
BP and CO↑

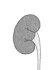 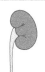

- RAAS↑ leading to vasoconstriction and the reabsorption of sodium and water
- Increased osmolality of the blood will trigger the release of ADH from posterior pituitary, urine output↓
- With more water conserved, blood volume is increased

Box 35.2 Passive leg raise.
Source: NICE, 2013.

- Passive leg raise can transfer a volume of around 300–500 mL of venous blood from the lower body toward the right side of the heart, mimicking a fluid challenge
- A positive clinical response to passive leg raise confirms volume depletion

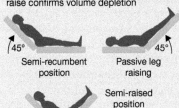

Semi-recumbent position | Passive leg raising — 45°

Semi-raised position reduces risk of aspiration — 45° 45°

Table 35.2 Management of hypovolaemia. Source: NICE, 2013. (updated 2017)

ABCDE assessment	• Are there clinical signs of hypovolaemia? (see Box 35.1) • Responsive to passive leg raise? • Is NEWS ≥ 5 ?
Stage 1	Identify cause of deficit and give fluid bolus of 500 mL of crystalloid solution (sodium content in range of 130–154 mmol/L)
Stage 2	Reassess: if required give up to 2000 mL in incremental doses of 250–500 mL
Stage 3	**Reassess: does the patient still have signs of shock?** **IF YES:** seek expert help **IF NO:** administer maintenance fluid of: • 25–30 mL/kg/day of water • 1 mmol/kg/day of sodium, potassium, chloride • 50–100 g/day of glucose Adjustments may need to be made for the elderly, obese patients or those with renal impairment **But:** • If abnormal fluid or electrolyte balance still persists: estimate deficits (or any excesses) and check for organ dysfunction, malnutrition, high nasogastric, stoma or urinary output losses and underlying infection (obtain stool sample) • **Seek expert help and re-estimate requirements**

Acute and Critical Care Nursing at a Glance, First Edition. Edited by Helen Dutton and Jacqui Finch
© 2018 John Wiley & Sons, Ltd. Published 2018 by John Wiley & Sons, Ltd.
Companion website: www.ataglanceseries.com/nursing/acutecare

Fluid distribution within the body

In a male adult of 70 kg there will be approximately 42 L of fluid in the body. Of this, approximately 24 L will be contained in the intracellular compartment and 18 L will be in the extracellular compartments (Chapter 27). Loss of volume from any one of these compartments can lead either directly or indirectly to a reduction in circulating volume.

Hypovolaemia: causes and pathophysiology

Hypovolaemia may occur for a number of different reasons depending on the type of body fluid lost (Table 35.1). Direct losses arise as a result of whole blood loss (as in haemorrhage), or plasma depletion (as in substantial burns). In contrast, indirect losses (where plasma has diffused from the intravascular to the extracellular space causing interstitial fluid loss) may develop following excessive sweating, severe diarrhoea and vomiting, or increased stoma or urinary output. Homeostatic responses will endeavour to compensate for all of these losses (Figure 35.1), but, depending on the severity and duration of the problem, they may be insufficient to prevent **hypovolaemic shock.**

Shock begins when the intravascular volume has been decreased by 15% or more. The result is reduced tissue perfusion and inadequate oxygen delivery to the cells, leading to impaired cellular metabolism. **Aerobic** (with oxygen) processes for the production of ATP (energy) will be replaced by the inferior **anaerobic** (without oxygen) metabolism. Lactic acid, a by-product of anaerobic metabolism, develops and accumulates within the body, causing a drop in pH, further impairing the oxygen-carrying capacity of the blood. Should the problem continue and the pathology be unresolved, other detrimental changes will ensue. Cells will become damaged, the sodium–potassium pump fails and cellular oedema and leakage will develop. As blood flow in the capillaries becomes more sluggish, the clotting cascade is activated initiating a procoagulant state.

Clinical presentation and patient assessment

Prompt recognition of hypovolaemic shock by the nurse is vital (Box 35.1). Failure to do so will quickly result in organ or **haematological dysfunction** or even death. Assessment of the patient must be systematic using the ABCDE format[1] and observing for key abnormal parameters:[2]

- **Airway** patency must be determined, as reduced oxygenation could quickly impair the patient's level of consciousness.
- **Breathing** may also be affected, with increased respiratory rate (>20 breaths/min). This is a result of hypoxaemia and also as a compensatory mechanism for the increasing metabolic acid, both detectable on ABG analysis. The presence of an elevated serum lactate level will also indicate tissue hypoperfusion as a result of lactic acid formation. Others signs of respiratory distress may also be visible such as the use of accessory muscles owing to the increased work of breathing.
- **Circulation** is inadequate, the patient may be pale in appearance and, depending on the severity of fluid loss, **peripheral cyanosis** and/or **central cyanosis** may be present. The lips and tongue will be dry and the skin will have poor turgor with loss of elasticity. The nurse may also note that the patient's skin is cold (especially peripherally) and possibly clammy to the touch. In addition, the capillary refill time may exceed 2 s as a result

of impaired perfusion. Patients with minor skin burns though will feel warm and dry. As dehydration is a feature the patient may complain of feeling weak and thirsty. Classic signs of shock may be evident with an initial tachycardia, and later hypotension with a systolic pressure of <100 mmHg. The pulse pressure may also be narrowed owing to vasoconstriction raising the diastolic pressure. The jugular venous pressure will be reduced as will the central venous pressure if the latter is being measured. Fluid responsiveness can be predicted by positive response to a **passive leg raise** of 45° (Box 35.2), with intravenous fluid resuscitation commenced as indicated.[2] Palpitations may be reported requiring cardiac monitoring and the possibility of arrhythmias secondary to electrolyte disturbance may also be present. Potassium loss in particular is commonly seen in severe diarrhoea. Haematemesis (blood in vomit) can be due to oesophageal varices, with blood also lost through malena (blood in the stool), both requiring urgent investigation.

- **Disability**: assessment may reveal impaired level of consciousness due to hypoxaemia. Pain may be an issue due to the injury (for example a burn, or trauma [Chapter 44] may be the reason for fluid/blood loss) or poor tissue perfusion may be the cause of discomfort. Blood glucose levels may be altered, with loss of circulating volume causing impaired glucose delivery to the tissues. However, in contrast, poor uptake of glucose by the cells may lead to hyperglycaemia and insulin resistance.
- **Exposure**: the nurse assesses the patient's temperature which may well be decreased with the loss of volume. Wounds or other injuries which may be the cause of the hypovolaemia should also be observed and, if clotting is affected, signs of bruising and petechial rashes noted. Burns in particular will need specialist assessment to ascertain the severity of the patient's condition and help determine treatment (Chapter 43).

Nursing management: key priorities

An ABCDE approach should again be used when managing a hypovolaemic patient, with maintenance of the patient's airway and target oxygen saturation level a first priority. As circulation is insufficient, close monitoring of vital signs and fluid balance is required, with timely administration of intravenous fluids as prescribed. Optimal fluid, electrolyte and glucose management should adhere to NICE guidelines (2013, updated 2017) (Table 35.2).[2] The choice of fluid administration has been hotly debated in the literature. Historically, colloid was favoured for its volume expanding capacity, but there is a general consensus now that there is little advantage over crystalloid solution, with no evidence of colloids having a positive impact on patient outcomes. Colloid use may be detrimental for some individuals, with albumin shown to increase mortality in patients with traumatic brain injury. Currently, 'balanced crystalloids' (physiologically similar to body fluid), such as Plasma-Lyte, are favoured to treat hypovolaemia. Normal saline 0.9% may be used, however, as there is no conclusive evidence to suggest it is not appropriate.[3] In cases of direct haemorrhage, blood and blood product replacement is necessary, with bleeding sources identified and halted in a timely manner. Specialist fluid regimes are required for patients with burns (Chapter 43). The presence, patency and security of large bore intravenous access is important to ensure prompt fluid replacement. Deterioration in level of consciousness must be promptly recognised and reported by the nurse, with action taken to secure the airway. The integrity of the skin needs to be preserved (especially when diarrhoea is present or the patient is immobile).

36 Acute circulatory failure 4: obstructive

Box 36.1 PE risk factors

- Deep vein thrombosis (DVT)
- Previous DVT or PE
- Active cancer
- Recent surgery, hospitalisation, long distance travel, or leg immobilisation
- Obesity
- One or more significant medical conditions
- Age > 60 years

Figure 36.1 DVT, PE and infarction

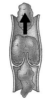

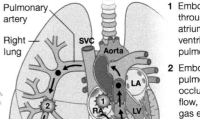

Blood clot forms in a deep vein in the leg. Emboli break off and travel via the vena cava and right ventricle to the pulmonary vessels

Unilateral calf swelling which is warm and erythematous are signs of a DVT. Most patients with DVT have no symptoms!

Pulmonary artery

Right lung

SVC

Aorta

LA

RA

LV

RV

IVC

Embolus

Possible area of infarct
No gaseous exchange as no blood flow

1 Embolus travelling through right atrium, to right ventricle then pulmonary artery

2 Embolus lodged in pulmonary artery occludes blood flow, and impairs gas exchange. Alveolar collapse follows. Area of lung distal to the embolus may die

Figure 36.2 Chest injury causing R tension pneumothorax and lung collapse. Air accumulated in pleural space causes compression of lung, heart and major vessels

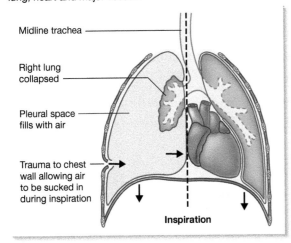

Midline trachea

Right lung collapsed

Pleural space fills with air

Trauma to chest wall allowing air to be sucked in during inspiration

Inspiration

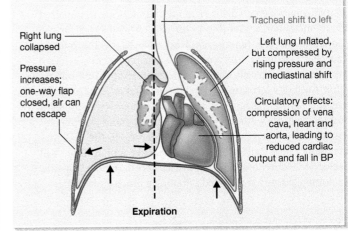

Right lung collapsed

Pressure increases; one-way flap closed, air can not escape

Tracheal shift to left

Left lung inflated, but compressed by rising pressure and mediastinal shift

Circulatory effects: compression of vena cava, heart and aorta, leading to reduced cardiac output and fall in BP

Expiration

Figure 36.3 Cardiac tamponade compressing the heart, reducing cardiac output

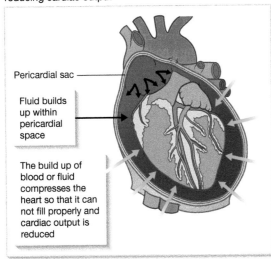

Pericardial sac

Fluid builds up within pericardial space

The build up of blood or fluid compresses the heart so that it can not fill properly and cardiac output is reduced

Figure 36.4 Emergency needle decompression site for right-sided tension pneumothorax

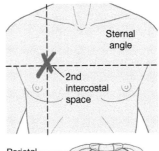

Sternal angle

2nd intercostal space

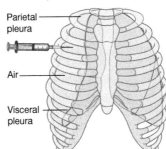

Parietal pleura

Air

Visceral pleura

Box 36.2 Tension pneumothorax (risk factors/causes)

- Trauma/chest injury; most common cause
- Chest surgery
- Pneumothorax
- Positive pressure ventilation
- COPD

Box 36.3 Cardiac tamponade (risk factors/causes)

- Chest trauma (blunt or penetrating)
- Caused inadvertently by invasive procedures such as cardiac surgery
- Myocardial rupture postinfarction
- Pericarditis (inflammation of the pericardium), pericardial effusion
- Dissecting thoracic aortic aneurysm

Acute and Critical Care Nursing at a Glance, First Edition. Edited by Helen Dutton and Jacqui Finch
© 2018 John Wiley & Sons, Ltd. Published 2018 by John Wiley & Sons, Ltd.
Companion website: www.ataglanceseries.com/nursing/acutecare

Shock occurs when the supply of blood from the circulation is insufficient to meet the metabolic requirements of organs and tissues. **Obstructive shock** is caused by an **obstruction to blood flow**, preventing blood from **returning to or from the right and/or left ventricle**. Any mechanical impediment that prevents diastolic filling of the ventricles, leads to a significant fall in cardiac output. Not all view this as a separate category, considering obstructive causes under cardiogenic shock. In common with all types of shock, effective treatment relies on early recognition using NEWS to assess risk of clinical deterioration. If left untreated obstructive shock can quickly lead to cardiac arrest. Initial treatment will usually be supportive in nature, such as oxygen administration and monitoring, until expert help is available. Invasive supportive therapies such as intubation and mechanical ventilation may also be required necessitating transfer to a higher level of care.

Pulmonary embolism

Pulmonary embolism (PE) results from obstruction within the pulmonary arterial vasculature. Risk factors are identified in Box 36.1. The emboli can be caused by:

- **Thrombosis** (blood clot usually in veins of the legs).
- **Fat** – following long bone fracture or orthopaedic surgery.
- **Amniotic fluid** – liberated during labour.
- **Air** – following central vein cannulation or bronchial trauma.
- **Sepsis** – from an infected central catheter, for example.

The most common source of emboli is **deep vein thrombosis** (DVT). **Thrombotic emboli**, broken off from a larger clot, lodges in the pulmonary vasculature (Figure 36.1). This impedes the exchange of gases across the alveolar capillary membrane, resulting in hypoxaemia. Large emboli may obstruct the flow of blood through the pulmonary vessels, causing lung tissue to die. Left ventricular blood volume (preload) and cardiac output are reduced. A large emboli, or multiple smaller emboli, may result in sudden death. **Venous thromboembolism** (VTE) encompasses both PE and DVT. Patients are regularly assessed for VTE risk, using tools such as the Wells Score.[1] VTE prophylaxis is achieved with antiembolus stockings and anticoagulation with low molecular weight heparin (LMWH) (such as enoxaparin or fondaparinux).[1]

Assessment, investigation and management

The nurse using the ABCDE approach, should note symptoms such as: dyspnoea, pleuritic chest pain (on inspiration) ↑RR, circulatory instability with ↑HR, and evidence of DVT (only clinically evident in 15% of PEs). Additional symptoms such as a cough or **haemoptysis** may also be present. Urgent medical referral is required so diagnostic scans such as computerised tomographic pulmonary angiography (CTPA) and bloods for **D-dimers** are completed. If PE is confirmed, parenteral anticoagulation with LMWH is continued for at least 5 days. Close cardiovascular monitoring is required.

Tension pneumothorax

Tension pneumothorax is the build-up of air within the pleural space.[2] This is usually due to a pleural or lung laceration. Air is able to enter the pleural space in inspiration, but cannot leave during expiration (Figure 36.2). A 'one-way valve' effect leads to a progressive pressure build-up in the pleural space, displacing the mediastinum and obstructing venous return to the heart. Causes are identified in Box 36.2. Tension pneumothorax is associated with a high mortality, and should be diagnosed within the initial minutes of a trauma assessment.[2]

Assessment investigations and management

Using the ABCDE approach, the nurse will see that the patient with a tension pneumothorax has chest pain, and is in considerable respiratory distress. The hyperexpanded chest moves little with respiration and breath sounds are absent on the affected side; ↑RR and profound hypoxaemia are evident and 15 L of oxygen via a non-rebreathe mask is required. Positive pressure ventilation such as CPAP or NIV exacerbates the 'one-way valve' effect, hastening deterioration, so must be stopped if in use. Tracheal deviation is a late sign as the pressure in the mediastinum compresses and moves the thoracic organs: urgent assistance is required at this time. **Juglar venous distension** (JVD) is evident and CVP would be raised if monitored. Tachycardia, with a falling BP alongside cool and clammy peripheries and a falling urine output, may be noted. The patient may quickly lose consciousness.

Tension pneumothorax can only be relieved by urgent removal of the trapped air by a competent healthcare professional, before CXR confirmation.[3] This is achieved by either **emergency needle decompression** (Figure 36.4), or inserting a tube into the pleural space, with a one-way valve system allowing air to escape but not re-enter. An underwater seal drain may also be used (Chapter 19 and Figure 19.3).

Cardiac tamponade

Cardiac tamponade is caused by accumulation of fluid in the pericardial space (Figure 36.3). Causes are identified in Box 36.3. The pericardial sac is unable to expand to accommodate extra fluid, so this results in compression of the heart, leading to a reduced cardiac output. Slow fluid accumulation enables the pericardial sac to gradually stretch, holding volumes of up to 1 L. If the fluid collections occur rapidly and acutely, then even a small amount of extra fluid gives severe problems. One common incidence of tamponade is after heart surgery. Postoperative bleeding may not clear sufficiently due to either a blocked pericardial drain, or excessive bleeding. This may necessitate further surgery to remove the blood clot, or stop the bleeding.

Assessment investigations and management

Cardiac tamponade is usually caused by trauma or cardiac surgery, and can be recognised by three classical signs, known as Beck's Triad: hypotension, due to the decreased stroke volume; JVD due to the increased pressure in the right ventricle; and muffled heart sounds due to fluid inside the pericardium. The nurse should suspect tamponade in the acutely unwell patient with these signs and a clinical history highlighting risk. Cardiac tamponade requires removal of the fluid which has accumulated. This is achieved via pericardiocentesis, a skilled procedure in which a needle or drain is inserted into the pericardial space under ultrasound guidance, to aspirate/drain the fluid. Emergency surgery may be required.

37 Acute circulatory failure 5: heart failure

Table 37.1 Symptoms, signs and diagnostic tests for HF

	Diagnostic tests (see also Chapter 26)
Symptoms • Breathlessness • Fatigue • Oedema • Orthopnoea	**Blood tests** Raised B-type natriuretic peptide (BNP) or N-terminal pro-B-type natriuretic peptide (NT-proBNP)
Signs • Crackles heard on lung auscultation • Raised JVP	**Echocardiogram** Evaluated how much blood the ventricle is pumping, checking heart valves and heart wall movements for abnormalities

Box 37.1 Causes of HF

- Hypertension
- High output failure: pregnancy, thyrotoxicosis, liver cirrhosis, septic shock
- Arrhythmias: tachy/bradyarrhythmias, intraventricular conduction problems
- Myocardial disease: cardiomyopathies (dilated, hypertrophic, restrictive), myocarditis
- Coronary artery disease: myocardial infarction
- Heart valve disease: ageing, e.g. calcification; infective endocarditis, congenital

Table 37.2 New York Heart Association (NYHA) functional classification describing severity of HF

NYHA 1	Ordinary physical activity does not cause undue fatigue or dyspnoea
NYHA 2	Slight limitation of physical activity Comfortable at rest, but activity causes fatigue or dyspnoea
NHHA 3	Marked limitation of physical activity Comfortable at rest, but less than ordinary activity causes fatigue or dyspnoea
NYHA 4	Unable to carry out any physical activity Symptoms at rest

Figure 37.1 The patient with CCF

Chronic fatigue and lethargy

Increased pressure in the lung vasculature irritates lungs causing chronic cough. Wheezing may also be present

Pleural effusion: an excess of fluid in the pleural space. Patient has difficulty expanding lungs and feels short of breath

Anorexia-reduced appetite due to reduced peristalsis, and nausea

Urine output reduces due to poor renal perfusion and RAAS activation

Abdominal swelling due to ascites. This is a build-up of fluid between the peritoneal layers, caused by an increase in pressure in the venous system due to RV failure.

Oedema and ascites are caused by fluid retention. Daily weights are useful to monitor fluid retention in patient with CCF

Paroxysmal nocturnal pulmonary oedema can occur. This may be relieved by sitting up, and dangling legs over the side of the bed

Acutely:
pulmonary oedema, with water surrounding and entering the alveoli, can occur due to rising pulmonary venous pressure (caused by LV failure). Patient becomes hypoxaemic and distressed (acute HF), requiring urgent intervention

Work of breathing is increased due to reduction in lung compliance. Patient feels short of breath

Neither LV or RV are pumping effectively; hypertrophy of myocardium enlarges heart. A reduction in cardiac output and tissue perfusion causes organ damage with renal and liver dysfunction

Oedema: swelling in ankles, legs and sacrum. Caused by increased pressure in the venous system due to RV failure

Figure 37.2 Acute LVF causing pulmonary oedema

2 As LV pressure ↑ pressure of blood increases in the pulmonary vasculature

4 Frothy sputum - pink or white: pulmonary oedema

Aorta

Lung

Lung

Alveolar air space

CO_2 CO_2

O_2 O_2

Fluid

Right ventricle

Left ventricle

Myocardial infarct

3 ↑ Pulmonary pressure causes plasma water to move into alveolar air space

1 Damage to LV, eg. myocardial infarction. Left ventricle severely impaired, unable to pump effectively, pressure rises

Figure 37.3 Physiological responses to reduced cardiac output in heart failure

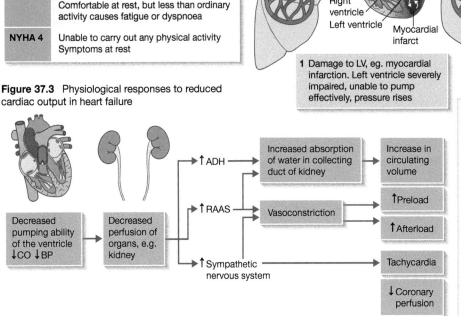

Decreased pumping ability of the ventricle ↓CO ↓BP

Decreased perfusion of organs, e.g. kidney

↑ADH → Increased absorption of water in collecting duct of kidney → Increase in circulating volume

↑RAAS → Vasoconstriction → ↑Preload

→ ↑Afterload

↑Sympathetic nervous system → Tachycardia

↓Coronary perfusion

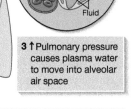

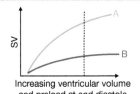

Increasing ventricular volume and preload at end diastole

Frank–Starling curve describes an ↑ SV with ↑ volume in the ventricle at end of diastole (normal heart curve A) In HF myocardium is damaged, this relationship fails and SV and CO fall. ↑LV volume does not increase CO as effectively as in the healthy heart. It may actually decrease CO and give rise to pulmonary oedema (failing heart, curve B)

Acute and Critical Care Nursing at a Glance, First Edition. Edited by Helen Dutton and Jacqui Finch
© 2018 John Wiley & Sons, Ltd. Published 2018 by John Wiley & Sons, Ltd.
Companion website: www.ataglanceseries.com/nursing/acutecare

Circulatory failure as a result of **acute heart failure** reduces cardiac output and perfusion pressure, resulting in inadequate tissue perfusion. Heart failure (HF) can be chronic or acute, left-sided, right-sided or bilateral and due to either systolic or diastolic dysfunction. The diagnosis of HF is made when the patient complains of a number of signs and symptoms, with evidence of a cardiac abnormality found on blood tests and/or cardiac imaging (Table 37.1). HF is seen as a syndrome rather than a diagnosis, so the cause of the failure needs to be determined.[1] Problems leading to HF are outlined (Box 37.1). Many people experience chronic heart failure, with occasional acute decompensation requiring hospital admission. Whatever the cause of HF, nurses should be able to recognise the signs of acute heart failure, instigate appropriate monitoring, escalating care to enable prompt diagnosis and treatment.

Heart failure: how does it happen?

Systolic dysfunction

Predominantly a problem of left ventricular systolic dysfunction (**LVSD**), it is caused by the inability of the LV myocardium to contract effectively, reducing the amount of blood (or SV) ejected. In health about 60% of the blood (**ejection fraction**) in the ventricle is ejected, but in HF the ejection fraction can fall to 20% or less. Failure of the LV in systole is caused by a number of problems, such as **myocardial infarction** or **cardiomyopathy**.

Diastolic dysfunction

During diastole the LV heart muscle relaxes and fills with the blood returned via the pulmonary veins. In diastolic failure the LV heart muscle thickens or hypertrophies, and/or becomes very stiff, caused by conditions such as hypertension. This means that less blood enters the ventricle and even though the ventricle can contract effectively, the SV is still reduced. This is referred to as HF with preserved ejection fraction (**HFPEF**).

Right-sided heart failure

Failure of the right ventricle (RV) is often precipitated by failure of the LV. The pressure in the pulmonary capillaries rises with the failure of the LV to eject blood forward into the systemic circulation. Rising pulmonary capillary pressure increases the RV work (↑afterload) in ejecting its stroke volume. The RV dilates to accommodate the larger volumes, then fails to contract effectively. Chronic respiratory problems such as COPD, increase RV afterload via hypoxic vasoconstriction of pulmonary arteries, causing RV heart failure (or **cor pulmonale**).

Bilateral or congestive heart failure

Also called congestive cardiac failure (CCF), this refers to chronic heart failure (CHF) involving both the RV and LV. Symptoms of CHF are outlined in Figure 37.1.

Sympathetic and hormonal responses

Autoregulatory systems to maintain blood pressure (Chapter 24) are activated by the poor cardiac output of HF (Table 37.3), but result in increasing the heart's workload by:
- Fluid retention: increasing preload, raising pulmonary vascular pressures and causing pulmonary oedema.
- Vasoconstriction: increasing afterload and heart work, decreasing SV, cardiac output and organ perfusion.

Heart failure management

NICE (2010 and 2014)[2,3] have published guidance on the management of heart failure that can be accessed at http://www.nice.org.uk. Administration of medications such as ACEI, beta blockers and diuretics (Chapter 24), improves heart function by reducing heart work and expelling excess fluid. Daily weights, in conjunction with an accurate record of fluid intake (which may be restricted) and output, helps prevent fluid overload. Heart failure can be classified according to patient symptoms (Table 37.2).

Acute decompensated heart failure

Rapid onset of symptoms, or changes in existing symptoms, mark the onset of acute heart failure. This is referred to as decompensated HF as normal compensatory mechanisms have failed. The patient often presents in acute respiratory distress, feeling intense anxiety, fearing that they are drowning.[4] Coughing up pink (blood-stained) frothy sputum is a feature of acute pulmonary oedema (Figure 37.2). Alternatively, a gradual worsening of symptoms and oedema may occur. Some present with signs of low cardiac output: low BP, cool peripheries, new mental confusion and low urine output. Each presentation requires detailed assessment, using NEWS to help identify risk of deterioration and guide care escalation.

Nursing care and management

Care escalation ensuring rapid symptom relief is a priority, with a calm confident approach to reassure the anxious patient. Immediate interventions[3] consist of:
- **Sitting patient upright** supported with pillows as BP allows. Give **supplemental oxygen** to achieve target saturations, 15 L via a non-rebreath mask may be indicated.
- **Intravenous diuretic** as prescribed, often **furosemide** a potent loop diuretic. Monitor urine output. Consider inserting an urethral catheter for accurate measurement if response to diuretic poor.
- **Opiates** such as morphine 2.5–5 mg IV are not routinely offered, but may be of benefit with heightened anxiety.

If response to initial therapy is poor **cardiogenic shock** may be present and at least **level 2 care** is indicated for additional support[3] such as:
- **Non-invasive ventilation** for hypercapnic respiratory failure. Continuous monitoring of SpO_2 and regular ABG analysis is required. Intubation and ventilation may be necessary.
- **Inotropic and or vasoactive support** to increase perfusion pressure and cardiac output (Chapter 24). This medication is given via a volumetric pump, through a central line, with the patient on continuous ECG, arterial and CVP monitoring (Chapter 28).
- **Intravenous nitrates** (such as glyceryl trinitrate) may be beneficial if myocardial ischaemia, hypertension or heart valve disease present.
- If response remains poor, multiple organ support in a level 3 environment is required.

Nurses working in acute care environments need skills of recognising acute decompensated heart failure, with the confidence to escalate as appropriate in order to provide safe and effective level 2 or 3 care.

38 Principles of cardiac surgery

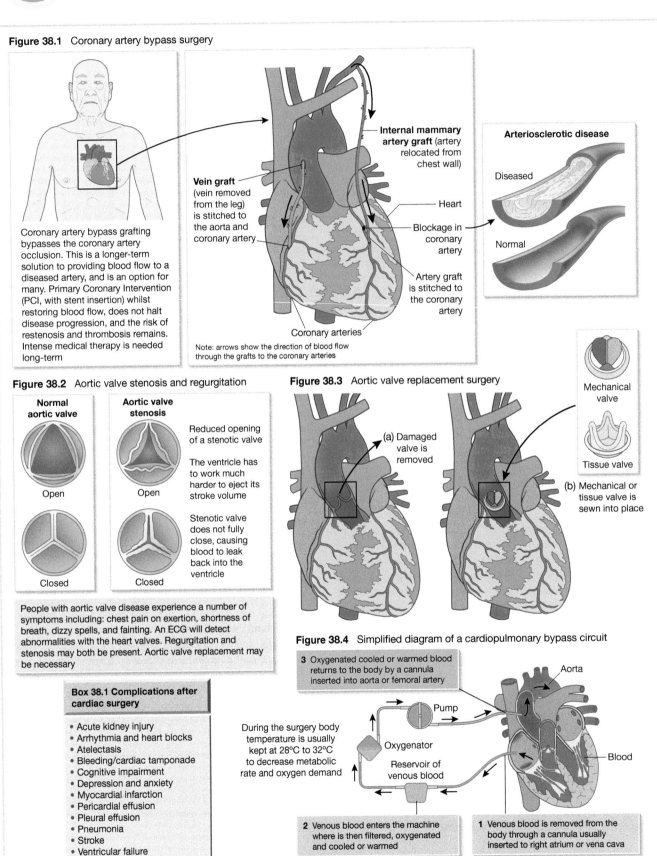

Figure 38.1 Coronary artery bypass surgery

Coronary artery bypass grafting bypasses the coronary artery occlusion. This is a longer-term solution to providing blood flow to a diseased artery, and is an option for many. Primary Coronary Intervention (PCI, with stent insertion) whilst restoring blood flow, does not halt disease progression, and the risk of restenosis and thrombosis remains. Intense medical therapy is needed long-term

Internal mammary artery graft (artery relocated from chest wall)

Vein graft (vein removed from the leg) is stitched to the aorta and coronary artery

Heart

Blockage in coronary artery

Artery graft is stitched to the coronary artery

Coronary arteries

Note: arrows show the direction of blood flow through the grafts to the coronary arteries

Arteriosclerotic disease

Diseased

Normal

Figure 38.2 Aortic valve stenosis and regurgitation

Normal aortic valve

Open

Closed

Aortic valve stenosis

Open

Closed

Reduced opening of a stenotic valve

The ventricle has to work much harder to eject its stroke volume

Stenotic valve does not fully close, causing blood to leak back into the ventricle

People with aortic valve disease experience a number of symptoms including: chest pain on exertion, shortness of breath, dizzy spells, and fainting. An ECG will detect abnormalities with the heart valves. Regurgitation and stenosis may both be present. Aortic valve replacement may be necessary

Figure 38.3 Aortic valve replacement surgery

(a) Damaged valve is removed

Mechanical valve

Tissue valve

(b) Mechanical or tissue valve is sewn into place

Box 38.1 Complications after cardiac surgery

- Acute kidney injury
- Arrhythmia and heart blocks
- Atelectasis
- Bleeding/cardiac tamponade
- Cognitive impairment
- Depression and anxiety
- Myocardial infarction
- Pericardial effusion
- Pleural effusion
- Pneumonia
- Stroke
- Ventricular failure

Figure 38.4 Simplified diagram of a cardiopulmonary bypass circuit

3 Oxygenated cooled or warmed blood returns to the body by a cannula inserted into aorta or femoral artery

Aorta

Pump

During the surgery body temperature is usually kept at 28°C to 32°C to decrease metabolic rate and oxygen demand

Oxygenator

Reservoir of venous blood

Blood

2 Venous blood enters the machine where is then filtered, oxygenated and cooled or warmed

1 Venous blood is removed from the body through a cannula usually inserted to right atrium or vena cava

Acute and Critical Care Nursing at a Glance, First Edition. Edited by Helen Dutton and Jacqui Finch
© 2018 John Wiley & Sons, Ltd. Published 2018 by John Wiley & Sons, Ltd.
Companion website: www.ataglanceseries.com/nursing/acutecare

Whilst many cardiac conditions can be managed with medical therapy, surgery is sometimes necessary. Common cardiac operations performed in adults are **coronary artery bypass grafting** (CABG) and **heart valve surgery**.

Coronary artery bypass grafting

CABG is performed in patients with significant narrowing of one or more coronary arteries to relieve angina, prevent myocardial infarction and sudden cardiac death. CABG improves the flow of blood to the area of myocardium affected by a coronary artery stenosis by >50%. During surgery a healthy blood vessel is taken from the leg, forearm or chest and grafted to the diseased coronary artery to create an alternative route for the blood flow around the atherosclerotic blockage. Either veins or arteries may be used as conduits for CABG. The most commonly used blood vessels are saphenous veins and the internal thoracic (mammary) artery (Figure 38.1).

Heart valve surgery

Valve surgery is performed to repair or replace diseased heart valves and is often combined with CABG. Valve regurgitation and stenosis are the most common problems requiring surgical intervention. Regurgitation results when the valve doesn't close tightly causing blood to leak back through the valve. Stenosis occurs when a valve doesn't open fully due to calcium deposits or scarring (Figure 38.2). Repair is common for mitral and tricuspid valves, while the aortic valve is usually replaced (Figure 38.3). Aortic stenosis, due to age-related progressive calcification is the most frequent type of heart valve disease in older adults, necessitating valve replacement.

Two types of replacement valve are used:
- Biological: preserved human or animal (bovine, porcine) tissues. Last 10–15 years and are more suitable for older patients.
- Mechanical: made of stainless steel, titanium, carbon and ceramic. Last longer than tissue valves but require lifetime anticoagulation with warfarin to prevent valve thrombosis and thromboembolism.

Surgical approaches

Open heart surgery usually requires stopping the heart and using cardiopulmonary bypass (CPB). A procedure that involves a **cardiopulmonary bypass machine** is called 'on pump' surgery. The CPB pump is often referred to as a heart–lung machine or 'the pump'. Figure 38.4 shows the CPB circuit. The machine takes over the function of the heart and lungs during surgery, maintaining the circulation of blood and supplying oxygen to organs and tissues.

CABG surgery can also be performed on a beating heart without cardiopulmonary bypass, so-called 'off-pump' surgery. This approach reduces recovery times and is often less painful, but is still under evaluation for its potential benefits over 'on pump surgery'.

Nursing management postsurgery

Initially the patient will require intensive care, often with a short period of ventilation. Haemodynamic instability may necessitate cardiac output monitoring and the use of inotropes, vasoactive drugs, or mechanical assist devices such as temporary pacing or an intra-aortic balloon pump. Within a few hours transfer to level 2 /HDU may be appropriate. Regular patient assessment is a crucial part of nursing care, enabling prevention and early detection of complications related to surgery and cardiopulmonary bypass (Box 38.1). Monitoring includes pulse oximetry, respiratory rate, ECG, blood pressure, central venous pressure, fluid balance, temperature, arterial blood gas analysis and assessment of neurological function.

Optimising respiratory function

Oxygen therapy is usually required in the first 24–48 h following surgery to maintain SpO_2 within target range. Hypoxaemia may occur due to atelectasis. Physiotherapy, encouraging deep breathing and coughing exercises, incentive spirometry and application of NIV via face mask, improves respiratory function, re-expanding collapsed alveoli. Early mobilisation depends on good pain management, encouraging the patient to sit out of bed as soon as possible. This is important in prevention and treatment of pulmonary complications.

Optimising cardiac function

Ensuring good tissue perfusion with haemodynamic stability are the main aims of postoperative care. Fluid therapy with crystalloids and colloids is used to ensure adequate volume supply and to improve heart function requiring close attention. Hourly recording of urine output monitors renal function. Recognising and managing electrolyte imbalance is necessary to decrease the incidence of arrhythmias, replacing potassium and magnesium as required. Arrhythmias and conduction blocks are managed with antiarrhythmic drugs, cardioversion or temporary pacing.

Pain management

Effective pain management is crucial in ensuring patients' comfort, promoting early mobilisation to reduce complications. Pain experienced following sternotomy is limited to the first few postoperative days and is usually successfully managed with PCA or oral pain medications, such as paracetamol. Leg incision pain from the harvest of saphenous veins is reported by patients as more intense, often affecting mobility.

Surgical wound care

Sternal wound infection is a serious complication leading to increased length of stay, mortality and care costs. Wound dressings are left for 48 h and aseptic non-touch techniques are used when changing the dressing to reduce sternal wound infections. Hyperglycaemia postoperatively needs to be promptly managed, to achieve normoglycaemia. Deep sternal wound infections are treated surgically or with vacuum-assisted closure therapy. Nurses should advise patients to limit lifting, and support the chest whilst coughing to prevent sternal instability or wound breakdown.

Psychological and emotional support

Many patients experience anxiety, mood changes and depression during the recovery period. Nurses play a vital role in providing psychological and emotional support for patients and their relatives by addressing fears and concerns, offering explanations, reassurance and advice. Patient education should focus on addressing risk factors for heart disease and strategies to help patients and their family members to adjust to a healthy lifestyle including smoking cessation, stress reduction, diet, physical activity and treatment compliance.

39 Physiology of the gastrointestinal system

Figure 39.1 Anatomy of the GI tract. Source: Peate I. and Nair M., 2011. Reproduced with permission of John Wiley & Sons.

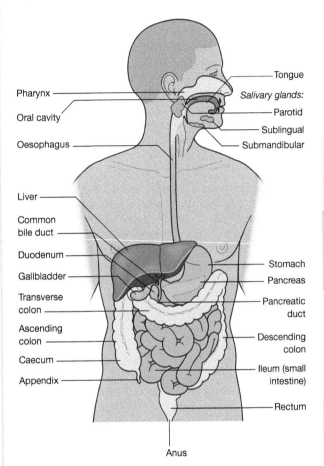

- Tongue
- Pharynx
- Oral cavity
- Oesophagus
- *Salivary glands:*
  - Parotid
  - Sublingual
  - Submandibular
- Liver
- Common bile duct
- Duodenum
- Gallbladder
- Transverse colon
- Ascending colon
- Caecum
- Appendix
- Stomach
- Pancreas
- Pancreatic duct
- Descending colon
- Ileum (small intestine)
- Rectum
- Anus

Figure 39.2 Digestive juices, enzymes and hormones

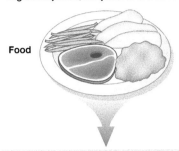

Food

(a) Salivary glands	• Amylase: an enzyme to begin the digestion of starches • Sodium bicarbonate to increase pH and optimise amylase • Mucus and water
(b) Stomach	• Pepsin: an enzyme to digest proteins • Hydrochloric acid to decrease pH • Intrinsic factor to promote later Vitamin B12 absorption • Mucus and water • Gastrin: a hormone to stimulate gastric juice
(c) Pancreatic	• Proteases to digest proteins: trypsin, chymotrypsin • Collagenase • Elastase • Lipases to digest fats • Amylase to digest starches • Sodium bicarbonate to increase pH • Mucus and water
(d) Intestinal mucosa	• Sodium bicarbonate to increase pH • Mucus and water • Gastric inhibitory peptide and secretin: both inhibit gastric secretion • Cholecystokinin-pancreozymin: stimulates pancreatic juice and bile ejection from the gallbladder

Figure 39.3 Anatomy of the liver

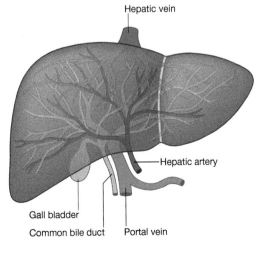

- Hepatic vein
- Hepatic artery
- Gall bladder
- Common bile duct
- Portal vein

Table 39.1 Key functions of the liver

Secretion of bile	Bile is made of bile salts, pigments and cholesterol. The bile salts aid in the digestion of fats and bile is also a pathway for the excretion of bilirubin (the haem portion of old erythrocytes)
Metabolism	• Breaks down stored glycogen (glycogenolysis) to increase availability • Converts amino acids into plasma proteins (albumin, fibrinogen and some globulins) • Utilises amino acids for gluconeogenesis resulting in ammonia production. Converts this together with ammonia from bacteria in the intestines into urea • With vitamin K, synthesises clotting factors: II ,VII, IX, and X. • Also produces clotting factors: I, V, XI, XII and XIII • Breaks down fatty acids in (triglycerides, phospholipids and cholesterol) into energy (adenosine triphosphate). Also processes fatty acids into ketone bodies when glucose is not available
Storage	• Glucose as glycogen, amino acids, fat soluble vitamins: A, D, E and K (absorbs latter from GI tract), vitamin B12 and iron
Detoxification	• Absorbs drugs to be excreted in the bile or urine • Breaks down ethanol to acetic acid and then acetyl-CoA for metabolism • Breaks down some hormones

Acute and Critical Care Nursing at a Glance, First Edition. Edited by Helen Dutton and Jacqui Finch
© 2018 John Wiley & Sons, Ltd. Published 2018 by John Wiley & Sons, Ltd.
Companion website: www.ataglanceseries.com/nursing/acutecare

The gastrointestinal tract

The gastrointestinal (GI) tract consists of the mouth, part of the pharynx, oesophagus, stomach, small and large intestines and the rectum. Accessory organs are the liver, gallbladder and pancreas (Figure 39.1). Together, these areas of the alimentary system are responsible for ingesting, digesting, absorbing food and then eliminating the waste products.

Anatomy and physiology of key gastroinestinal organs

Once food has been ingested, mastication with the aid of salivary gland secretions (Figure 39.2a) will propel the bolus into the hollow, muscular **oesophagus**. Peristaltic action here will move it on through the **cardiac sphincter** into the **stomach** where it will mix with gastric juice (Figure 39.2b) to form a soup-like substance called **chyme**. Very little absorption takes place in the stomach because the epithelial cells found here are impermeable to most substances. However, its mucous cells can absorb some water, fatty acids and significantly, drugs like aspirin and 20% of alcohol. From the stomach, the chyme will pass through the pyloric sphincter to the **duodenum**, the first part of the small intestine. In the duodenum, intestinal juices, water and mucus are joined by pancreatic secretions (Figure 39.2d). Together these facilitate the intestinal absorption of the constituents in the chyme, by the villi and microvilli. Microvilli are known as the 'brush border' due to their fine, brush-like appearance. In the **jejunum,** the second part of the small intestine, glucose, amino acids, water and fat soluble vitamins and 80% of any alcohol is absorbed. In the **ileum**, the third part of the small intestine, Vitamin B12 and bile salts are soaked up. In total, the small intestine is 3 m in length and is the major site of digestion. The large intestine is 1.5 m long and is composed of the **appendix**, the **caecum** and the four areas of the **colon** (ascending, transverse, sigmoid and descending). The major function of the mucosa here is to absorb more water, secrete mucus and generate faeces for elimination via the final 17–20 cm of the alimentary tract, the **rectum**. This structure, terminating in the anal canal, expels the waste products of digestion when receptors in the mucosa are stimulated by colonic peristalsis. Although this is primarily a reflex action, voluntary inhibition of defaecation is possible.

Finally, covering most of these digestive structures, is a membrane called the **peritoneum**. The **parietal layer** of this sheet of serous tissue lines the abdominal cavity and the **visceral layer** forms the outer coating of the organs. In several places the peritoneum has folds and extensions within it and these are called the **mesentery**, the **transverse mesocolon** and the **greater** and **lesser omentum**. Their collective purpose is to bind abdominal organs together, whilst allowing free movement.

Anatomy and physiology of the accessory organs of the gastrointestinal tract

The **liver**, a large organ weighing up to 1.6 kg, is located under the right diaphragm and attached to the anterior abdominal wall. The large right lobe, and the much smaller left lobe, receive blood from two vessels. The hepatic artery delivers oxygenated blood, whilst the hepatic portal vein brings deoxygenated blood containing absorbed nutrients from the gut such as drugs and toxins.

Small capillaries or *sinusoids,* with their permeable, endothelium-lined walls play a key role in the delivery of oxygen and absorbed substances to the **hepatocytes** (the functional units of the liver). The sinusoids also contain Kuppfer cells (specialised phagocytes), which have bactericidal properties and are important for bilirubin production and lipid metabolism.

The hexagonal-shaped hepatocytes, composed of specialised epithelium, have many vital functions within the body, not all of them directly related to digestion such is the complexity of the liver as an organ (Figure 39.3 and Table 39.1). One function is to produce bile, and adjacent to the hepatocytes are the **bile canaliculi** through which the bile is drained away into the bile ducts and hepatic duct. From here it will meet resistance at the closed **sphincter of Oddi** (which prevents reflux of duodenal contents) and then pass into the common bile duct on its way to the gallbladder.

The **gallbladder** is a 7–10 cm pear-shaped organ that is attached to the undersurface of the liver by connective tissue. Its function is to store the bile arriving from the liver via the bile and hepatic ducts. Able to hold up to 50 mL of bile at any one time, the gallbladder will concentrate the bile up to 10 times more than its original strength. The wall of this organ is composed of serous, muscular and mucous layers. It contracts when food is being digested in the stomach and intestines; this will then open the sphincter of Oddi and eject the bile into the duodenum.

The **pancreas** is a 15–20 cm organ that lies deep within the abdomen, behind the stomach. A fish-like structure, its head is touching the duodenum whilst its tail is in contact with the spleen. The tissue of the pancreas is glandular, with 98% of it being classified as **exocrine** and this means that it has ducts to carry secretions to specific locations. The grape-like cells found here secrete over a litre of pancreatic juice daily (Figure 39.2c), which is emptied into the duodenum, firstly via the pancreatic duct and then via the common bile duct.

Amongst the exocrine units of the pancreas, there are clusters of **endocrine** cells known as pancreatic islets or more commonly the **'islets of Langerhans'**. Tissue that is endocrine in nature is capable of internal secretion directly into the blood, without the use of a system of ducts. Hormones are released in this way and in the pancreatic islets there are different types of hormone-producing cells. Firstly, the **alpha cells** which secret **glucagon,** a polypeptide hormone that initiates a rise in blood glucose. When the blood glucose level is low in the body, glucagon stimulates the liver to breakdown **glycogen** (glucose that is stored for later use). If, conversely, the blood glucose is too high, the **beta cells** will release insulin which increases the uptake and use of glucose by the body thus lowering the blood level. A third group, the **delta cells,** will produce **somatostatin**. This complex hormone (also made in other areas of the body, including the hypothalamus) exerts a general inhibitory effect. In the pancreas it is capable of inhibiting both glucagon and insulin release and, in addition, it is thought to reduce intestinal absorption. Finally, the **gamma cells** of the islets produce pancreatic polypeptides and these regulate appetite.

The organs of the GI tract therefore regulate digestive processes. However, if dysfunction should occur with any of these, it can lead to physiological disturbances such as infection, sepsis, bleeding, hypovolaemia and electrolyte imbalance. Clinical deterioration will ensue, resulting in the patient requiring acute and/or emergency care (Chapter 40).

40 Acute medical and surgical gastrointestinal problems

Box 40.1 Intestinal obstruction

- Intestinal content, gas and fluid builds up behind the obstruction

- Bowel wall distends and pressure increases

- Oedema forms and capillaries in the bowel lumen become permeable, with fluids leaking into the peritoneal cavity. Intravascular volume and electrolyte loss ensues. Pressure is placed on the diaphragm reducing respiratory capacity

- Gut bacteria move through the leaky bowel wall (translocation) leading to peritonitis and toxin release

Figure 40.1 Possible assessment findings in acute gastrointestinal disorders

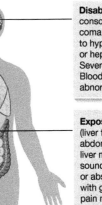

Airway: may be compromised due to the presence of blood and the development of hypoxaemia

Breathing: rate may be increased due to pressure on the diaphragm, metabolic acidosis and pain. Pleural effusion in pancreatitis

Disability: impaired consciousness leading to coma may develop secondary to hypoxaemia, hypercarbia or hepatic encephalopathy. Severe pain may be present. Blood glucose level may be abnormal

Exposure: may look jaundiced (liver failure), have a distended abdomen with increasing girth, liver may be palpable. Bowel sounds may be high pitched or absent. **Acute abdomen** with guarding (tenseness) and pain may be present. Bruising (Grey Turner's and Cullen's sign) may be present with pancreatitis

Circulation: BP reduced due to sepsis, or hypovolaemic shock, may have visible blood loss, vomiting and/or diarrhoea. Electrolyte imbalance can impair cardiac function, with arrhythmias or ischaemic changes. Liver dysfunction can lead to abnormal blood clotting. Pancreatitis will cause raised serum lipase and amylase. Blood lactate level may be raised. Acute kidney injury may develop secondary to poor kidney perfusion

Figure 40.2 (a) Laparoscopy. (b) Laparotomy

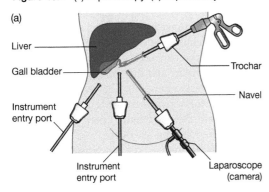

(a)

Liver
Gall bladder
Instrument entry port
Trochar
Navel
Instrument entry port
Laparoscope (camera)

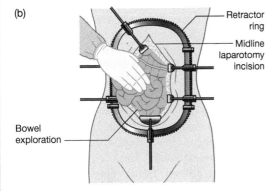

(b)

Retractor ring
Midline laparotomy incision
Bowel exploration

Figure 40.3 Types of colectomy

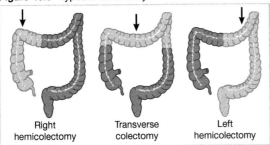

Right hemicolectomy | Transverse colectomy | Left hemicolectomy

Table 40.1 Specific nursing care of the patient with acute GI dysfunction

A	• Maintain airway: risk of obstruction from haemorrhage and vomiting
B	• Monitor SpO_2 readings and if required, administer oxygen therapy as prescribed according to target saturation levels • Measure respiratory rate reporting if outside normal range • Monitor for signs of respiratory distress: grunting, nasal flaring, lip pursing • Observe sputum which may be bloodstained or infected, send a sample as appropriate • Auscultate chest for added breath sounds, such as crackles or wheezes that might indicate infection • Observe for equal lung expansion, unilateral movement may indicate presence of pleural effusion (common in pancreatitis) • Ensure arterial blood gases are checked if respiratory distress evident
C	• Check skin turgor for signs of dehydration • Monitor BP and HR for signs of hypovolaemia, including temperature for signs of sepsis • Keep patient nil by mouth as directed • Administer intravenous crystalloid or colloid as prescribed • Administer blood and blood products as prescribed • Insert nasogastric tube (on medical instruction only, owing to the possibility of varices), to reduce distension and nausea • Measure urine output, reporting if < 0.5 mL/kg/h • Maintain an accurate fluid balance chart, reporting imbalances • Monitor electrolyte status and report and replace losses as prescribed • May require continuous ECG monitoring • Check that serum lactate level, CRP and clotting status are monitored for abnormalities
D	• Assess level of consciousness; pupil reaction may be compromised in hepatic encephalopathy • Monitor blood glucose levels, report abnormalities and replace glucose or start prescribed insulin regime as required • Assess pain and administer analgesia as prescribed
E	• Observe skin and sclera for jaundice and skin for bruising • Check NEWS, and seek advice/escalate care as appropriate

Acute and Critical Care Nursing at a Glance, First Edition. Edited by Helen Dutton and Jacqui Finch
© 2018 John Wiley & Sons, Ltd. Published 2018 by John Wiley & Sons, Ltd.
Companion website: www.ataglanceseries.com/nursing/acutecare

Many disorders affect the organs of the GI tract, both acute and chronic in nature. Nurses need to recognise possible assessment findings for patients with acute GI problems to escalate care in a timely manner, reducing risk of deterioration (Figure 40.1).

Main organs of the gastrointestinal tract: acute disorders

The main organs of the GI tract can be affected by many problems. These may be due to weakened structures, herniation, leakage, obstructions, malignancies or infection. Two specific conditions require immediate attention: haemorrhage and obstruction.

Upper or lower gastrointestinal tract bleeding

Upper GI haemorrhage, carrying a 10% mortality, can originate from the stomach or duodenum and may be due to peptic or duodenal ulceration. Infection with *Helicobacter pylori* is often found to be the cause. This gram-negative bacterium lives in epithelial walls weakening them and exposing the mucosal layer to gastric secretions which then leads to their erosion. **Oesophageal varices** occur secondary to liver disease. Bleeding from the **lower GI tract** (commencing at the jejunum), is often due to inflammatory disease such as **ulcerative colitis**. Patients with GI bleeding will present with **haematemesis**, vomiting bright red blood or dark 'coffee grounds' (digested blood), particularly where problems occur higher up the GI tract. The presence of tarry **malaena** stools, with their characteristic offensive smell, indicates that blood has passed through the GI tract. Whilst for lower lesions, **haematochezia** or the passing of bright red blood from the rectum occurs. In all cases **endoscopic procedures** are required (within the first 24 h from onset of bleeding) to determine the location and cause of the problem. The patient's physiological response to the haemorrhage and how it will be managed, depends largely on how much blood has been lost, with some patients developing hypovolaemic shock quite quickly (Chapter 35). Numerical scoring systems exist for determining the severity of a GI bleed and these consider clinical parameters including: the patient's age, haemoglobin, vital signs and the presence of comorbidities such as pre-existing hepatic or cardiac disease. NICE (2012)[1] recommends the use of the **Glasgow-Blatchford score** pre-endoscopy and the **Rockall score** postprocedure.

Treatment for GI bleeding depends on the exact cause, but for peptic and duodenal ulceration includes: further endoscopic intervention such as dilute adrenaline injection to vasoconstrict the bleeding area, pharmacological administration in the form of **proton pump inhibitors** to suppress gastric acid production (e.g. omeprazole) and the use of **tranexamic acid** to control bleeding. Surgery is rarely required but, if necessary, a **vagotomy**, **pyloroplasty** or gastroduodenal reconstruction is performed. A **laparotomy** will be required if perforation of the gut occurs.

Intestinal obstruction

Causes include: **adhesions**, hernia, tumour, **volvulus**, **paralytic ileus**, **diverticular** or inflammatory disease. Nurses need to be aware of the common pathophysiology (Box 40.1). Diagnosis can be made by abdominal X-ray, **barium studies**, **ultrasound** and **colonoscopy**.

Abdominal surgery such as laparoscopy or laparotomy may be carried out as part of an exploratory operation (Figure 40.2).

Surgery to relieve the obstruction, including hemicolectomy, transverse colectomy (Figure 40.3) or **Hartmann's procedure** with the formation of a colostomy may be required.

Accessory organs of the gastrointestinal tract: acute disorders

Acute liver failure

Acute liver failure is potentially life threatening and can occur as a result of: a viral infection like hepatitis (A,B,C,D or E); poisoning with drugs (e.g. paracetamol) or toxins (certain fungi); metabolic or vascular disorders (such as shock). High blood pressure develops in the portal venous system (portal hypertension) and this impedes blood flow. Collateral blood vessels in the oesophagus, abdominal wall and rectum open between the portal and systemic veins, bypassing the obstructed ones. Over time this can lead to several problems. Collateral blood vessels, still subject to the high pressure of the portal system, become distended (forming varices) and rupture leading to severe haemorrhage. The patient's spleen will also become enlarged. **Ascites** (fluid in the peritoneal cavity) will develop as will **hepatic encephalopathy**. Blood that would normally pass through the liver for detoxification is shunted away via the collateral vessels and gives substances like ammonia (normally removed by the liver) access to the brain. Confusion may lead to coma if severe and ultimately death. The patient may have other manifestations of liver disease (all related to the organ's inability to carry out its normal functions – see Chapter 39) including jaundice due to obstruction of the bile duct, coagulopathy due to lack of clotting factors, oedema as a result of impaired plasma protein production and lastly abnormal protein, fat and glucose metabolism (where hypoglycaemia is a significant problem). Management includes prevention of bleeding by **sclerosing** or banding varices, administration of vasopressors, and use of the **Sengstaken–Blakemore tube** for balloon tamponade. For recurrent bleeding the insertion of a trans-intrahepatic portosystemic shunt (TIPS) to reduce portal blood pressure may be required.

Acute pancreatitis

This is most commonly caused by gallstones (the close proximity of the gallbladder inflames the pancreas) or alcohol (secondary to GI irritation causing spasm). In both cases the pancreas autodigests. The powerful pancreatic enzymes (Chapter 39) leak into the tissue and become activated, breaking the organ down and affecting its normal functions (Chapter 39), causing inflammation, haemorrhage and necrosis. These toxic enzymes, together with inflammatory mediators, are then released into the blood initiating a severe systemic disorder, with multiple organ dysfunction. Diagnosis is made by biochemical analysis, abdominal ultrasound and CT scan. Endoscopic retrograde cholangio-pancreatogram (ERCP) may also be performed to look at the biliary and pancreatic ducts, but carries the risk of further inflaming the pancreas. Treatment includes suppression of pancreatic function, analgesia, countering the shock and inflammatory processes and maintenance of homeostasis.

Whatever the cause, the patient with GI dysfunction may become acutely unwell with an 'acute abdomen'. Assessment and recognition of problems is important to prevent deterioration and skilled care is required to promote recovery (Table 40.1).

41 Physiology of the renal system

Figure 41.1 (a, b) Anatomy of the urinary tract. Source: Peate I., *et al.*, 2014. Reproduced with permission of John Wiley & Sons.

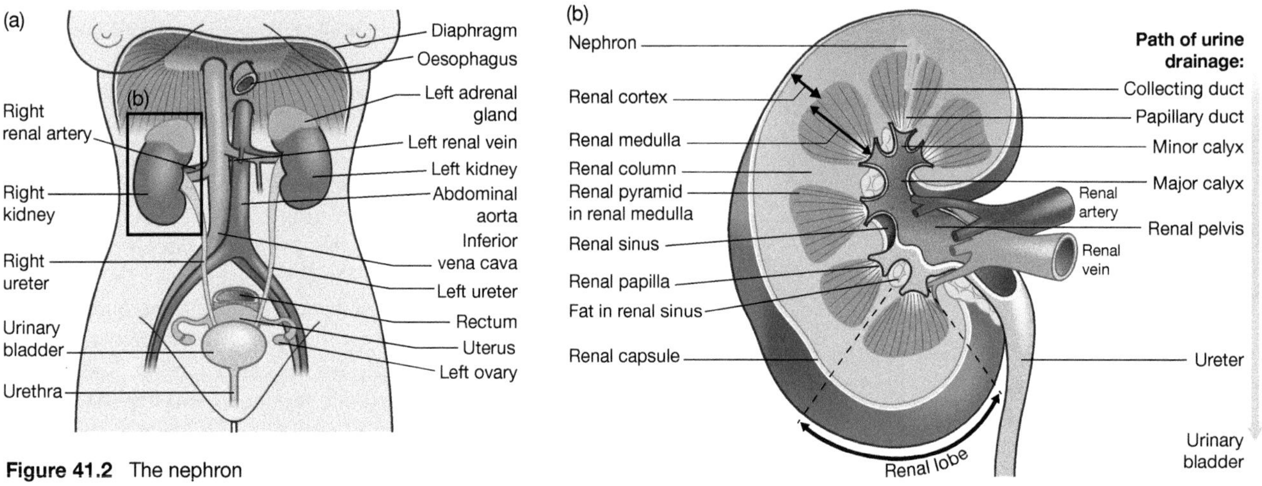

(a)
- Diaphragm
- Oesophagus
- Left adrenal gland
- Left renal vein
- Left kidney
- Abdominal aorta
- Inferior vena cava
- Left ureter
- Rectum
- Uterus
- Left ovary

- Right renal artery
- Right kidney
- Right ureter
- Urinary bladder
- Urethra

(b)
- Nephron
- Renal cortex
- Renal medulla
- Renal column
- Renal pyramid in renal medulla
- Renal sinus
- Renal papilla
- Fat in renal sinus
- Renal capsule

- Renal lobe

Path of urine drainage:
- Collecting duct
- Papillary duct
- Minor calyx
- Major calyx
- Renal artery
- Renal pelvis
- Renal vein
- Ureter
- Urinary bladder

Figure 41.2 The nephron

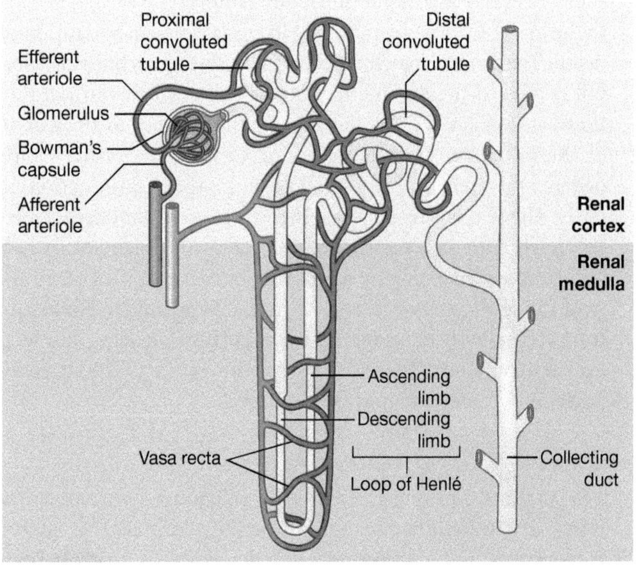

- Efferent arteriole
- Glomerulus
- Bowman's capsule
- Afferent arteriole
- Proximal convoluted tubule
- Distal convoluted tubule
- Ascending limb
- Descending limb
- Vasa recta
- Loop of Henlé
- Collecting duct
- **Renal cortex**
- **Renal medulla**

Figure 41.3 The glomerular filtration layer. Source: Peate I., *et al.*, 2014. Reproduced with permission of John Wiley & Sons.

- Basement membrane
- Capillary endothelium
- Capillary
- Foot processes of podocyte of glomerular capsule
- Plasma
- Filtrate in capsular space
- Fenestration
- Slit diaphragm
- Filtration slit

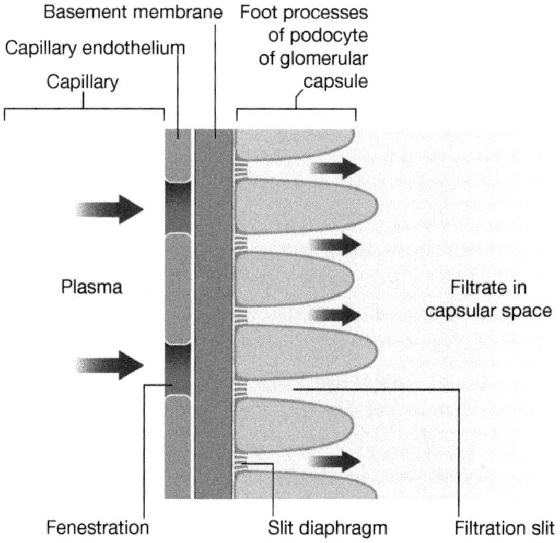

Figure 41.4 Tubular filtration, reabsorption and secretion

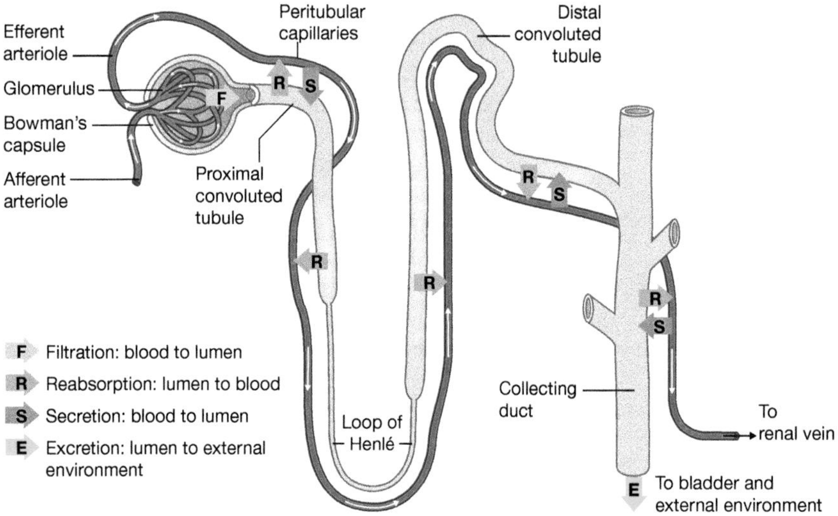

- Efferent arteriole
- Glomerulus
- Bowman's capsule
- Afferent arteriole
- Proximal convoluted tubule
- Peritubular capillaries
- Distal convoluted tubule
- Loop of Henlé
- Collecting duct
- To renal vein
- To bladder and external environment

- **F** Filtration: blood to lumen
- **R** Reabsorption: lumen to blood
- **S** Secretion: blood to lumen
- **E** Excretion: lumen to external environment

Figure 41.5 Normal urine

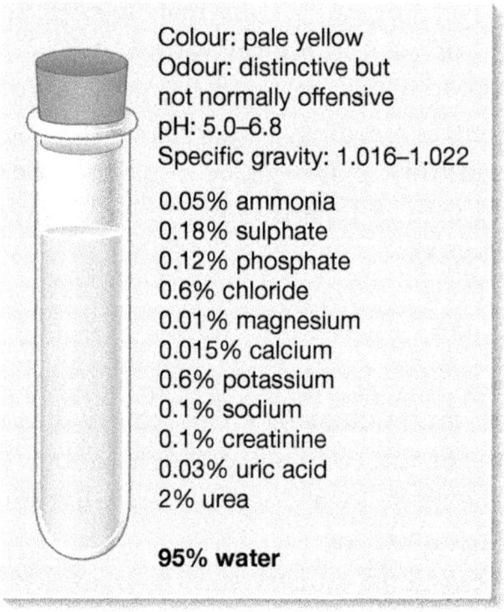

Colour: pale yellow
Odour: distinctive but not normally offensive
pH: 5.0–6.8
Specific gravity: 1.016–1.022

0.05% ammonia
0.18% sulphate
0.12% phosphate
0.6% chloride
0.01% magnesium
0.015% calcium
0.6% potassium
0.1% sodium
0.1% creatinine
0.03% uric acid
2% urea

95% water

Acute and Critical Care Nursing at a Glance, First Edition. Edited by Helen Dutton and Jacqui Finch
© 2018 John Wiley & Sons, Ltd. Published 2018 by John Wiley & Sons, Ltd.
Companion website: www.ataglanceseries.com/nursing/acutecare

Urinary tract

The kidney, ureters, bladder and urethra are structures of the renal system (Figure 41.1a). The kidneys, located either side of the vertebral column, are approximately 11 cm in length, 6 cm in width and 4 cm in depth. Each kidney has three layers: the renal fascia composed of connective tissue which attaches the kidney to the posterior abdominal wall, a covering of protective fat and a tough fibrous layer. The ureters, blood vessels, lymphatics and nerve supply enter and exit at the **hilum** of each kidney (Figure 41.1b). The ureters, composed of three layers (mucous, muscular and fibrous) convey urine by peristalsis from the collecting space at the top of each ureter (the renal pelvis) to the bladder. The bladder is an expandable, muscular collecting bag. Contraction is regulated by the parasympathetic nervous system and emptied by voluntary relaxation of the external sphincter muscle. The urethra, of varying length (short in the female and longer in the male) leads from the floor of the bladder or **trigone** to outside of the body. Voiding of urine takes place when about 300 mL has accumulated, with a minimum of 500 mL to about 1.5 L of urine formed in 24 h.

Functional unit: the nephron

There are approximately one million nephrons per kidney. Figure 41.2 shows the glomerulus, blood flow through the nephron, and the nephron structures. The **glomeruli** and parts of the renal tubules lie in the **renal cortex,** the outer section of the kidney (Figures 41.1b and 41.2). The inner vascular area called the **renal medulla** consists of the **loops of Henle,** the vasa recta (the network of blood vessels round the loop) and portions of the **collecting ducts.** It is in this medullary region that urine is effectively concentrated.

Applied physiology

The kidneys have a key role in maintaining homeostasis in the body and when renal function is impaired systemic effects are soon seen. Functions of the kidneys include:
- Excretion of waste products.
- Regulation of body fluids and electrolytes.
- Acid base (pH) balance.
- Hormone production:renin (the starting point of the RAAS) and erythopoietin for the production of red blood cells (or erythrocytes).

The production of urine and regulation of fluid and solute balance is achieved by filtration and tubular reabsorption and secretion.

Filtration

This process occurs in the glomerulus. Filtration occurs when fluid and the substances in it are forced through a membrane under pressure. In the kidney, the blood and all of its constituents are pushed by arterial pressure through the glomerulus and into the Bowman's capsule via the glomerular–capsular membrane. This consists of three layers (endothelial, basement membrane and podocyte)which collectively allow unwanted substances through the filter, whilst retaining essential body constituents such as blood cells and medium to large proteins such as albumin (Figure 41.3). These larger molecules are repelled by the negative electrical charge of the filtration membrane, and the pores in the filtration layers are too small for them to pass through. If protein is detected in the urine, this could be a sign of damage to the filtration membrane, possibly caused by infection. In contrast, smaller molecular weight substances such as urea, can pass easily though the membrane and into the filtrate. Successful filtration depends on adequate kidney perfusion and a healthy glomerulus, giving a normal **glomerular filtration rate (GFR)** of 105–125 mL/min.

Tubular reabsorption

A large volume of filtrate passes from the glomerulus to the Bowman's capsule and then to the **proximal convoluted tubule (PCT)**. Most of the reabsorption of solute occurs here, via active transport mechanisms using ATP (e.g. glucose) and the passive mechanisms, diffusion and osmosis: 65% of sodium, the major extracellular cation and 65% of potassium, the major intracellular cation, is reabsorbed here. Other electrolytes such as calcium, phosphate, glucose, amino acids and water are also partially or wholly reabsorbed in this section of the nephron (Figure 41.4). When the filtrate leaves the PCT, it is still quite dilute, but it progresses through the loop of Henle where concentration begins. The formation of osmolality gradients between the ascending and descending limbs assists this process. From here the filtrate will pass into the distal tubule and collecting duct where further refinements are made,with additional water reabsorption taking place under the influence of **vasopressin** (antidiuretic hormone). The constituents and characteristics of urine are shown in Figure 41.5. In health, normally about 1000–1500 mL of concentrated urine is produced per day.

Tubular secretion

Tubular secretion involves the movement of substances from the blood into the tubular fluid where they can be excreted (Figure 41.4). The distal and collecting tubules excrete potassium, hydrogen and ammonium ions. The release of the hormone **aldosterone** from the **adrenal cortex** leads to the reabsorption of sodium ions from the filtrate into the extracellular space and the excretion of potassium.

The kidneys regulate the body pH, helping to maintain the normal range of pH 7.35–7.45. Increasing numbers of hydrogen ions (H^+) increase acidity. Hydrogen ions (H^+) are transported out of the blood when blood H^+ increases and ammonium ions (NH_4^+) are secreted into tubule fluid from tubule cells. The kidneys excrete the 'fixed acids' produced by metabolic processes. The kidneys **'buffer'** strong acids or strong bases to produce either a weaker acid or a weaker base, so that less hydrogen ions are generated, thereby protecting the body from large swings in pH. The kidney has three buffering systems:
- Bicarbonate (extracellular and the main buffer).
- Proteins (intracellular).
- Phosphate (intracellular).

Buffering alone, however, cannot regulate the pH of the blood due to the constant generation of H^+ from cellular metabolism. The kidneys must therefore also secrete H^+. For every H^+ excreted, a sodium ion (Na^+) and a bicarbonate ion (HCO_3^-) will be reabsorbed. In summary, these processes regulate the blood pH and prevent harmful changes in acidity. The lungs also contribute to maintaining pH balance by excreting carbon dioxide (from carbonic acid), reducing hydrogen ions. Both systems work together to prevent a harmful change in pH.

42 Acute kidney injury

🚩

Risk factors in AKI
- Chronic renal disease
- History of AKI
- Existing cardiac or liver disease
- Existing neurological/cognitive impairment
- Diabetes
- History of urological obstruction
- Age > 65 years
- Increasing NEWS
- **Hypovolaemia**
- **Use of nephrotoxic drugs**
- **Sepsis**
- **Use of iodinated contrast media**

Table 42.1 Classification of AKI. Source: Bellomo R., et al., 2004.

RIFLE	Clinical measurements	AKIN	Clinical measurements
Risk	Increased creatinine × 1.5 GFR decreased > 25% Urine output < 0.5 mL/h/kg for 6 h	Stage 1	Increased creatinine × 1.5–2.0 from baseline Urine output < 0.5 mL/h/kg for 6 h
Injury	Increased creatinine × 2 GFR decreased > 50% Urine output < 0.5 mL/h/kg for 12 h	Stage 2	Increased creatinine × 2.0–3.0 from baseline Urine output < 0.5 mL/h/kg for 12 h
Failure	Increased creatinine × 3 GFR decreased > 75% Urine output < 0.3 mL/h/kg for 24 h or anuria for 12 h	Stage 3	Increased creatinine > 3.0 from baseline Urine output < 0.3 mL/h/kg for 24 h or anuria for 12 h
Loss	Loss of renal function for more than four weeks		
End stage	End-stage kidney disease		

Figure 42.1 Causes of AKI

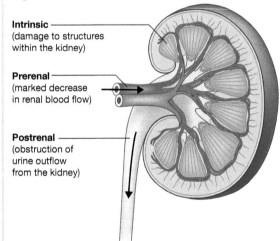

Intrinsic (damage to structures within the kidney)

Prerenal (marked decrease in renal blood flow)

Postrenal (obstruction of urine outflow from the kidney)

Normal serum ranges:
Urea: 2.5–6.6 mmol/L
Creatinine: 55–120 µmol/L

Box 42.1   KDIGO criteria for AKI.
Source: KDIGO, 2012.

- Increase in serum creatinine ≥ 26.5 µmol/L within 48 h
  OR
- Increase in serum creatinine to ≥ 1.5 times baseline occurring within the previous seven days
- Urine volume < 0.5 mL/kg/h for 6 h

Figure 42.2 Possible problems for patients with AKI

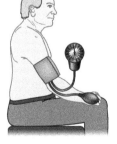

Elevated serum urea with risk of uraemic syndrome (seizure, coma, cardiac arrest)

Risk of pulmonary oedema, due to fluid retention

Risk of anaemia due to haemopoietic disturbance

Risk of cardiac arrhythmia due to rising level of K+ (> 6 mmol/L)

Risk of haemodynamic instability with fluid imbalance

Risk of peripheral oedema, due to fluid retention, and possibly protein loss

Potential haematuria and proteinuria

Abnormal serum and urinary sodium

Risk of metabolic acidosis

Box 42.2   Investigations

- Urinalysis
- Haematology and biochemistry
- Microscopy and culture
- Radiological investigation: ultrasound and angiography
- Renal biopsy

Acute and Critical Care Nursing at a Glance, First Edition. Edited by Helen Dutton and Jacqui Finch
© 2018 John Wiley & Sons, Ltd. Published 2018 by John Wiley & Sons, Ltd.
Companion website: www.ataglanceseries.com/nursing/acutecare

Risk factors for acute kidney injury

Acute kidney injury (AKI), is characterised by a sudden, but sometimes reversible, disruption to renal function. The 2009 NCEPOD report noted an incidence of AKI in 13–19% of people admitted to hospital, especially in older patients.[1] All patients admitted to hospital as an emergency, regardless of clinical condition, require: assessment for renal dysfunction risk factors, electrolyte monitoring, track and trigger scoring of physiological parameters and consultant review within 12 h of admission. Prevention, detection and optimal management of patients at risk of acute kidney injury is essential.[2] Acute care nurses need to understand the signs and of risk factors associated with AKI (see red flag box) as these are exacerbated by late recognition and, inappropriate or delayed treatment. Normally around 1L to 2L of urine is produced in 24 h. A minimum of 0.5–1 mL/kg/h is required to indicate good renal perfusion and function with, for example, a person weighing 70 kg, producing between 35 and 70 mL/h of urine.

Definition of acute kidney injury

AKI is defined as low urine output (oliguria) accompanied by rising serum creatinine. For normal ranges see illustration page opposite. The severity of AKI is dependent on the duration of the problem and degree to which abnormal biochemistry is evident. The RIFLE and the AKIN criteria (Table 42.1) describe levels of renal impairment,[3,4] whilst the KDIGO criteria (Box 42.1) refines the staging by highlighting more specific time frames.[5] Causes of AKI fall into three categories: prerenal, intrinsic and postrenal (Figure 42.1).

Pathophysiology and clinical presentation

Prerenal or 'volume responsive'

In acute illness, the cause of AKI may be a result of a prerenal problem. Loss of circulating volume or reduced perfusion secondary to cardiac problems, or renovascular disorders, could cause a prerenal problem. In these circumstances, urine output is reduced due to the combined effects of sympathetic nervous system activation and the RAAS. This leads to vasoconstriction with water and electrolyte conservation, in an attempt to restore the circulating volume. In a prerenal presentation the kidneys are able to conserve and concentrate urine. Serum sodium and potassium may rise and acidosis may occur due to metabolic derangement, but there is no actual damage to the nephrons. Urine produced is unlikely to contain any abnormalities, even though it will be concentrated with a high specific gravity. As the name implies, this form of renal dysfunction normally responds well to careful fluid resuscitation. When the kidneys remain poorly perfused, however, prolonged ischaemia can lead to permanent damage to the nephrons.

Intrinsic kidney injury

Intrinsic damage to the kidney often occurs with severe renal hypoperfusion, but also with other disorders including:
- Renal disease such as a glomerular infection.
- Systemic disease such as sickle cell.
- Nephrotoxicity: with NSAIDs (e.g. ibuprofen), or aminoglycoside antibiotics (e.g. gentamycin).

In response to these insults an inflammatory process is initiated that can lead to **acute tubular necrosis** (death of tissue in the renal tubules), shedding of tubular cells and blockage of the tubular lumen. Casts appear in the urine and urinalysis may reveal haematuria or proteinuria. The kidney loses the ability to concentrate urine, evident by an increased urinary sodium loss. Electrolyte, fluid and pH imbalance occurs, risking heart rhythm and breathing problems. Renal failure causes **uraemia**, with increased risk of blood disorders, **encephalopathy**, gastrointestinal disturbance and **pericarditis**.

Postrenal impairment

Caused by an obstruction anywhere in the renal tract below the kidneys, this leads to increased pressure in the glomerulus with the formation of **hydronephrosis**. Urine starts to back up in the ureters, pelvises and calyces, causing dilatation and damage to the nephrons. As this process continues, serum and urinary biochemistry indicate actual damage to renal parenchyma, as with intrinsic renal damage.

Principles of nursing management

Patients with AKI, whatever the cause, require close monitoring with timely care escalation. NEWS does not trigger on low urine output, but the lack of trigger point should not prevent concern being raised. If renal dysfunction is suspected, specific investigations (Box 42.2) enable the exact nature and extent of the problem to be determined. Clinical deterioration is a risk (Figure 42.2), so excellent nursing care and management is required. This includes:
- Awareness of risk factors for AKI.
- **Recognition and reporting of oliguria, or a urine output <0.5 mL/kg/h.**
- Knowledge of normal serum ranges of urea and creatinine.
- Awareness and cessation of nephrotoxic drugs, plus therapeutic drug dosing for altered kinetics in renal impairment.
- **Breathing.** Monitoring SpO_2, respiratory rate and effort of breathing. Respiratory function may deteriorate owing to pulmonary oedema occurring secondary to fluid overload.
- Recognition and reporting of changes in circulatory status that may lead to prerenal AKI, or cause intrinsic renal failure.
- Close monitoring of **circulatory** status, including urine output and accurate recording of fluid balance. Risks associated with IV fluids and diuretic therapy must be understood. In general diuretics should be avoided in AKI.
- Knowledge of normal serum K^+ range and other blood results, commencing continuous cardiac monitoring if there is a risk of cardiac arrhythmias. Administering therapy to lower serum potassium as prescribed.
- Individual assessment is required by a dietician of patients' nutritional needs, with the aim of providing 25–35 kcal/kg/day.

Patients with ongoing AKI, failing to respond to initial therapy, may require additional monitoring and support in level 2 or 3 care. The **airway** may be compromised due to changes in neurological status caused by encephalopathy. **Breathing** interventions such as oxygen therapy or additional support may be required. Additional **cardiovascular** support with the administration of vasopressor and inotropic therapy to increase cardiac output and renal perfusion, if volume resuscitation has failed to do so, may be necessary. Timely referral to a consultant renal physician for specialist management, such as dialysis or possibly haemofiltration in a higher level of care, may be required.

43 Burns: immediate care

Figure 43.1 Lund and Browder chart. Source: Hettiaratchy S. and Papini R., 2004. Reproduced with permission of BMJ Publishing Ltd.

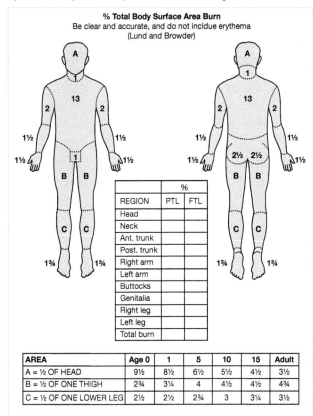

% Total Body Surface Area Burn
Be clear and accurate, and do not incldue erythema
(Lund and Browder)

REGION	%	
	PTL	FTL
Head		
Neck		
Ant. trunk		
Post. trunk		
Right arm		
Left arm		
Buttocks		
Genitalia		
Right leg		
Left leg		
Total burn		

AREA	Age 0	1	5	10	15	Adult
A = ½ OF HEAD	9½	8½	6½	5½	4½	3½
B = ½ OF ONE THIGH	2¾	3¼	4	4½	4½	4¾
C = ½ OF ONE LOWER LEG	2½	2½	2¾	3	3¼	3½

Figure 43.2 Palmer method. Patient's palm, fingers closed = 1% total body surface area (TBSA)

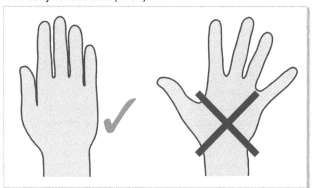

Table 43.1 Burn depths

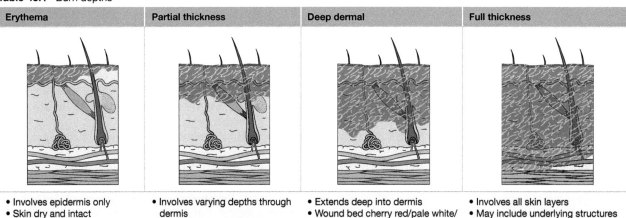

Erythema	Partial thickness	Deep dermal	Full thickness
• Involves epidermis only • Skin dry and intact • No blisters • Hyperemic → erythema • Rapid blanching • Very painful	• Involves varying depths through dermis • Skin integrity damaged → blisters present/have been present • Wound bed pink/red/mottled/speckled • Moist with moderate exudate • Brisk capillary refill • Very painful • Sensitive to air and temperature	• Extends deep into dermis • Wound bed cherry red/pale white/creamy • Staining/speckling of coagulated blood vessels • Drier appearance • Hairs pull out easily • Diminished capillary refill → sluggish/no blanching • Reduced sensation → sensitive to deep pressure but not pinprick	• Involves all skin layers • May include underlying structures • Wound bed white/cream/black/brown/waxy/leathery appearance • Usually painless

Acute and Critical Care Nursing at a Glance, First Edition. Edited by Helen Dutton and Jacqui Finch
© 2018 John Wiley & Sons, Ltd. Published 2018 by John Wiley & Sons, Ltd.
Companion website: www.ataglanceseries.com/nursing/acutecare

Introduction

Burn injuries are a unique form of trauma and even small burns may present as a challenge to most healthcare professionals due to the complex physical and psychological changes that can occur. In the UK approximately 175 000 people attend accident and emergency departments every year with burns and around 13 000 of these will require admission. The management of the majority of these injuries are by healthcare professionals outside the burns speciality. An accurate assessment of the burn-injured patient is paramount to ensure timely and effective treatment. For those patients who have sustained a major burn injury, trauma management guidelines apply (Chapter 44). However, further specific considerations for burn injuries also need to be recognised and managed accordingly.

First aid

All burn injuries seen within the first 3 h of injury should be given appropriate first aid to significantly reduce pain and oedema, and decrease the inflammatory response. This reduces the amount of fluid resuscitation required and improves the speed of wound healing, thus reducing burn scarring. This consists of:

- **Stopping the burning process:**
  - Removing hot clothing/putting out flames/irrigating chemicals.
- **Cooling the burn wound:**
  - Irrigate under cool running water for 20 min.
  - Difficult areas to irrigate, use cold wet towel/gauze.
  - Do not use ice or ice water.

Burns first aid focuses on cooling the burn wound, but due to the risk of hypothermia you must also keep the patient warm. Use clean, dry blankets, warmed humidified oxygen and a warm air-heating blanket. Remember, cool the wound; warm the patient.

Airway

It is essential to identify the difference between an airway- and breathing-related inhalation injury, as the management is significantly different. For an airway injury look for:

- Visible full thickness burns to the face or neck.
- A change in the voice/cry or hoarseness.
- Erythema or oedema to the tongue or uvula.
- Later signs may include dyspnoea, tachypnoea or stridor.

These must be treated prophylactically with airway protection, oxygenation and treatment of bronchospasm. If in doubt, intubate, but do not cut the endotracheal tube.

Breathing

A patient may encounter breathing-related inhalation injuries from inhalation of soot, inhalation of toxic substances (most commonly carbon monoxide), circumferential burns to the chest that restrict chest expansion or steam inhalation that damages the lower airway. Signs and symptoms include burns or soot in the mouth, nose or pharynx, singed nasal hairs or soot in the sputum, altered level of consciousness, dyspnoea or tachypnoea. Significantly, signs and symptoms may initially be absent; therefore, a history of entrapment in an enclosed space or an explosion at the scene should raise a high index of suspicion for potential inhalation injury. These patients should be monitored and treated expectantly, according to their symptoms. Oxygen (10–15 L) should be administered via a non-rebreathe oxygen mask.

Circulation

Intravenous access should be gained, preferably through unburnt skin. Patients who have sustained a burn of >15% total body surface area (TBSA) require intravenous fluid resuscitation. Patients should be given warmed crystalloids using the Parkland formula[1] which is used to calculate the fluid requirements from the time of injury.

Parkland formula for calculating intravenous fluids in burns 2–4 mL crystalloids × kg × %TBSA (over 24 h):

- Half in the first 8 h (from time of injury)
- The remainder over the next 16 h

The formula is a guide for fluid resuscitation and therefore it is essential to monitor urine output to establish its effectiveness. Patients with burns >20% TBSA should be catheterised and a minimum urine output of 0.5 mL/kg/h should be maintained.

Burn wound assessment

The area and depth of the burn will indicate the severity of the wound. The area is described as the percent of total body surface area burnt (%TBSA). The most commonly recognised method of assessing the %TBSA is the rule of nines which divides the body's surface area into multiples of nine to allow for a quick estimation of the size of the burn. For this reason, it is predominantly used in the prehospital environment. The Lund and Browder Chart (Figure 43.1) should be used in the hospital environment.[1] It is more detailed, with specific percentages that remain the same regardless of the age of the patient, as well as lettered areas that are calculated, using the incorporated table, according to their age. For smaller burns the palmer method (Figure 43.2) may be used. The patient's palm and fingers, with fingers closed, equates roughly to 1% TBSA.

The depth of the burn is divided into four categories: erythema, superficial partial thickness, deep dermal and full thickness (Table 43.1). Erythema is not included in TBSA calculation and can be managed with soothing moisturisers if required. If blisters are present or develop, the blistered area is then calculated as a partial thickness burn. Partial thickness burns should be cleaned and dressed with a non-adhesive contact layer, an absorbable secondary dressing and secured. The dressing should be changed every 2–3 days or if the dressing becomes wet, peels or falls off or there are signs of infection. Any deep dermal or full thickness burn should be discussed with and referred to the local burns unit.

Burns referral

Nationally, the criteria for referring patients to local burns services vary. It is important to check the local guidelines local guidelines. In general, burns that meet the following criteria should be considered for referral: >2% TBSA, deep dermal or full thickness, special areas such as face, hands, feet, genitals or major joints, electrical or chemical burns, circumferential to limbs, trunk or neck, burns with inhalation injury and those not healed within 2 weeks.

44 Major trauma

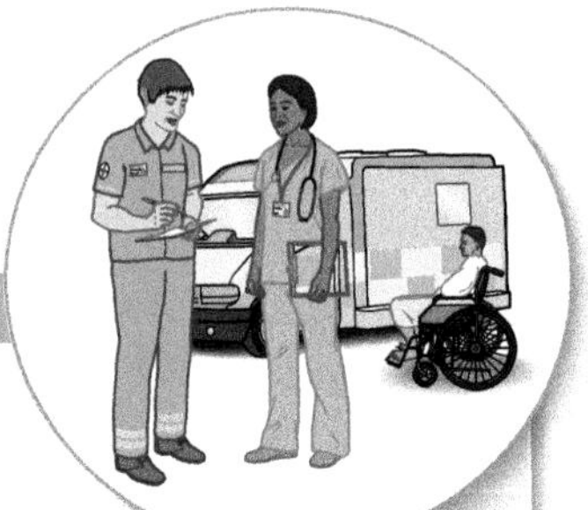

Table 44.1 NATMIST handover

		Example
N	Name	"This is Tom Lee"
A	Age	"He is 29 years old"
T	Time of injury	"Injuries sustained at 10:30 hours"
M	Mechanism of injury	"He was the restrained driver in a car-versus-car head-on, road traffic collision travelling at 40 miles per hour. He self-extricated"
I	Injuries sustained	"He has a suspected open fracture to his right tibia/fibia and a 5 cm laceration to his forehead. No other complaints of pain"
S	Signs and symptoms	"Airway is patent, no loss of consciousness. His oxygen saturations are 99% on 15 L of oxygen via a non-rebreathe facemask. His blood pressure is 120/80, heart rate 90, respiration rate 18, temperature 36.9°C, He has full sensation and movement of all limbs and strong peripheral pulses"
T	Treatments given	"I have placed a sterile dressing to the head laceration. I have cannulated his right arm and given 5 mg of intravenous morphine. I have splinted his leg with a box splint. Any questions?"

Box 44.1 AMPLE history

A	Allergies
M	Medications
P	Past medical history
L	Last ate and drank
E	Events leading

Box 44.2 Full spinal immobilisation

- Tailor the approach to each individual patient Use spinal immobilisation devices with caution in patients who are:
  - uncooperative
  - agitated
  - distressed
  - children
- It may be better to allow them to find a position in which they are comfortable
- Fit a semirigid collar correctly sized for the patient. Unless:
  - has a compromised airway
  - known spinal deformities (e.g. ankylosing spondylitis)
- Reassess the airway post collar application
- Place patient on a scoop stretcher or vacuum mattress
- Secure head with head blocks and tape

Table 44.2 Spinal injury risk factors. Source: NICE, 2016, NG41.

In general	Full in-line spinal immobilisation if...	A patient is at high risk of spinal injury if...	A patient is at low risk of spinal injury if...	Do not immobilise the cervical spine if:
Protect the whole spine with manual in-line immobilisation (MILS) and restrictive movement at all times	• Distracting injuries • Under the influence of drink or drugs • Confused or uncooperative • Reduced level of consciousness • Spinal pain • Hand or foot weakness • Altered or absent sensation in the hands or feet • Priapism • History of spinal problems including surgery or spinal conditions	They have one of the following factors: • They are over 65 years of age • Fall from > 1 m or five steps • Fall onto head • Paresthesia in upper or lower limbs	They have one of the following factors: • Involved in a minor rear-end motor vehicle collision • Comfortable in seated position • Been ambulatory since time of injury • No midline cervical spine tenderness • Delayed onset neck pain **AND** • Unable to actively rotate neck 45° to the left and right	They have low risk factors: • Are pain free • Can rotate neck 45° left and right

Figure 44.1 ATOM-FC mnemonic

A T O M F C

Airway
Audible bubbling, gurgling, wheeze, stridor or snoring
Treat: airway manoeuvres (Chapters 8, 9) May need surgical airway (Chapter 10)

Tension pneumothorax
Air under pressure in the pleural space following injury
Signs: respiratory distress, distended neck veins, reduced breath sounds, increased resonance, deviated trachea, hypotension
Treat: open thoracotomy followed by chest drain insertion (Chapter 36)

Open pneumothorax
A large open chest wound and collapsed underlying lung
Signs: absent or reduced breath sounds, respiratory distress, surgical emphysema, wound
Treat: cover with occlusive dressing and observe for signs of tension pneumothorax

Massive haemothorax
Large volume of blood in the lung
Signs: shock, reduced/absent air entry, dull percussion
Treat: large bore IV access, fluid and chest drain

Flail chest
Two or more ribs broken in two or more places.
Signs: paradoxical chest movement, pain, increased breathing rate
Treat: epidural or nerve block. Close monitoring for worsening respiratory function. Intubation and ventilation may be required

Cardiac tamponade
Blood in the pericardium constricting the heart's action
Signs: shock (HR↑ BP↓ RR↑), distended neck veins. Ultrasound may identify pericardial fluid
Treat: depends on clinical status but may require urgent thoracotomy (Chapter 36)

Acute and Critical Care Nursing at a Glance, First Edition. Edited by Helen Dutton and Jacqui Finch
© 2018 John Wiley & Sons, Ltd. Published 2018 by John Wiley & Sons, Ltd.
Companion website: www.ataglanceseries.com/nursing/acutecare

Major trauma is a leading cause of death and disability in all age groups worldwide. It is categorised by its mechanism into blunt (e.g. falls, road traffic collisions) or penetrating injury (stabbings, shootings). Initial management utilises the ABCDE approach to identify and treat life-threatening injuries, active haemorrhage, shock and coagulopathy. Guidelines for trauma management have been issued by NICE (2016)[1,2]

Communication

Practitioners should elicit a NATMIST (Table 44.1) and AMPLE handover[3] (Box 44.1) from prehospital emergency services, witnesses and/or relatives as soon as possible after hospital admission.

Catastrophic haemorrhage

Haemorrhage causes 40% of trauma-related deaths. Rapid control of catastrophic haemorrhage is the immediate priority in trauma and can be achieved quickly by applying dressings, direct pressure and elevating the wound. Tourniquets and haemostatic dressings may be used if simple measures fail to stop bleeding. A pelvic binder should be applied to patients with suspected pelvic fracture with signs of shock.

Assessment and management

Airway with inline spinal immobilisation

Cervical spine injury occurs in 2% of trauma patients and should be assumed in patients with significant risk factors (Table 44.2). Manual inline stabilisation (MILS) should be used to immobilise the spine in these patients (Box 44.2). The patency of the airway should be established and maintained using basic and advanced airway manoeuvres (Chapters 8 and 9). The presence of vomit, blood in the mouth, neck wounds, neck swelling, facial fractures, stridor, gurgling or altered level of consciousness should alert the practitioner to potential airway compromise. Due to the risk of hypoxia, high-flow oxygen (10–15 L/min) should be administered to all self-ventilating patients via a non-rebreathe facemask, with assessment at regular intervals.

Breathing

Identification of life-threatening injuries begins with examination of the neck and chest for deformities, bruises, wounds, unequal movement and surgical emphysema in addition to normal breathing assessment (Chapter 13). The six life-threatening thoracic injuries can be remembered using the mnemonic ATOM-FC[4] (Figure 44.1). Specialist teams may use ultrasound to augment physical assessment to confirm diagnosis of thoracic injury. Practitioners should note that ultrasound may identify but not exclude injury. A CXR or ultrasound scan should be considered in respiratory compromise as part of the immediate assessment. Patients considered to be stable, responding to treatment and in the absence of severe respiratory distress should be considered suitable for CT scan to identify injuries.

Circulation

Haemorrhagic shock is a failure of oxygen delivery to the tissues resulting in ischaemia and cell death as a consequence of acute blood loss. Blood loss can occur internally or externally and assessment should focus on identifying unrecognised or inadequately controlled bleeding. Blood loss can occur in the chest, retroperitoneum, abdomen, long bones, and the pelvis. Practitioners should regularly assess and document vital signs to identify patient deterioration or improvement, making the team immediately aware of any changes in status. The patient who is unstable, fails to respond to treatment or rapidly deteriorates should be transferred for immediate surgery to control haemorrhage. The adequacy and need for tourniquets should be reassessed and if not required removed to prevent neurovascular injury. If bleeding has not stopped then they should remain in place until surgical control of the bleeding has been achieved. Peripheral intravenous access should be established to facilitate fluid replacement and blood samples. If peripheral access is unsuccessful then intraosseous or central venous access should be achieved. Blood (25 mL) is required for: blood type, full crossmatch, full blood count, urea, electrolytes, clotting screen, glucose, venous blood gas for lactate and venous oxygen levels.

Lethal triad

Serious injury can lead to the development of the lethal triad: coagulopathy, acidosis and hypothermia. In the cold, acidotic patient, blood clotting is impaired (coagulopathy). Coagulopathy also develops in response to severe tissue injury and shock. If left untreated hypoperfusion, ischaemia, organ dysfunction, multiple organ failure and death ensues.

Volume resuscitation

Volume resuscitation should restore and maintain perfusion of the vital organs. In patients who are bleeding, fluid resuscitation should be titrated to ensure a palpable radial pulse using crystalloids. Blood transfusion using a fixed ratio of 1 unit of red blood cells and 1 unit of plasma should be commenced in accordance with the hospital's haemorrhage protocol and continued until physiologically stable. Fluids should be warmed to treat hypothermia. Intravenous tranexamic acid, a haemostatic agent that inhibits blood clot breakdown, should be administered in patients with suspected or active bleeding. The first dose should be administered as soon as possible but not more than 3 h after initial injury.

Dysfunction of the central nervous system

Check and record the Glasgow Coma Scale (GCS) and pupil response (Chapter 47). Pain should be assessed, recorded and managed (Chapter 5).

Exposure and environment

The environment should be warm enough to maintain normal body temperature. The patient should be fully undressed to allow a full head-to-toe assessment and detailed examination. Three blankets, one over the thorax, one over the midriff and one over the legs, allows progressive exposure and assessment whilst maintaining dignity. Patients who are hypothermic should be actively warmed.

If wound contamination is suspected, intravenous antibiotics may be administered in accordance with hospital guidelines.

Fractures

The orthopaedic team should review fractures as soon as possible. Limbs should be frequently assessed for pulses, movement and sensation. Traction or splinting should be applied and the limb elevated where possible. Open fractures should be covered with a saline-soaked dressing and prophylactic antibiotics given within 1 h of injury.

Ongoing care

After assessment the trauma team leader should have an impression of injuries sustained and a plan of ongoing care. The patient may need an interhospital transfer to a major trauma centre, or an intrahospital transfer to operating theatres, the ICU, the trauma or observation ward.

45 Resuscitation

Figure 45.1 Overview of incidence and outcome of cardiac arrest from the UK National Cardiac Arrest Audit (2011–13). Source: Nolan J., *et al.*, 2014. Reproduced with permission of Elsevier.

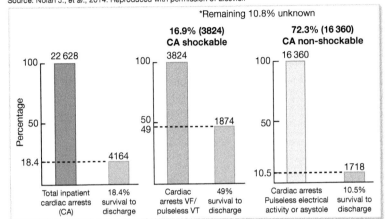

*Remaining 10.8% unknown

16.9% (3824) CA shockable

72.3% (16 360) CA non-shockable

Figure 45.2 In-hospital resuscitation. Source: RCUK, 2015. Reproduced with permission.

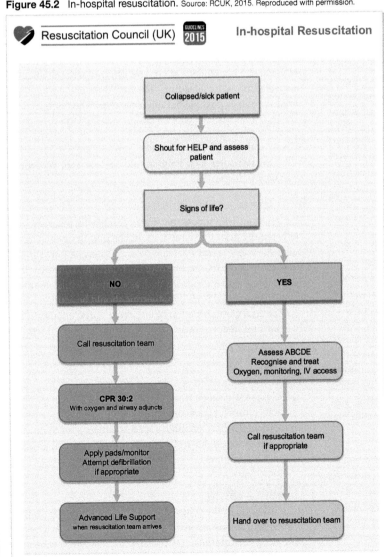

Resuscitation Council (UK) GUIDELINES 2015 **In-hospital Resuscitation**

Collapsed/sick patient

Shout for HELP and assess patient

Signs of life?

NO — Call resuscitation team → CPR 30:2 With oxygen and airway adjuncts → Apply pads/monitor Attempt defibrillation if appropriate → Advanced Life Support when resuscitation team arrives

YES — Assess ABCDE Recognise and treat Oxygen, monitoring, IV access → Call resuscitation team if appropriate → Hand over to resuscitation team

Figure 45.3 (a) Chest compressions should start as soon as possible.
(b) Use airway adjuncts and oxygen as soon as they are available.
(c) Continue with chest compressions whilst defibrillator pads are positioned

(a)

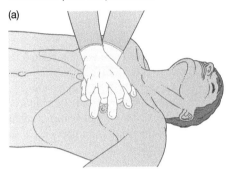

(b)

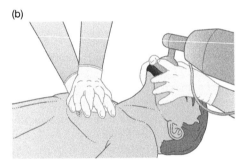

(c)

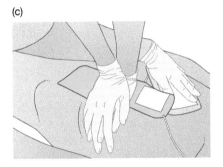

Figure 45.4 Shockable and non-shockable rhythms, and reversible causes of cardiac arrest. Source: RCUK, 2015. Reproduced with permission.

Shockable rhythms VF/pulseless VT	Non-shockable rhythms PEA/Asystole
Four Hs: • Hypoxia • Hypovolaemia • Hypo/hyperkalaemia/ metabolic • Hypothermia	Four Ts: • Thrombosis, coronary or pulmonary • Tension pneumothorax • Tamponade – cardiac • Toxins

Figure 45.5 Advanced life support algorithm. Source: RCUK, 2015.
Please see Appendix.

Acute and Critical Care Nursing at a Glance, First Edition. Edited by Helen Dutton and Jacqui Finch
© 2018 John Wiley & Sons, Ltd. Published 2018 by John Wiley & Sons, Ltd.
Companion website: www.ataglanceseries.com/nursing/acutecare

Preventing cardiopulmonary arrest

Previous chapters have discussed physiological problems leading to patient deterioration. Cardiac arrest (CA) rarely happens 'out of the blue', with about 80% of patients showing signs of clinical deterioration before collapse. Acute care tools that help detect deterioration, such as the NEWS[1], supports nurses in their assessment and recognition of those who are most at risk. Nurses may also intuitively feel that their patient is unwell, noticing small changes in behaviour such as agitation, subtle changes in respiratory and cardiovascular status, and/or peripheral circulations, alteration in mentation, and an increase in patient pain and anxiety.[2] These signs are important elements of patient assessment, and any cause for concern should prompt care escalation. Response to deterioration needs to be timely and appropriate with support from teams such as the CCOT probably reducing adverse events such as CA, ICU admissions and increasing survival.[3] Incidence and survival rates for CA are shown in Figure 45.2. The low survival to discharge(18.4%) emphasises the need to prevent CA occurring.

Resuscitation guidelines

The Resuscitation Council UK (RCUK) update and publish guidelines every 5 years, available from https://www.resus.org.uk. Practitioners need to keep regularly updated and practice skills of cardiopulmonary resuscitation (CPR), details of which are fully outlined by RCUK.[3] When CA occurs, four key priorities called the 'chain of survival' increase the chances of a successful outcome. These consist of:

- Early recognition and call for help.
- Early CPR to buy time.
- Early defibrillation, to restart the heart.
- Good postresuscitation care.

The **in-hospital resuscitation algorithm** is shown in Figure 45.1:

- Practitioner safety is a primary consideration: check area for danger and don protective clothing when possible.
- On approaching a collapsed patient call for help whilst you begin your assessment. Try and rouse the patient by shouting their name, and gently shaking their shoulders.
- If there are **no signs of life, call the resuscitation team on the universal UK arrest number 2222,** clearly stating hospital ward and location, or **ensure that the call is/has been made.**
- **Commence chest compressions** at a rate of 100–120/min (Figure 45.3a), using airway adjuncts and oxygen as they become available (Figure 45.3b) giving two breaths to every 30 cardiac compressions.
- Apply pads for the automatic external defibrillator, minimising compression interruptions (Figure 45.3c). **Defibrillation** is attempted if appropriate, or continue CPR until the team arrives.

The **Adult Advanced Life support (ALS) algorithm** guides the team in patient management. **Early defibrillation** for shockable rhythms (VF and pulseless VT, see Chapter 31 Figure 31.2 a&b) is associated with increased survival.[3] The nurse will support the team as the ALS algorithm is followed see Appendix Figure 45.5. This may involve activities such as continuing cardiac compressions, assisting the anaesthetist with airway management, checking and recording of emergency drugs, or making the patient's notes available to the resuscitation team. Any **reversible causes** of CA need to be identified and treated promptly (Figures 45.4 and 45.5). Extra equipment such as chest drains or intravenous fluids may be required. The nurse also has a key role in supporting relatives, whether they are present at the arrest, or waiting away from the clinical area.

Postresuscitation care commences on return of spontaneous circulation (ROSC), and urgent transfer to a level 3 unit is required. Physiological parameters are optimised to maximise recovery, often requiring multiorgan support. The quality of care at this stage significantly influences outcome, particularly for neurological recovery. With good care 40–50% of patients who are not conscious when transferred to ICU post CA, survive to hospital discharge, many with only minor cognitive impairment.[3]

Unfortunately, many who suffer CA will not survive. The senior doctor present has the legal responsibility for the decision to stop treatment, taking into account the views of the team. A team debrief allow worries to be expressed and constructive feedback for the team.

Presence of relatives

It has been increasingly common for family to be present during resuscitation activities. This is not without controversy and has stimulated worldwide debate. In recent years American and European guidelines have advocated giving family members the opportunity to be present,[4] but there is a lack of established policies.[5] Benefits of family presence include:

- An increased understanding by the family of the patient's condition, helping them to come to terms with the death, enabling a healthier bereavement process.
- The chance to speak to and touch their loved one for the last time;many relatives feel presence with their love done is important.
- They can see that everything possible to be done, was done.

Staff attitudes vary, but studies indicate that nurses may have a higher level of support for family presence than physicians. Disadvantages of family presence include:

- Watching the resuscitation event could be stressful and traumatic, especially without adequate staff support.
- Their presence may affect staff performance, as anxiety increases with the feeling of being watched.
- Families' misinterpretation of events may cause further stress.

Many healthcare practitioners support the presence of family at the end of life, perceiving it to be normal and desirable. It then seems natural to include relatives in an event that is likely to result in their loved one's death. Support through the process is essential. Principles to help guide healthcare professionals[6] through this emotive situation include:

- Make clear that the choice to stay or go is entirely theirs.
- Acknowledge that this is stressful and difficult.
- Try and be with the relatives whatever their decision.
- Give clear and simple explanations throughout.
- Offer them the chance to touch the patient when possible.
- Be honest in your answers; it is OK to say that you are not able to answer questions such as 'Will he live?' or 'Will she have brain damage?', but that you will keep them informed at all stages.

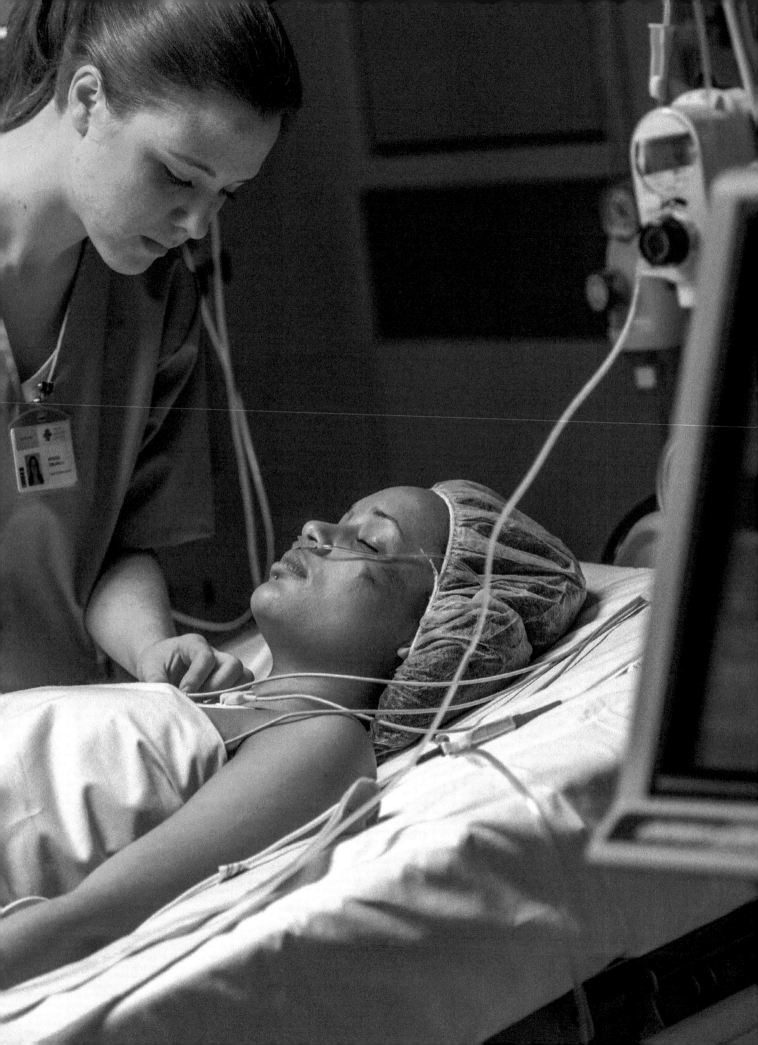

Disability: patients with neurological impairment

Part 5

Chapters

46 Physiology of the brain   100
47 Neurological assessment   102
48 Neurological impairment   104
49 Drug overdose and poisoning   106
50 Acute endocrine problems   108

46 Physiology of the brain

Figure 46.1 Major divisions of the brain. Source: Peate I., *et al.*, 2014. Reproduced with permission of John Wiley & Sons.

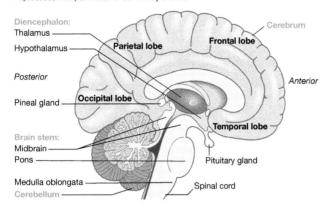

Diencephalon:
Thalamus
Hypothalamus
Parietal lobe
Frontal lobe
Cerebrum
Posterior
Anterior
Pineal gland
Occipital lobe
Temporal lobe
Brain stem:
Midbrain
Pons
Pituitary gland
Medulla oblongata
Spinal cord
Cerebellum

Figure 46.3 Cranial nerves. Source: Peate I., *et al.*, 2014. Reproduced with permission of John Wiley & Sons.

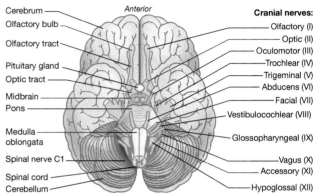

Cerebrum
Olfactory bulb
Olfactory tract
Pituitary gland
Optic tract
Midbrain
Pons
Medulla oblongata
Spinal nerve C1
Spinal cord
Cerebellum
Anterior
Posterior

Cranial nerves:
Olfactory (I)
Optic (II)
Oculomotor (III)
Trochlear (IV)
Trigeminal (V)
Abducens (VI)
Facial (VII)
Vestibulocochlear (VIII)
Glossopharyngeal (IX)
Vagus (X)
Accessory (XI)
Hypoglossal (XII)

Diencephalon
This lies between the cerebrum and the midbrain and consists of two key sections, the **thalamus** and **hypothalamus**. The thalamus is responsible for recognising sensations (pain, temperature and touch), emotional response to unpleasant stimuli, arousal or alertness and complex reflex movements. The hypothalamus has many functions, including control of autonomic activity, hormone production, sleep regulation, appetite and maintenance of body temperature.

Cerebrum
The surface of this structure is the **cerebral cortex** and it is divided into two halves, the right and left hemispheres, connected by the white matter of the corpus callosum. Each hemisphere is further partitioned into five lobes: frontal, parietal, temporal, occipital and insula. These different sections of the cerebrum have many functions and these include motor and sensory activity, language, memory and, in conjunction with the Reticular Activating Centre in the brain stem, the control of consciousness.

Brain stem
This consists of the medulla, the midbrain and the pons. Essential sensory, motor and reflex activity occurs here. In the **medulla**, nuclei regulate respiratory, cardiac and vasomotor activity, as well as non-vital reflexes such as vomiting and coughing. In the **midbrain** there are reflex centres for the 3rd and 4th cranial nerves. Similarly in the **pons** there are reflex centres for the 5th, 6th, 7th and 8th cranial nerves as well as the pneumotaxic centre which assists with respiratory control.

Cerebellum
This centre together with the cerebral cortex controls coordinated muscle movement. This area is also responsible for controlling balance and posture.

Figure 46.2 Spinal nerves

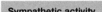

Cervical nerves
C1
C2
C3
C4
C5
C6
C7
C8
Thoracic nerves
T1
T2
T3
T4
T5
T6
T7
T8
T9
T10
T11
T12
Lumbar nerves
L1
L2
L3
L4
L5
Sacral/coccygeal nerves
S1
S2
S3
S4
S5
Coccygeal nerve
Conus medullaris
Cauda equina

Table 46.1 Autonomic nervous system

Sympathetic activity	Parasympathetic activity
• Dilates airways, increases rate and depth of respiration • Increases heart rate and myocardial contractility • Dilatation (beta effect) and constriction (alpha effect) of coronary blood vessels • Dilatation of skeletal muscle • Constriction of blood vessels in digestive tract with decreased peristalsis, decreased pancreatic secretion • Increased glycogenolysis • Bladder relaxation • Pupil dilatation	• Constriction of bronchioles • Decreased heart rate and myocardial contraction • Increased peristalsis • Increased secretion of tears • Increased secretion of saliva • Increased secretion of pancreatic enzymes and insulin • Contraction of bladder • Contraction of pupil

Figure 46.4 The neuron. Source: Peate I., *et al.*, 2014. Reproduced with permission of John Wiley & Sons.

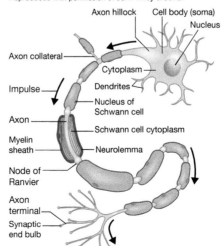

Axon hillock
Cell body (soma)
Nucleus
Axon collateral
Cytoplasm
Impulse
Dendrites
Nucleus of Schwann cell
Axon
Schwann cell cytoplasm
Myelin sheath
Neurolemma
Node of Ranvier
Axon terminal
Synaptic end bulb

Figure 46.5 Synaptic transmission

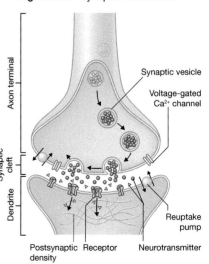

Axon terminal
Synaptic vesicle
Voltage-gated Ca²⁺ channel
Synaptic cleft
Dendrite
Postsynaptic density
Receptor
Neurotransmitter
Reuptake pump

Acute and Critical Care Nursing at a Glance, First Edition. Edited by Helen Dutton and Jacqui Finch
© 2018 John Wiley & Sons, Ltd. Published 2018 by John Wiley & Sons, Ltd.
Companion website: www.ataglanceseries.com/nursing/acutecare

Gross structure

The nervous system is composed of two key areas: the central nervous system (consisting of the brain and spinal cord) and the peripheral nervous system (made up of the nerves and their branches).

Within the **central nervous system**, the brain itself has four major divisions: cerebrum, diencephalon, cerebellum and brain stem (Figure 46.1). It is one of the largest organs in the body, weighing about 1.4 kg. Owing to its delicacy and importance it requires careful protection, hence the three layers of the meninges guarding it. These consist of the tough, fibrous outer layer of the dura mater, with its inward extensions into other parts of the brain (falx cerebri, falx cerebelli and the tentorium cerebelli), the central web-like structure of the arachnoid mater and finally the innermost, transparent layer (closest to the brain and containing blood vessels) called the pia mater. The meningeal layers continue down the spinal cord, eventually terminating in the periosteum of the coccyx.

There are several gaps between the layers of the meninges and these include the epidural, subdural and subarachnoid spaces. Their purpose is to cushion brain tissue further with fat, connective tissue, serous and cerebrospinal fluid. Around 140 mL of circulating CSF is found here and in the ventricles of the brain. This substance, formed by the separation of fluid from blood in a network of capillaries emerging from the pia mater called the choroid plexuses, is essential to brain health. It not only protects brain tissue, but also provides (together with the blood), nutrients and a means of monitoring internal physiological changes in the body. Raised carbon dioxide levels, for example, can be detected in the CSF and initiate homeostatic responses to increase respiration and thereby regulate the body's pH.

Blood supply to the brain is via the internal carotid and vertebral arteries, with the internal jugular veins returning venous blood to the heart. Passage of harmful substances to brain tissue is prevented by the blood–brain barrier (BBB). This is composed of tight junctions that seal the endothelial cells of brain capillaries which, aided by chemical secretions from neuroglia, regulate movement of blood constituents allowing some to pass through to brain tissue and others not.

The spinal cord, approximately 45 cm in length, extends from the foramen magnum in the inferior aspect of the occipital lobe to the first lumbar vertebra. The two key functions of the cord are:
- Provision of conduction routes to and from the brain; ascending tracts convey sensory information whilst descending tracts conduct motor impulses.
- Serving as a centre for spinal reflexes.

Conduction of sensory and motor impulses to and from the spinal column occurs via bundles of nerve roots projecting from either side of it. The fibres of the dorsal nerve root transmit sensory impulses to the cord, whilst the ventral nerve root fibres convey motor information out of it. These nerve roots join to form spinal nerves. There are 31 pairs of spinal nerves (Figure 46.2) and these are components of the **peripheral nervous system**, together with the cranial nerves (Figure 46.3). There are 12 pairs of cranial nerves and they originate from the undersurface of the brain, mostly from the brain stem.

The **autonomic nervous system**, part of the peripheral nervous system, regulates involuntary sensory and motor pathways. There are two distinct divisions: the sympathetic and the parasympathetic branches and both are made up of nerves, ganglia and plexuses (Table 46.1). Sympathetic stimulation occurs as a result of stress and is sometimes referred to as 'fight or flight' response. Environmental factors such as being afraid or physiological impairment such as critical illness may cause it to be evoked. In contrast, the parasympathetic response creates a state of relaxation in the body and opposes sympathetic actions. The sympathetic branch is known as **adrenergic** and its chemical neurotransmitter **noradrenaline** binds to alpha- and beta-adrenergic receptor sites found in the muscle and in target organs. The parasympathetic branch is known as **cholinergic** and its chemical neurotransmitter **acetylcholine** binds to the two types of cholinergic receptor sites, **nicotinic** and **muscarinic**, also found throughout the body (see also Chapter 24).

Functional units

There are two main types of cells in the nervous system: **glia,** of which there are five types (astrocytes, microglia, ependymal, oligodendrocytes and Schwann cells) and **neurons**. Collectively the different types of glia serve to provide the brain with nutrients and protective substances which cushion it and prevent tissue damage from trauma and other inflammatory processes. Neurons, of which there are an estimated 100 billion in the human brain, specialise in conducting nervous impulses or 'action potentials'. These are waves of electrical activity that travel along the surface of each neuron's plasma membrane and are initiated through a series of changes in ionic balance.

Each neuron consists of a cell body, an axon and a varying number of thread-like extensions called dendrites (Figure 46.4). The axon conducts impulses away from the cell body, the dendrites towards it. The speed at which impulses are conveyed depends on the size of the axon and whether or not it is covered in a fatty, white myelin sheath. White matter of the nervous system is myelinated, with faster conduction of impulses, whilst grey matter is not. Neurons can be afferent in nature (sensory), efferent (motor) or interneuron (conducting impulses from afferent to efferent neurons) and information is conveyed via routes of conduction such as the basic reflex arc. In this case, sensory input is processed via afferent neurons to the CNS and then to effector neurons for initiation of a response.

The point at which nerve information is transmitted from one 'presynaptic' neuron to another 'postsynaptic' neuron is called the 'synapse' and this can be electrical or chemical in nature (Figure 46.5). Electrical synapses occur where two cells are joined end to end and this arrangement is common in cardiac muscle cells, with action potentials continuing along the cells as if they were one body. In contrast, chemical synapses require neurotransmitters to send information between neurons. Large molecule transmitters like neuropeptides and small molecule transmitters like acetylcholine, amines (plus their subclass catecholamines) and amino acids are all released from the tiny vesicles of the 'synaptic knob' of each presynaptic neuron to initiate the transmission of information.

47 Neurological assessment

Table 47.1 AVPU – the patient's response

Alert	Eyes are already open or they open in response to the nurse's voice. The patient is orientated to time and place and recalls own name
Voice	Eyes may or may not be open, but the patient does not always give correct answers to questions like 'Do you know where you are?'
Pain	Eyes may or may not be open, but there is no response to the nurse's voice or being gently shaken. May localise, flex or extend to trapezius pinch
Unresponsive	Eyes are closed and there is no response to voice, being gently shaken or to trapezius pinch or supraorbital ridge pressure

Figure 47.1 Testing for pain

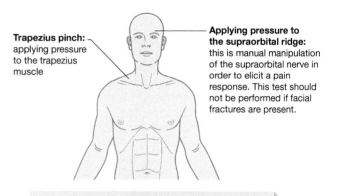

Trapezius pinch: applying pressure to the trapezius muscle

Applying pressure to the supraorbital ridge: this is manual manipulation of the supraorbital nerve in order to elicit a pain response. This test should not be performed if facial fractures are present.

With both tests, start by applying soft pressure and then increase. Apply pressure for no more than 10 s

Figure 47.2 Face, arm, speech, time (FAST) test for stroke

Face
Has the patient's face fallen on one side? Can the patient smile?

Arm
Can the patient raise both arms and keep them there?

Speech
Is the patient's speech slurred?

Time
to call 999 or medical emergency team in hospital if you see any one of these signs

Figure 47.3 Pupil assessment: shape, size, symmetry and reaction

1 mm 2 mm 3 mm 4 mm 5 mm 6 mm

Examine the shape, size and symmetry of the pupils – they should be round, equal and about 2.5 mm.
Shine a bright light into each eye one at a time, from the outer aspect, and look for pupil constriction in both eyes (consensual reaction)

Table 47.2 Glasgow coma scale

Eyes opening: E	Verbal response: V	Motor response: M
4: Spontaneously	**5:** Orientated, communicating normally	**6:** Obeys commands
3: Only to voice	**4:** Disorientated conversation	**5:** Localises – brings hand to the source of pain
2: Only to pain	**3:** Incoherent words or incomprehensible sounds	**4:** Withdraws to pain: patient bends arm to the source of the pain but can't locate it
1: None	**2:** Sounds only	**3:** Decorticate posture: flexion to pain
	1: None	**2:** Decerebrate posture: extension to pain
		1: None
E +	**V** +	**M**

For example:
4 + 5 + 6 = 15 = Total score

Stick your tongue out and now put it back in

Lift your arm and now put it down

Any drop in GCS score should be reported immediately

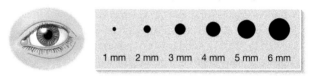

Pain (supraorbital pressure)

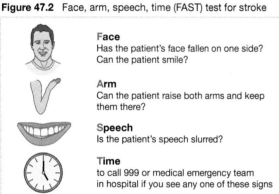

Types of motor response
Flexed
Plantar flexed   Internally rotated   Flexed   Adducted
Decorticate rigidity

Extended   Adducted
Plantar flexed   Flexed   Pronated
Decerebrate rigidity

Acute and Critical Care Nursing at a Glance, First Edition. Edited by Helen Dutton and Jacqui Finch
© 2018 John Wiley & Sons, Ltd. Published 2018 by John Wiley & Sons, Ltd.
Companion website: www.ataglanceseries.com/nursing/acutecare

Disability

Disability is a vital part of the ABCDE assessment process. It reveals both primary and secondary neurological problems and thus enables prompt therapeutic intervention which, in many cases, can be life-saving.

Assessment of impaired consciousness

Firstly, the patient's level of consciousness (LOC) needs to be determined. The LOC is controlled by the reticular activating system (Chapter 46) and two distinct components of LOC are thought to exist: **arousal**, indicating how awake an individual is, and **awareness** which determines cognitive function and the extent to which the patient is able to recognise and respond to the general environment. Impaired consciousness may occur for a variety of reasons, including: primary injuries to the brain secondary to trauma or vascular accident; hypoxaemia; acidosis; infective disorders; status epilepticus; hypothermia; biochemical and metabolic disturbances; drug overdose; and poisoning. For some people rapid deterioration will occur requiring equally fast and accurate assessment, in the first instance the use of the **AVPU scale**[1] (Table 47.1), is recommended. This will reveal whether the patient is fully alert, verbalises appropriately, responds to pain (Figure 47.1) or doesn't respond to anything. Signs and symptoms of stroke (Chapter 48) should always be looked for, using the Face, Arm, Speech and Time (FAST) test (Figure 47.2).

Glasgow Coma Scale

The **Glasgow Coma Scale** (GCS)(Table 47.2) is commonly used to monitor deficits if neurological impairment is established.[2] Depending on the severity of the patient's condition, ongoing monitoring using this scoring system may be required as frequently as every 15–30 min. This internationally used tool scores between 3 and 15, with 3 being the worst score and 15 the best. It is a standardised method of assessing the patient's LOC and effectively communicating findings. Some subjectivity is associated with its use, but this does seem to correlate with the level of the user's clinical experience.[3] The scale examines three behavioural responses giving useful information in diagnosing central and peripheral nervous system defects:
- The first area to be assessed is **eye opening**, testing arousal and degree of general alertness.
- The second is **verbal response**, testing awareness, by monitoring whether or not the patient can speak and, if so, how effectively.
- The third is **motor response**, reviewing how much and in which way the patient responds to a spoken command or a physical stimulus. A variety of motor responses may be seen (Table 47.2).

When assessing GCS in all three areas it is important to note factors that may invalidate the assessment process: firstly, the patient's ability to hear, secondly whether the language being spoken can be understood in order to obey commands and finally the presence of any pre-existing state of confusion. New confusion may be acute and part of the current pathophysiology, but pre-existing confusion may be due to problems such as dementia.

Assessing pupillary response

A useful adjunct to the GCS is pupil assessment (Figure 47.3). By shining a bright and focused light into each of the patient's eyes, the third cranial nerve (oculomotor) can be assessed. This nerve emerging from the midbrain is one of three cranial nerves that control muscular movement of the eyes. In response to light an intact oculomotor nerve will cause pupillary constriction. Before testing the pupils, the nurse should ensure that the area is not too brightly lit, as this will affect the response seen. Be aware of conditions which may alter pupil response, such as pre-existing eye disease, e.g. cataracts. Certain medications, e.g. opiates, will cause pupils to constrict, whilst inotropic and vasopressor agents will cause dilation. When testing pupils, always be alert to the presence of a prosthetic eye! In general, the nurse should carefully monitor and record the size, shape and symmetry of the pupils, together with the speed of their reaction to light. Report any difference in pupil size and sluggish or unequal reactions, as this may indicate serious impairment.

Assessment of the vital signs

As part of the **ABCDE assessment** process the nurse should take especial care to recognise the *specific* changes that may occur in the vital signs as a result of neurological impairment. The rate, rhythm and depth of breathing may be altered by damage having occurred to the diencephalon, midbrain, pons and/or medullary regions of the brain. Cheyne–Stoke respirations (crescendo breathing followed by apnoea) can occur as a result of dysfunction in diencephalic structures. Breathing may also be affected by the presence of **pulmonary oedema**, commonly seen in patients with subarachnoid haemorrhage (SAH), due to neural disturbance. Another significant sign of CNS impairment seen in raised intracranial pressure is **Cushing's triad**. This is characterised by bradycardia, a widened pulse pressure with an elevated systolic pressure and irregular respirations. The patient's temperature should be closely monitored too, as neurological injury to the hypothalamus usually results in an initial hyperthermia (which may be quite severe) and in turn may lead to desaturation secondary to increased oxygen consumption.

Assessment of fluid balance

Patients with CNS impairment are also at risk of fluid and electrolyte disorders which may not only worsen their neurological condition, but in some cases lead to haemodynamic instability. Direct or indirect (ischaemic) damage to the hypothalamus and/or the pituitary gland can lead to **diabetes insipidus** or **syndrome of inappropriate ADH**. In both cases the patient experiences problems with fluid balance and disruption to serum sodium levels can occur (Chapter 50). Another condition that can occur following brain injury (traumatic or spontaneous) is **cerebral salt wasting**. This is due to extracellular fluid depletion and thought to be secondary to a tubular defect in sodium transport. With this problem the patient will become hypovolaemic and hyponatraemic. The nurse must therefore carefully assess patients with a brain insult for fluid balance and electrolyte status on a daily basis, reporting and documenting any abnormalities promptly so that appropriate treatment can be initiated.

Assessing blood glucose

The brain needs a constant supply of glucose, as it has no capacity to store it. Vigilance with blood glucose monitoring is required as hypoglycaemia quickly results in neurological impairment and unless remedied swiftly will lead to coma and death (Chapter 50). Hyperglycaemia is similarly detrimental as it can increase brain lactate levels, cause acidosis and is particularly harmful in cases of stroke. A normal blood glucose level is in the range of 4.0–6.0 mmol/L, rising to around 7.8 mmol/L within an hour or so of eating a meal.

48 Neurological impairment

Figure 48.1 Transient ischaemic attack (TIA)

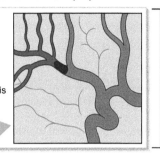

TIA: A mini stroke
Signs and symptoms:
• Numbness of face
• Difficulties with speech
• Limb weakness/paralysis
• Visual disturbances

Figure 48.2 Stroke

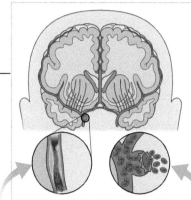

Sign and symptoms of a stroke:

• Depressed LOC/collapse
• Facial weakness or numbness
• Difficulty speaking
• Difficulty walking
• Paralysis or numbness
  on one side
• Visual disturbances
• Papilloedema
• Neck stiffness
• Severe headache
• Difficulty swallowing

TIA treatment:
• Aspirin 300 mg daily
  (or Clopidogrel as
  a substitute)
• Lifestyle advice:
  blood pressure, diet
• Brain imaging (CT scan)
• Carotid scanning:
  stenosis or occlusion
• Possible carotid
  endarterectomy and
  carotid stenting

Remember!
Always have
emergency equipment
checked and ready
to use in case of
rapid patient
deterioration

Ischaemic stroke:
Urgent CT scan within 24 h but if
designated 'immediate' – within 1 h
Treatment:
• Thrombolysis with intravenous alteplase
  within 3–5 h or antiplatelet treatment
  (NICE 2012, 2015)
Main risk: Haemorrhage

Haemorrhagic stroke:
Urgent CT scan within 24 h but if
designated 'immediate' – within 1 h
Treatment:
• Reversal of anticoagulation: blood
  products (NICE 2012, 2015)
• Surgical evacuation or, if too
  severe, palliation

Table 48.1 Specific nursing care of a patient with neurological impairment

A	• Maintain airway: may need to use airway adjuncts such as NPA (intubation is required if GSC ≤ 8) • Assess cough reflex, use suction to remove oropharyngeal secretions
B	• Position at 30°, head raised to reduce risk of hospital-acquired pneumonia • Measure RR and pattern, report if ≤ 8 or > 20 • Monitor SpO_2, maintain within target saturation range. Administer oxygen as prescribed • Consider need for arterial blood gas measurements, $\downarrow PaO_2$ and $\uparrow PaCO_2$ will both increase ICP • Auscultate chest for adventitious sounds (crackles may indicate pulmonary oedema or aspiration pneumonia)
C	• Monitor HR, BP, mean arterial BP and CRT • Maintain MAP within 60–90 mmHg for good cerebral perfusion • Evaluate fluid balance, ensure adequate fluid intake and urine output > 0.5 mL/kg/h • Administer diuretic therapy as prescribed to reduce ICP if required (e.g. mannitol) • Administer drugs as prescribed: thrombolysis, anticoagulants, antibiotics, steroids • Monitor temperature: warm or cool the patient as required. Initiate septic screen if pyrexia or infection suspected

D	• Record GCS (on admission: ½ hourly for 2 h, 1 hourly for 4 h and then 2 hourly) (NICE 2003, 2014)
	• Assess pain and administer analgesia as prescribed
	• Monitor pupil response: should be equal in size, and briskly respond to light. Report any changes immediately
	• Monitor blood glucose. Use sliding scale insulin as prescribed to maintain within target range of 7–10 mmol/L
	• Observe for twitching or early signs of seizures. Report and administer anticonvulsant therapy as prescribed
	To reduce the risk of raised ICP:
	DO: – Elevate the head of the bed to 30°. If the patient has spinal injury or it is suspected, tilt bed
	       – Log roll (keep body in alignment when turning)
	DO NOT: – Turn the patient's head to the side sharply or flex the hips or knees
	       – Tie tapes around the face or neck constricting blood flow

E	• Observe for wounds and bleeding (latter may be spontaneous) • Observe skin for rashes • Ensure affected limbs are placed comfortably, work with physiotherapist in ensuring range of passive movements met • Assess skin integrity, using pressure-relieving devices as required. Change position frequently • Ensure nutritional needs are met, enteral feeding via nasogastric tube may be required

Acute and Critical Care Nursing at a Glance, First Edition. Edited by Helen Dutton and Jacqui Finch
© 2018 John Wiley & Sons, Ltd. Published 2018 by John Wiley & Sons, Ltd.
Companion website: www.ataglanceseries.com/nursing/acutecare

Neurological impairment may occur as a result of a variety of problems that directly or indirectly impair the central or peripheral nervous systems. Of most concern are those conditions that can quickly lead to an altered level of consciousness and have the potential to cause permanent neurological damage.

Cerebrovascular accident

Cerebrovascular accident (CVA) or stroke is one of the most common causes of sudden deterioration in neurological function, detectable by use of the acronym FAST (Chapter 47). General risk factors include: age, male gender, genetic predisposition, ethnicity (Asian or Afro-Caribbean), pre-existing hypertension and diabetes. There are two main types of stroke:

- **Ischaemic.**
- **Haemorrhagic.**

Ischaemic strokes account for 85% of CVAs. This typically occur as a result of progressive occlusion of the larger arteries (often the carotids) with atherothrombotic plaques.

Warning signs of progressive blood vessel narrowing include a diminished carotid pulse, a **carotid bruit** (a noise heard over the carotid pulse on auscultation, caused by turbulent blood flow) and **transient ischaemic attack** (TIA) which may cause neurological deficit for up to 24 h (Figure 48.1). TIA should be treated promptly as it often heralds a major ischaemic stroke, with severe hypoperfusion of the areas that the affected blood vessels serve. As ischaemic stroke usually leads to infarction of the cerebral cortex, the patient will also experience equal losses of motor and sensory function. Embolic stroke caused by the sudden impaction of a blood clot in a small cerebral artery is similar to ischaemic stroke. Patients with atrial fibrillation (see Chapter 31, Figure 31.1c) are at risk from embolic stroke.

Haemorrhagic events occur when small blood vessels in the brain rupture, secondary to chronic hypertension or vascular defects. Patients who are being anticoagulated are at risk, such as those prescribed thrombolysis, warfarin or heparin. A subarachnoid haemorrhage, if occurring spontaneously, is also classed as a **stroke syndrome**,[1] caused by bleeding into the cerebrospinal fluid secondary to a ruptured aneurysm or arteriovenous malformation. Rebleeding and vasospasm are common complications of this type of brain haemorrhage.

Patients with stroke present with characteristic neurological deficits or FAST (Chapter 47), but require specific investigations and management depending on the type of stroke sustained (Figure 48.2).[1,2,3]

Infection

The CNS can become infected by bacteria, viruses or fungi amongst other colonising agents. In **meningitis** the pia mater, the arachnoid mater, the subarachnoid space, ventricular system and the CSF are all affected. Patients have severe headaches, neck stiffness, photophobia, **Brudzinski's sign** (when the head is flexed the hips and knees also flex) and **Kernig's sign** (pain caused by first flexing and then straightening the knees of a supine patient). Seizures and loss of consciousness may occur. The patient will be pyrexial, tachycardic and, with meningococcal disease, have a petechial rash (small, red or purple spots that are non-blanching). Specific medical treatment includes prompt administration of antibiotics (benzylpencillin is the drug of choice). Encephalitis, also a febrile illness, is viral in origin (e.g. herpes simplex) and has a similar presentation to meningitis, but no rash is present. Antiviral therapy such as acyclovir will be required to manage this condition.

Seizures

Seizures are commonly caused by epilepsy (electrical instability), drug toxicity or metabolic disturbances such as abnormal electrolytes. They may be brief in nature or they may be sustained, in which case neurological damage can occur. Seizure can lead to loss of airway. If prolonged it may also deprive cells of oxygen, causing impaired ATP production and increased intracellular calcium levels leading to neuronal death. Significant haemodynamic instability may develop too with hypertension, pyrexia, acidosis, hyperkalaemia and hypoglycaemia. Respiratory function may also be affected by the presence of pulmonary oedema secondary to intense vasoconstriction. Specific treatment will consist of anticonvulsant therapies, usually in the form of benzodiazepine and phenytoin administration.

Trauma

Most neurological injury, whether it be to the head or spine, occurs as a result of high velocity impact and falls. **Primary brain injury** may initially be in the form of fractures (linear, depressed, compound, comminuted or the more severe basal skull fracture), contusion (bruising) or major intracranial haemorrhage (open or closed). The latter can be **epidural** in nature (bleeding between the dura mater and the skull), **subdural** (blood accumulating between the brain and the dura) or **intracerebral** (a dense collection of blood in brain tissue). **Secondary brain injury** occurs as a result of raised intracranial pressure (ICP), hypoperfusion and hypoxaemia and these mechanisms lead to death in over 50% of cases of severe head trauma.[1] In many cases, **surgical intervention** will be urgently required. This may take the form of **craniotomy** or **hemicraniotomy** (where a bone flap is temporarily removed) or **decompressive craniectomy** (where the bone flap is removed but not replaced, therefore allowing the brain to swell).[4]

Raised intracranial pressure

Normal ICP is less than 15 mmHg and in all types of severe brain illness or injury it can rise, leading to significant neuronal damage. The **Monro–Kellie hypothesis** states that the three constituents of the cranium (approximately 80% brain, 10% CSF and 10% blood) are incompressible, so an increase in one must be offset by a decrease in the others. In health, this is achieved by two homeostatic mechanisms: movement of cerebral venous blood into the systemic circulation and increased reabsorption of CSF. However, in illness or injury, if the ICP continues to rise (with a haematoma, for example), these processes are overwhelmed. The pressure that is building up will start to compress brain tissue and cause impaired cerebral perfusion. It is important to note that mean arterial pressure minus ICP is equal to cerebral perfusion pressure. As blood flow and oxygenation decreases ischaemic injury occurs and this contributes to shifting of brain matter. **Transtentorial herniation** or 'coning' may occur and this is where the brain is squeezed through intracranial structures under pressure. Brain stem death will follow and this is characterised by irreversible coma and an inability to breathe spontaneously.

A prioritised approach, using the ABCDE format, should always be employed to assess the patient and deliver evidence-based care (Table 48.1), whatever the cause of neurological impairment.

49 Drug overdose and poisoning

Table 49.1 Other types of poisoning

Toxin	Route	Effect
Fungi	Ingested	GI disturbances followed by hepatorenal failure
Organophosphates and carbamate pesticides used in agriculture **Pesticide**	Ingested, inhaled, cutaneous exposure	Leads to the accumulation of the parasympathetic autonomic nervous system neurotransmitter acetylcholine at the neuromuscular junction, causing bradycardia, salivation, tremor, urination, vomiting, diarrhoea and miosis
Carbon monoxide	Inhaled	Depression of the CNS. Patient will have a cherry pink skin owing to the formation of carboxyhaemoglobin
Other noxious gases	Inhaled	Airway obstruction, bronchial hyperreactivity producing asthma-like symptoms
Corrosive agents	Ingested	• Perforation of GI organs • Mediastinitis • Peritonitis • Multiple organ dysfunction

Box 49.1 History taking

- What are the names of the drug(s)or poison(s) taken?
- How much and when?
- What are the initial signs and symptoms?
- Is there chronicity of use?
- Are there any pre-existing diseases?

Figure 49.1 Key diagnostic investigations

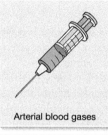

Arterial blood gases

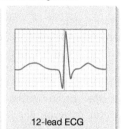

12-lead ECG

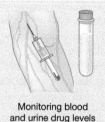

Monitoring blood and urine drug levels

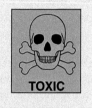

TOXIC

Toxicology screening

Table 49.2 Specific patient assessment

A	• Observe for choking and listen for signs of an obstructed airway such as stridor • Observe for vomit and foreign substances around the mouth • Action appropriately using suction, airway adjuncts and calling for help
B	• Monitor SpO_2 for desaturation, use supplemental oxygen to keep within target range • Observe for increased or decreased RR, shallow or deep breaths, added breath sounds
C	• Observe patient colour for cyanosis or excessive redness • Check central and skin temperature, perfusion with CRT • Carefully monitor fluid balance • Check record and score vital signs using NEWS to assess risk of deterioration
D	• Calculate GCS • Observe pupils for miosis (constriction of pupil) or mydriasis (dilation of pupil) and reaction to light. Report changes • Observe for seizures • Check blood glucose, maintain within normal range
E	• Observe for rashes and burns • Observe for abdominal signs and symptoms including guarding • Observe for needle marks or other injuries

Table 49.3 Clinical management strategies

Remember
- Maintain **a**irway
- Maintain effective **b**reathing and oxygenation
- Maintain good **c**irculation
- Maintain neurological **d**isability
- Maintain **e**xposure

Methods of treatment	Drugs/poisons
Limit absorption: activated charcoal	To absorb and bind ingested toxins, e.g. digoxin/aspirin Risks include vomiting and pneumonitis (inhalation)
Forced diuresis or urinary and serum alkalinisation	Increase urine production with IV fluid administration Alkaline urine helps excretion of drugs such as aspirin (salicylate) and phenobarbitone, by a process known as 'ion trapping'. Intravenous sodium bicarbonate is administered to reduce metabolic acidosis
Antidotes to specific drugs	• **Naloxone** for opiates • **Flumazenil** for benzodiazepines • **Glucagon** for insulin • **N-Acetylcysteine** for paracetamol (three continuous IV infusions with a total dose of 300 mg/kg being given over 21 h (Commission on Human Medicines, 2012).
Enhance elimination	• Administration of laxatives and whole bowel irrigation to clear the drug • Haemodialysis to clear low molecular weight, water-soluble, non-protein-bound agents like lithium
Other methods	• Skin decontamination for transdermal absorptions of toxins

For advice: UK healthcare professionals should contact the National Poisons Information Service **TOXBASE**

Acute and Critical Care Nursing at a Glance, First Edition. Edited by Helen Dutton and Jacqui Finch
© 2018 John Wiley & Sons, Ltd. Published 2018 by John Wiley & Sons, Ltd.
Companion website: www.ataglanceseries.com/nursing/acutecare

In the UK around 140000 people are admitted to hospital each year with poisoning. Many are minors, but of the adults most are aged 20–29 years. Although exposure to a number of toxins can occur, the ingestion of pharmaceutical agents is, in cases of poisoning, the single, most common reason for attendance at Emergency Departments. Analgesia, antidepressants and calcium channel blockers are historically amongst the common culprits, with a recent increase seen in the use of recreational drugs (including so-called 'legal highs') and medication sold on the internet for weight loss. There has also been a rise in the abuse of household products like air fresheners.[1] Whilst many cases of overdose and poisoning seen in the Emergency Department are as a result of self-harm, nurses should always be aware that **they too** can overdose patients when administering medication if they fail to follow local and national drug policies.

Drugs commonly taken in overdose

Drugs that can be purchased over the counter are easily available, and are a popular choice for overdose, with **paracetamol** (acetaminophen) being a prime example. When this is taken in excess (a fatal dose usually exceeds 140 mg/kg, but does vary with each individual), the normal metabolism of the substance is disrupted. Taken in moderation, the liver cytochrome P-450 system (a super protein that renders pharmacological metabolites inactive) enables conjugation of the drug with glutathione (an antioxidant). In overdose, a toxic metabolite (N-acetyl-p-benzoquinoneimine) forms and then accumulates, overwhelming the glutathione supply. Initially, only nausea and vomiting occurs, but unless treated within 72 h hepatic necrosis and failure develops. Prognosis is likely to be poor, especially if signs of multiple organ dysfunction are developing.

Aspirin

Aspirin (a salicylate), is another analgesic agent. Overdoses are less common now, but the mortality rate is 30%. The principle effect of aspirin toxicity is disordered cellular metabolism and impaired energy production. This leads to hypoxaemia and an initial metabolic acidosis (although depending on the dose taken, alkalosis may occur later as a result of severe vomiting). Other symptoms include coagulopathy secondary to prothrombin inhibition and impaired platelet function. Salicylate is also a powerful gastric mucosal irritant, so haematemesis may be a specific feature. In some patients, pulmonary oedema due to acute respiratory distress syndrome (ARDS) can also occur.

Antidepressants

These are widely prescribed and therefore often taken as an overdose. An excess of a tricyclic agent such as **amitriptyline** (increases the level of the neurotransmitters noradrenaline and serotonin) will lead to respiratory impairment, hypotension, hypothermia, hyperreflexia, arrhythmias, metabolic acidosis, and loss of consciousness. The less toxic and more commonly prescribed **selective serotonin re-uptake inhibitor** (SSRI) like citalopram (increases extracellular levels of serotonin), can still cause systemic illness if abused. GI disturbance, tachycardia, drowsiness and convulsions occur but in rare circumstances the life threatening **'serotonin syndrome'** may develop, leading to autonomic and neuromuscular instability, hyperthermia, rhabdomolysis, renal failure and clotting disorders.

Sedation and analgesia

There are many different types of **barbiturates** (e.g. phenobarbital)**, benzodiazepines** (e.g. diazepam), and **opioids** (e.g. morphine). Working on the CNS (as intended), if taken in overdose will severely depress consciousness, and impair respiration to the point of apnoea. A drop in blood pressure may occur due to vasodilation and the negative inotropy they can initiate. Arrhythmias and hypothermia are also common side effects. In contrast, **stimulants** lead to a very different clinical presentation. Those who have taken amphetamines, cocaine or ecstasy experience CNS excitation with catecholamine release, leading to intense vasoconstriction. Hypertension, tachycardia, myocardial ischaemia and haemorrhagic stroke are therefore common pathophysiological effects. Hyperkalaemia, rhabdomyolysis, pulmonary haemorrhage or even aortic dissection are also a possibility.

Cardiac drugs

When taken as an overdose, cardiac drugs will also have systemic effects, which vary according to the drug that has been taken. Digoxin, a cardiac glycoside (which increases contractility by enhancing intracellular calcium levels), can lead to GI disturbance and brady- or tachycardia. Whilst an overdose of a beta-adrenergic receptor blocking agent (beta blocker) will produce severe bradycardia and may cause bronchospasm. Propranolol, however, is most likely to cause coma and convulsions, whilst a sotalol overdose often results in hypokalaemia and ventricular tachyarrhythmias. Similarly, calcium channel blockers (drugs that block calcium transit through cell membranes) commonly cause GI and neurological disturbance. Verapamil and diltiazem are especially likely to cause cardiac depression, possibly leading to asystole.

Other types of overdose and poisoning

Other drugs that may be ingested in overdose include iron (for anaemia), which often has a poor prognosis due to the hepatorenal failure that ensues, and lithium (for the treatment of psychiatric disorder) which when overdosed causes major neurological disturbance. Ethanol (alcohol) is often consumed with an excess of drugs. Intoxication with this alone can lead to CNS depression with aspiration of gastric contents, metabolic acidosis and hypoglycaemia. Alcohol can also sometimes exacerbate the effects of drugs. The nurse should remember, however, that not all poisons ingested are drugs and not all poisons are ingested (Table 49.1).

History taking and patient assessment

History taking in drug overdose and poisoning is often challenging. The nurse should be aware that the patient may be unwilling to divulge information, may give incorrect details or be physically unable to communicate owing to impaired consciousness. Family members, other bystanders or ambulance personnel similarly may not be able to provide any useful particulars depending on the circumstances in which the patient has been found. If a history can be obtained it is important to ascertain certain key information (Box 49.1). Patient assessment by the nurse must also be systematic using an ABCDE approach, confirming which specific signs and symptoms are (or have been) present (Table 49.2). This will aid clinical investigation (Figure 49.1) and assist with diagnosis, ensuring the appropriate line of clinical management is adopted (Table 49.3).

50 Acute endocrine problems

Figure 50.1 Major endocrine glands

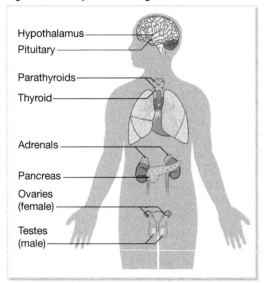

Hypothalamus
Pituitary
Parathyroids
Thyroid
Adrenals
Pancreas
Ovaries (female)
Testes (male)

Figure 50.2 Hypothalamus production and pituitary gland release of hormones

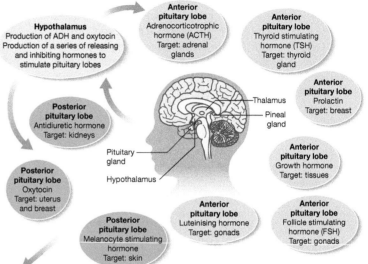

Hypothalamus
Production of ADH and oxytocin
Production of a series of releasing and inhibiting hormones to stimulate pituitary lobes

Anterior pituitary lobe
Adrenocorticotrophic hormone (ACTH)
Target: adrenal glands

Anterior pituitary lobe
Thyroid stimulating hormone (TSH)
Target: thyroid gland

Anterior pituitary lobe
Prolactin
Target: breast

Posterior pituitary lobe
Antidiuretic hormone
Target: kidneys

Thalamus
Pineal gland

Anterior pituitary lobe
Growth hormone
Target: tissues

Pituitary gland
Hypothalamus

Posterior pituitary lobe
Oxytocin
Target: uterus and breast

Posterior pituitary lobe
Melanocyte stimulating hormone
Target: skin

Anterior pituitary lobe
Luteinising hormone
Target: gonads

Anterior pituitary lobe
Follicle stimulating hormone (FSH)
Target: gonads

Table 50.1 Other key hormones

Hormone	Gland
Melatonin to control sleep/wake cycles	Pineal
Adrenaline and **noradrenaline** to target adrenergic receptors and control vasomotor tone
Cortisol to regulate metabolism and **aldosterone** to regulate sodium and potassium	Adrenal
Parathyroid hormone to regulate calcium	Parathyroid
Oestrogen, progesterone and **androgens** to regulate reproductive activity	Gonads
Thymosin for immunity	Thymus
Insulin and **glucagon** to regulate blood glucose	Pancreas

Table 50.2 Diabetic emergencies

Diabetic ketoacidosis	Hyperglycaemic hyperosmolar syndrome	Hypoglycaemia
Blood glucose > 13.9 mmol/L
Polyuria leading to dehydration and hypovolaemia
Polydipsia
Electrolyte deficits
Nausea, vomiting and abdominal pain
pH < 7.30: ketoacidosis/ ketonuria
Serum bicarbonate < 15 mmol/L
Kussmaul respiration: rapid and deep, as compensation for acidosis
Deteriorating conscious level	Blood glucose > 33.3 mmol/L
Polyuria leading to dehydration and hypovolaemia
Polydipsia
Vomiting
Electrolyte deficits
Hyperosmolality with serum readings > 320 mOsmol/kg
pH < 7.30 but no ketoacidosis
Absence of ketones in urine
Serum bicarbonate > 15 mmol/L
Deteriorating conscious level (seizures common)	Blood glucose < 3 mmol/l
Sweating, anxiety, palpitations, nausea (autonomic symptoms)
Tired, confusion impaired consciousness, seizures (neuroglycopenic symptoms)
Severity of presentation may be measured by using Gold or Clarke scoring systems[3]. Use to assess how aware patient is of symptoms of hypoglycaemia
Clinical management[3]:
A/B:
Maintain airway if compromised
Monitor respiratory rate
Monitor SpO$_2$, administer oxygen therapy to meet target saturations
C:
Monitor vital signs
Replace volume as prescribed IV (within 24 h and according to patient's needs) with isotonic saline: 0.9% NaCl
Glucose-containing fluid can be given once serum glucose reduced to 10–15 mmol/L, but not more than 2 L in 24 h
Monitor urine output
Monitor/replace electrolytes as required:
Target K$^+$: 4–5 mmol/L
Administer sliding scale insulin:
Target blood glucose: 5–8 mmol/L
Monitor serum ketone level
Monitor blood pH
Insert nasogastric tube if required
D:
Monitor conscious level hourly
Monitor blood glucose levels	**Clinical management:**
As for DKA, but:
C:
When replacing volume if serum sodium is normal or elevated hypotonic saline (0.45% NaCl) may be used
Serum K$^+$ may be lower than in DKA owing to the hyperosmolality shifting K$^+$ into cells, therefore ensure level is corrected sufficiently before insulin therapy commences
D:
Monitor for seizures	**Clinical management:**
A/B:
Maintain airway if compromised by loss of consciousness
Monitor respiratory rate
Monitor SpO$_2$ and administer oxygen therapy to meet target saturations
C:
Monitor vital signs, fluid balance and electrolyte levels
D:
Monitor conscious level
If the patient is conscious, administer an oral carbohydrate or apply prescribed Glucogel. If consciousness is impaired and the blood glucose is < 4 mmol/L administer prescribed: 50 mL of 10% glucose solution. Further doses can be given every minute until consciousness is regained or a total of 250 mL has been given (Resuscitation Council 2015)[4] The administration of intramuscular glucagon is another immediate treatment option for the unconscious patient[5]

Acute and Critical Care Nursing at a Glance, First Edition. Edited by Helen Dutton and Jacqui Finch
© 2018 John Wiley & Sons, Ltd. Published 2018 by John Wiley & Sons, Ltd.
Companion website: www.ataglanceseries.com/nursing/acutecare

The endocrine system consists of all the glands and organs in the body that produce hormones (Figure 50.1). These chemical transmitters bind to the hormone receptors of specific target cells and by working synergistically or antagonistically lead to a variety of physiological reactions. Owing to the existence of complex mechanisms for hormonal regulation, when dysfunction occurs many organs in the body are affected.

Hormonal influence and acute organ dysfunction

The hypothalamic–pituitary axis is important to consider. The hypothalamus, located in the brain just below the thalamus, is the major link between the endocrine and nervous systems and it has many functions. It receives sensory input from other parts of the brain as well as from internal organs, plus it regulates temperature, thirst, hunger, emotional response and sexual behaviour. The hypothalamus also regulates the pituitary gland and together the two structures produce many hormones (Figure 50.2 and Table 50.1). When either of these areas of the brain is affected by disease/injury or their target organs are damaged, hormonal disruption quickly occurs. Acute disorders may be observed in patients with anterior pituitary lobe dysfunction such as adrenal dysfunction.

Adrenal insufficiency can lead to acute deterioration. **Adrenocorticotrophic hormone** (ACTH) produced by the anterior pituitary, stimulates the adrenal cortex to secrete glucocorticoids such as **cortisol** (hydrocortisone). This has a major role in catecholamine synthesis and maintenance of blood pressure, glucose regulation and fatty acid metabolism. Should the adrenal glands actually be impaired, the production of **aldosterone** (a mineralocorticoid responsible for sodium reabsorption and potassium excretion) will also be reduced.

In contrast, excessive corticosteroid production results in **Cushing's syndrome** and if hyperaldosteronism is a feature, water retention and potassium loss will also occur.

In rare cases, a tumour of the adrenal medulla may develop (**phaeochromocytoma**). Very high levels of catecholamines are released into the blood, generating severe hypertension. Surgical removal of the tumour will be required.

Pituitary dysfunction may also lead to thyroid disorder, because the anterior lobe of the pituitary produces **thyroid stimulating hormone (TSH)**. This targets the thyroid gland resulting in an increase in **thyroxine** (T4) and **tri-iodothyronine** (T3). These hormones (made under the action of iodine and stored in the gland itself), have several functions including: increasing the basal metabolic rate (BMR), regulation of catecholamines, stimulation of sodium/potassium pump production, protein synthesis, fatty acid metabolism and assistance with human growth. Their release in excess causes **hyperthyroidism** whereby the patient experiences pyrexia, tachycardia, arrhythmias and possibly heart and liver failure. Management of this condition requires careful monitoring of cardiovascular parameters and the administration of pharmacological agents such as carbimazole 15–40 mg daily.[1] **Thyroid crisis or storm** requires emergency treatment with intravenous fluids, propranolol (a beta blocker) and hydrocortisone. Lastly, insufficient thyroid hormone secretion can lead to **hypothyroidism**. In rare cases this can progress to **myxoedema coma**, characterised by bradycardia, hypotension, hypoventilation and hypothermia. Thyroxine administration is required urgently.

Dysfunction of the posterior lobe of the pituitary can lead to **central diabetes insipidus (DI)** and **syndrome of inappropriate ADH (SIADH)**. With the former, there is a deficiency of **arginine vasopressin**, the antidiuretic hormone (made in the hypothalamus). Poor water reabsorption by renal tubules means that large amounts of dilute urine are produced resulting in hypernatraemia as the patient dehydrates and becomes hypovolaemic. Treatment will consist of water replacement and 1-deamino-8-D-arginine vasopressin (**DDAVP**) administration (1–4 μg daily if given via subcutaneous, intramuscular or intravenous route).[1] DI can be nephrogenic in origin too, but this occurs when the kidneys cannot respond to the ADH released by the pituitary. In SIADH there is excessive ADH secretion and this can lead to water retention. Haemodilution of solutes can occur and the serum sodium level may decrease low enough to cause coma. In such circumstances, water restriction and careful saline administration (0.5 mmol/h) will be required.[2]

Diabetic emergencies: a common endocrine problem

In health, glucose is regulated in the blood by the pancreas through insulin, glucagon and somatostatin secretion and by the liver via glycogenolysis and gluconeogenesis (Chapter 39). Patients with diabetes mellitus either type 1 (pancreatic atrophy and loss of beta cells with little or no insulin production) or type 2 (insulin resistance or decreased insulin production) may develop three specific complications (Table 50.2), each of which requires careful assessment and prompt, specific clinical management.[3,4]

Diabetic ketoacidosis

Diabetic ketoacidosis (DKA) often occurs either as a result of a raised metabolic rate (as with infection) or due to non-adherence to treatment regimes. The lack of insulin leads to two specific pathophysiological problems (Table 50.2):
• Hyperglycaemia secondary to increased glycogenolysis. This in turn affects the renal threshold for glucose causing an increase in osmotic pressure. Glycosuria and increased diuresis will follow which may be so severe as to cause hypovolaemia.
• Metabolic acidosis due to the breakdown of fatty acids and subsequent production by the liver of ketone bodies (a constituent of which is acetoacetic acid).

Hyperglycaemic hyperosmolar syndrome

Hyperglycaemic hyperosmolar syndrome (HHS) is similar to DKA in that hyperglycaemia as a result of insulin deficiency may lead to severe dehydration with an excessive water deficit (Table 50.2). Hyperketonaemia, however, is not commonly seen with HHS and this is thought to be due to lower circulating levels of hormones such as cortisol and **growth hormone** that can break down fats.

Hypoglycaemia

In diabetic patients this is often as a result of too much insulin, increased metabolic requirements or too little food. Excess alcohol consumption is a common cause of low blood glucose as it suppresses gluconeogenesis. In hypoglycaemia the hypothalamus senses the drop in blood glucose, leading to a sympathetic autonomic nervous system response, with sweating, raised HR, and possibly tremors. **Neuroglycopenia** (shortage of glucose in the brain) causes irritability and confusion and if untreated can lead to coma, brain damage and death (Table 50.2). In all diabetic emergencies, the nurse working in acute care needs to remember that early recognition and prompt management is vital if organ dysfunction (and in many cases death) is to be avoided.

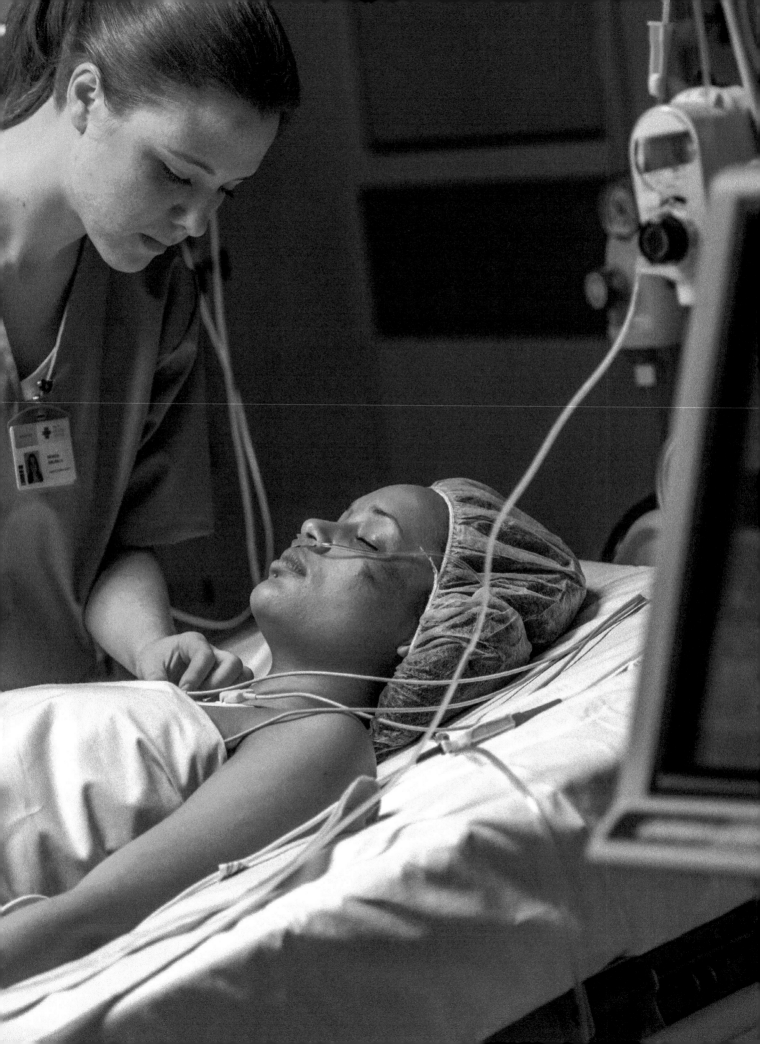

Exposure

Part 6

Chapters
51   **Skin integrity**   112
52   **Nutritional assessment and support**   114

51 Skin integrity

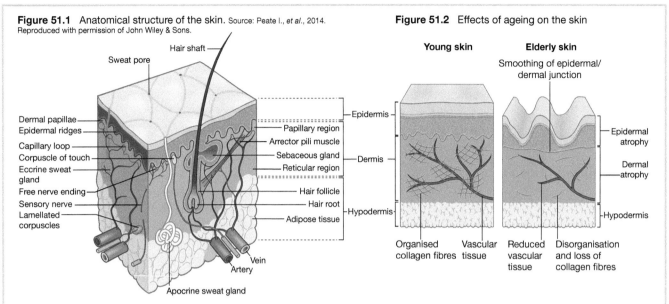

Figure 51.1 Anatomical structure of the skin. Source: Peate I., *et al.*, 2014. Reproduced with permission of John Wiley & Sons.

Hair shaft
Sweat pore
Dermal papillae
Epidermal ridges
Capillary loop
Corpuscle of touch
Eccrine sweat gland
Free nerve ending
Sensory nerve
Lamellated corpuscles

Epidermis
Papillary region
Arrector pili muscle
Sebaceous gland
Reticular region
Hair follicle
Hair root
Adipose tissue
Dermis
Hypodermis
Vein
Artery
Apocrine sweat gland

Figure 51.2 Effects of ageing on the skin

Young skin   Elderly skin
Smoothing of epidermal/dermal junction
Epidermis
Dermis
Hypodermis
Epidermal atrophy
Dermal atrophy
Hypodermis
Organised collagen fibres   Vascular tissue   Reduced vascular tissue   Disorganisation and loss of collagen fibres

Figure 51.3 Pressure ulcer classification

Stage 1   Stage 2   Stage 3   Stage 4
Skin
Fat
Muscle
Bone

Box 51.1 Stages of wound healing

- Haemostasis
- Inflammation
- Proliferation
- Maturation

Box 51.3 Treatment of wound – examples of dressing types

- Alginate/hydrofibre – for use on deep granulating wounds with moderate/heavy exudate
- Vapour permeable – for bacterial infection
- Vapour permeable or hydrocolloid – for low exuding wounds
- Hydrogel – for sloughy, necrotic wounds and cavity wounds

Note: No clear evidence as to the efficacy of one product over another when dressing wounds. Source: NICE, 2015.

Box 51.2 TIME principle in wound management

- Time management: debridement and clearing of slough
- Infection management
- Moisture management
- Edge management (of wound margins)

Box 51.4 Negative pressure wound therapy – vacuum-assisted closure

- Tissue viability specialist to advise on use
- **Vacuum-assisted closure** is a vacuum suction used for cavity or dehiscence surgical wounds
- It applies topical negative pressure which removes exudate and stimulates granulation
- It is not to be used on necrotic wounds or for treating anticoagulated patients who are at risk of bleeding

Figure 51.4 Visual infusion phlebitis (VIP) score. Source: Jackson A., 1997. Reproduced with permission from Andrew Jackson, IV Nurse Consultant, The Rotherham NHS Foundation Trust, UK.

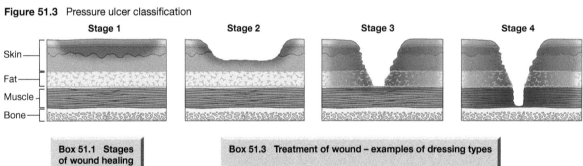

IV site appears healthy	0	No sign of phlebitis • Observe cannula
One of the following is evident: • slight pain near the IV site or • slight redness near the IV site	1	Possible first sign of phlebitis • Observe cannula
Two of the following are evident: • pain near the IV site • erythema • swelling	2	Early stage of phlebitis • Resite cannula
All of the following are evident: • pain along the path of cannula • erythema • induration	3	Medium stage of phlebitis • Resite cannula • Consider treatment
All of the following are evident and extensive: • pain along the path of cannula • erythema • induration • palpable venous cord	4	Advanced stage of phlebitis or start of thrombophlebitis • Resite cannula • Consider treatment
All of the following are evident and extensive: • pain along the path of cannula • erythema • induration • palpable venous cord • **pyrexia**	5	Advanced stage of thrombophlebitis • Initiate treatment • Resite cannula

Acute and Critical Care Nursing at a Glance, First Edition. Edited by Helen Dutton and Jacqui Finch
© 2018 John Wiley & Sons, Ltd. Published 2018 by John Wiley & Sons, Ltd.
Companion website: www.ataglanceseries.com/nursing/acutecare

Skin: function and structure

The skin is the largest organ in the body, responsible for 20% of its total weight and, together with the hair, nails and glands, it forms the integumentary system. The main function is protection, because skin can prevent environmental agents from causing harm, conserve fluids, assist with thermoregulation, participate in the production of vitamin D (required for the absorption of calcium and phosphate by the small intestine) and relay important information to the brain via touch and pressure. Three distinct layers of the skin exist: the **epidermis**, the **deeper dermis** and the **hypodermis** or subcutaneous layer of connective tissue (Figure 51.1).

Factors impairing skin integrity in acute illness

Skin integrity may be threatened by both intrinsic factors (related to the patient's condition) and extrinsic factors (originating from external sources) and a recognised risk assessment tool such as the Waterlow score should be used to determine if these are present.[1] Some patients are predisposed to skin impairment owing to the general state of their health and the pre-existence of medical disorders such as diabetes mellitus. Secondly, the skin of elderly patients will already be susceptible to breaking down, independent of any ill health. This is because there are many changes naturally occurring in skin as part of the ageing process (Figure 51.2). Finally, **inadequate nutrition** is a significant risk factor for impaired skin integrity (Chapter 52). An inability to meet dietary requirements can lead to loss of skin collagen and moisture, which in turn can cause wounds and delay healing.

Poor perfusion

Skin perfusion is a particular problem for many acutely ill patients. This may be as a result of physiological stress, where autonomic sympathetic stimulation constricts the arterioles in the skin, diverting blood away from it to the major organs. The administration of vasoactive drugs such as adrenaline and noradrenaline will also alter blood flow and increase the risk of skin ischaemia. Impaired perfusion may be as a result of pressure due to **immobility** and this poses many challenges for nursing staff, especially where **bariatric** (obese) patients are concerned. A **decubitus ulcer** (pressure ulcer), may form when there is a prolonged deficiency of blood flow to an area of the body, usually in tissue covering a bony projection such as the heels, buttocks or even the bridge of the nose subsequent to pressure from an oxygen mask. Over time, superficial abrasions can develop into more substantial tissue damage, and with poor healing properties necrosis may be the end result. Whilst the primary aim of care in these circumstances is to relieve pressure, mobilising the patient must be well planned and executed according to manual handling policy, as **friction and shearing injuries** can occur with poor technique. Patients with **altered sensory perception** are also at risk of skin damage, as neurological impairment may cause sensation loss, preventing the detection of pain or the effects of pressure on tissue.

Incontinence

Acutely unwell patients who are immobile will require continual assistance with elimination, as **excoriation** of the skin secondary to urinary and/or faecal incontinence can occur. The ammonia in urine and the digestive enzymes in faeces lead to the development of sore, inflamed skin which may cause irritation and become infected. Fungal infections like *Candida albicans* are encouraged by moist, warm conditions.

Infection

Skin integrity may be impaired by the number of **invasive sites** present. These may take the form of an indwelling cannula puncturing the skin, drains, urinary catheters, stomas or surgical wounds. Whilst all serving a clinical purpose, these points of entry into the body also provide a direct route for infection, which may progress to sepsis (Chapter 33). **Necrotising fasciitis**, whilst rare, can occur even in healthy individuals. This bacterial infection affecting bands of connective tissue around muscles, nerves and blood vessels (fascia) is most commonly caused by *Group A Streptococcus*. Extensive surgery to remove necrotic tissue may be required if septic shock and ultimately death is to be avoided.

Nursing assessment

Assessment of the skin should take a structured approach, beginning at the patient's head and progressing to the toes. Two techniques should be employed: **inspection** and **palpation**.

Inspection

An assessment of the patient's hair should also be made, noting its general health and the presence of any colonisation such as head lice, so appropriate treatment can commence. Skin colour changes should be observed: areas of redness are associated with inflammation; central or peripheral cyanosis is secondary to hypoperfusion; pallor due to shock or jaundice as a result of bilirubin accumulation (Chapter 40). Other visible signs of skin impairment may include rashes of infective, allergic or autoimmune origin, bruising, nodules, lumps, sites of malignancy such as melanoma, plus varied types of wounds. Early recognition of these disorders is vital for appropriate treatment to be commenced. Decubitus ulcers for example will be inspected and graded from one to four, according to their severity on the 2009 **EPUAP-NPUAPA classification system**,[2] the recommended assessment tool (Figure 51.3). With all wounds, the stage of healing (Box 51.1) will determine the specific specialist management required[1,5,6] (Boxes 51.2, 51.3 and 51.4). The sites of intravenous cannulae should also be closely inspected for signs of inflammation, infection and extravasation, with the **visual infusion phlebitis (VIP) score**[3] being recorded (Figure 51.4). This validated and highly recommended tool (devised by Nurse Consultant Andrew Jackson in 1997) can determine when an indwelling cannula should be removed.[4] Other indwelling devices like urinary catheters and nasogastric tubes should also be checked to ensure they are not causing pressure to adjacent skin. Lastly, the nurse should observe nailbeds on fingers and toes for abnormalities such as discolouration, or a misshapen appearance which may indicate infection.

Palpation

Palpation reveals important factors such as: temperature (hot with infection or cold with poor perfusion); the presence of moisture (for example, clammy as in most shocked states); the degree of turgor or elasticity (poor with dehydration); or the presence of oedema (some of which may be pitting leaving an indentation in the skin when pressure is applied for 5 s). Pressure to the nailbed can also be applied to determine the capillary refill time (normal is 2 s in duration); this may be prolonged in hypoperfusion. Touch can also determine the size, texture and symmetry of any lesions present even if these are not easily visible.

Nutritional assessment and support

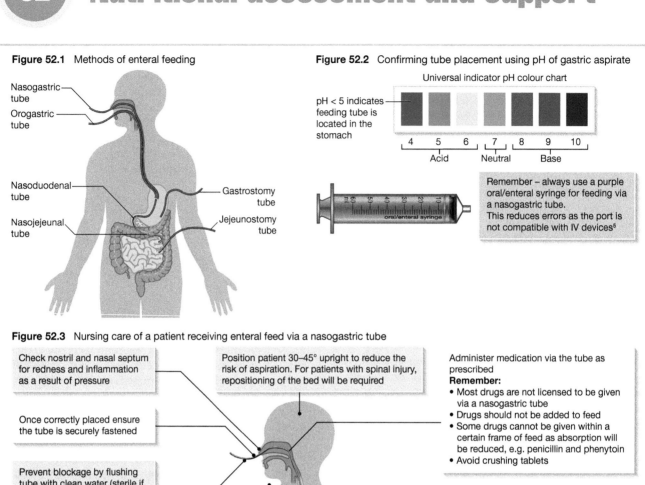

Figure 52.1 Methods of enteral feeding

Nasogastric tube
Orogastric tube
Nasoduodenal tube
Nasojejunal tube
Gastrostomy tube
Jejeunostomy tube

Figure 52.2 Confirming tube placement using pH of gastric aspirate

Universal indicator pH colour chart

pH < 5 indicates feeding tube is located in the stomach

4   5   6   7   8   9   10
Acid   Neutral   Base

Remember – always use a purple oral/enteral syringe for feeding via a nasogastric tube. This reduces errors as the port is not compatible with IV devices[5]

oral/enteral syringe

Figure 52.3 Nursing care of a patient receiving enteral feed via a nasogastric tube

Check nostril and nasal septum for redness and inflammation as a result of pressure

Once correctly placed ensure the tube is securely fastened

Prevent blockage by flushing tube with clean water (sterile if immunocompromised) pre and post-aspiration, feeding and medication. Volume of administration to be given according to dietetic advice

Observe infection control procedures at all times: strict hand hygiene is required

Administer feed as prescribed via an enteral feeding pump, using an enteral feeding giving set. Feed must be discarded after 24 h

Position patient 30–45° upright to reduce the risk of aspiration. For patients with spinal injury, repositioning of the bed will be required

Document feed and monitor volume of aspirate
Monitor fluid balance

Administer medication via the tube as prescribed
Remember:
• Most drugs are not licensed to be given via a nasogastric tube
• Drugs should not be added to feed
• Some drugs cannot be given within a certain frame of feed as absorption will be reduced, e.g. penicillin and phenytoin
• Avoid crushing tablets

Monitor patient's weight and monitor anthropometry: skinfold thickness and mid-arm muscle mass

Monitor blood glucose and electrolytes

Monitor bowel function:
• **In the event of constipation** conduct rectal examination as per policy and commence stool chart
• **In the event of diarrhoea** commence stool chart and take specimen for culture
Manage both conditions according to dietetic advice and local policy

Box 52.1 The patient with a gastrostomy tube

• A gastrostomy tube is for long-term enteral feeding
• Percutaneous endoscopic gastrostomy is one method of insertion
Remember:
• Only give liquid or soluble medication via this tube
• Always consult with the dietician regarding the following:
  – 2–3 weeks following insertion commence weekly rotation advancement of tube to avoid overgrowth of gastric tissue around it
  – Observe for oozing around stoma site and check that the fixation device is secure
  – Observe for overgranulation of site: take swab for culture if infection is suspected

Box 52.2 The patient requiring parenteral feed

• Intravenous feeding is used for patients who have digestive tract dysfunction
Remember:
• The nurse is required to be assessed as competent in the administration of parenteral nutrition
• Strict asepsis is required: premixed bags to be used whenever possible
• Feed should be given via a central line and a volumetric pump and it must be clearly labelled
• The administration set is to be changed every 24 h or, if using a 48 h infusion bag, according to local policy

Acute and Critical Care Nursing at a Glance, First Edition. Edited by Helen Dutton and Jacqui Finch
© 2018 John Wiley & Sons, Ltd. Published 2018 by John Wiley & Sons, Ltd.
Companion website: www.ataglanceseries.com/nursing/acutecare

Daily nutritional requirements in health

Good nutrition is essential to regulate the body's cell growth and repair. Carbohydrates, lipids and proteins (providing energy) and vitamins and minerals (catalysing metabolic reactions) are all essential nutrients, together with water. Sufficient intake of these can be achieved by consuming a healthy diet composed of largely starches, vegetables and fruit, with smaller portions of proteins and dairy and even smaller amounts of fats and simple sugars. Together these substances will provide the daily calorific requirements, currently estimated to be 2500 kcal for an adult male and 2000 kcal for an adult female.[1]

Malnutrition and the body's response to illness

NICE (2012) defines malnutrition as 'a state in which a deficiency of nutrients such as energy, protein, vitamins or minerals results in measurable adverse effects on body composition, function or clinical outcome'.[2] All individuals with a suboptimal diet are at risk, particularly those who are elderly with a reduced appetite, or who are unable to acquire and prepare food for themselves. Members of certain ethnic and subcultural groups may not eat all the recommended food types, thus predisposing them to malnutrition unless careful dietary adjustments are made. In acute and critical illness significant nutritional problems may occur. Firstly, the body experiences metabolic stress, especially with pyrexia, and this leads to increased energy expenditure and demand. Secondly, with hypoperfusion the cells are deprived of their normal energy sources and this leads to anaerobic metabolism and the production of lactic acid. This acidity creates a hostile environment for cells further impairing their growth, function and repair.[3] Periods of suboptimal nutrition lead to a state of starvation, with the body seeking alternative sources of energy, the first choice being protein from muscle. Patients who are hypermetabolic with sepsis or following trauma/burns injury are most at risk from this, with up to 25 g of nitrogen (metabolised protein) being lost per day. This can lead to severe muscle wasting, particularly in the form of skeletal muscle loss.

Nutritional assessment

The Care Quality Commission (2010) states that healthcare practitioners must ensure, in the interests of quality care, that all patients' nutritional needs are met.[4] Effective nutritional assessment is therefore required and should be carried out for all patients admitted to hospital and for those in the community. The assessment should be conducted using a validated assessment tool such as the **Malnutrition Universal Screening Tool (MUST)** and the findings clearly disseminated and documented.[2] This instrument calculates the risk of malnutrition by determining patients' body mass index (BMI), their percentage of unintentional weight loss and the effect of the disease process present. Any patient scoring two or above is deemed to be at high risk of malnutrition and in need of dietetic referral.

Providing nutritional support

Oral consumption of food should always be encouraged, as use of the digestive tract maintains its physiological integrity. However, for acutely ill patients who have anorexia, swallowing difficulties or impaired consciousness, an oral intake will not be possible and enteral or parenteral nutrition will be necessary. Enteral feeding can be accomplished via a number of different methods (Figure 52.1); the use of a fine-bore nasogastric tube being the most common. This is appropriate for patients who require short-term feeding of <4 weeks' duration. Passage of the tube is a skilled procedure, requiring the nurse to be assessed as competent to perform it independently. For patients with nasopharyngeal, laryngeal, oesophageal, or maxillofacial disorders or surgery, the procedure should be medically led as there may be anatomical derangement which would make the insertion particularly hazardous. For the same reason, a patient with a **facial or basal skull fracture** should **never** have a nasogastric tube inserted. If either of these injuries is a possibility (for example, with a trauma patient) they must be excluded radiologically prior to feeding. An orogastric tube can sometimes be used instead.

To prevent aspiration of any feed administered, it is essential to confirm that the enteral feeding tube is correctly placed.[5] Confirmation is by pH testing of the aspirate using pH indicator sticks, with a safe reading being <5.0 (Figure 52.2). If the patient is prescribed a proton pump inhibitor this can increase the pH value, so additional safety checks must be performed, with CXR seen as the gold standard measurement. Feeding regimes and types of feed prescribed will vary according to individual patient's dietary needs. In all cases it is important for the nurse to monitor accurately how much feed is being administered in conjunction with how much aspirate is being obtained; increasing amounts of aspirate indicate poor absorption. In these circumstances local policy will identify the steps to be taken next. These may include reduction in feed, replacement of some aspirated volume, or prokinetic therapy (such as metoclopromide) to enhance gastric emptying. All patients receiving enteral feed require specific nursing care in order to safely meet their nutritional needs and prevent any complications from occurring (Figure 52.3). For most patients, this type of short-term feeding will be sufficient but for those who experience ongoing problems, gastrostomy feeding (Box 52.1) or intravenous/parenteral nutrition (Box 52.2) will be required. With parenteral feeding, possible complications include infection, hyperglycaemia and **re-feeding syndrome**. The latter, which can also sometimes develop with oral and enteral feeding, occurs when carbohydrates are administered to a malnourished patient. Cellular fluid and electrolyte shifts occur, leading to severe depletion. In such cases specialist dietetic management will be required.

Nutritional support and rehabilitation

Good rehabilitation following an episode of critical illness depends on optimal nutrition and effective muscle exercise, with early mobilisation of the patient being a key feature. If physiotherapy and nurse-led active and passive limb movements are accompanied by effective feeding, it is not just the well-known problems of immobility such as pressure ulcer development and deep vein thrombosis that can be prevented. Combining these strategies will also assist the patient to regain muscle mass, strength and endurance, in preparation for going home.[6]

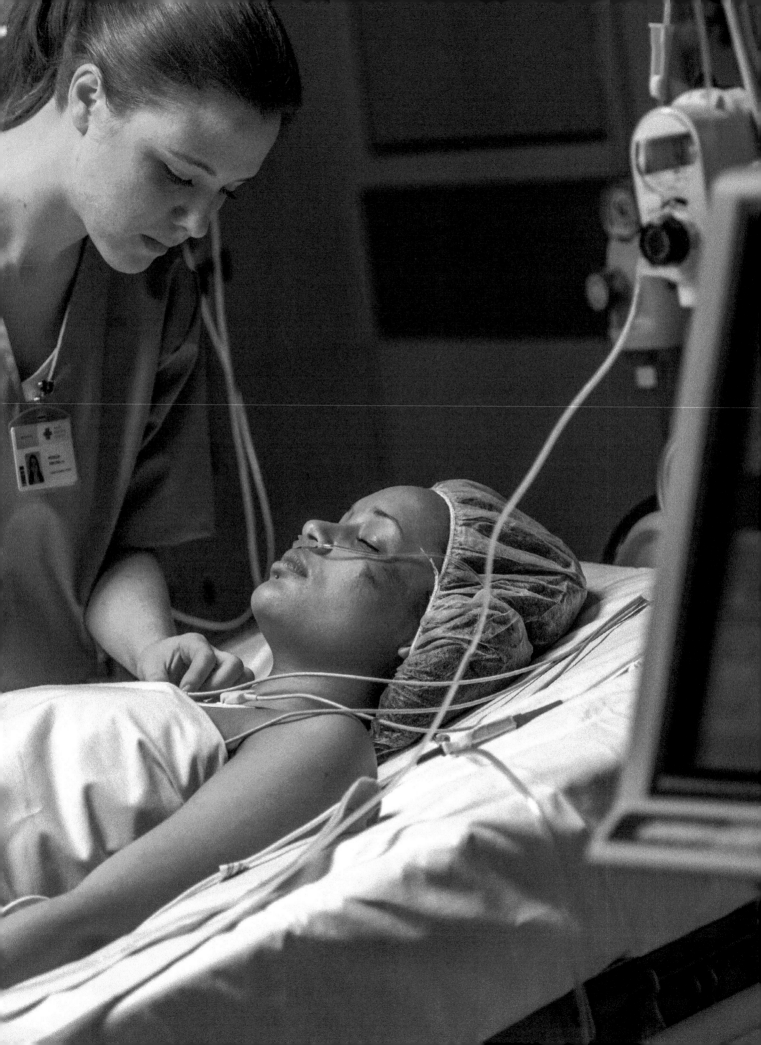

Decision making in acute and critical care

Part 7

Chapters

53 **Summary of decision making** 118
54 **Professional, legal and ethical considerations** 120
55 **Mental health concerns** 122
56 **Last days of life** 124

53 Summary of decision making

Figure 53.1 Processes to support decision making in practice

Prioritising/risk assessment

- Recognition of deterioration
- ABCDE assessment
- Early warning scores (e.g. NEWS)
- Pressure sore risk/falls risk/MUST

Ethico-legal issues

- Informed consent
- Safeguarding
- Human Rights
- Accountability
- Code of Conduct

Identifying problems/planning

- Writing diagnostic statements
- (Patient problems/needs)
- Development of care plan
- Setting short and long-term SMART goals

Using a systematic approach

- Nursing process frameworks, or models of nursing
- Nursing models describe the beliefs, values, and goals of nursing and the knowledge and skills needed to practise nursing. Examples include: Roper et al., 1996[6]; Orem 2001[7]

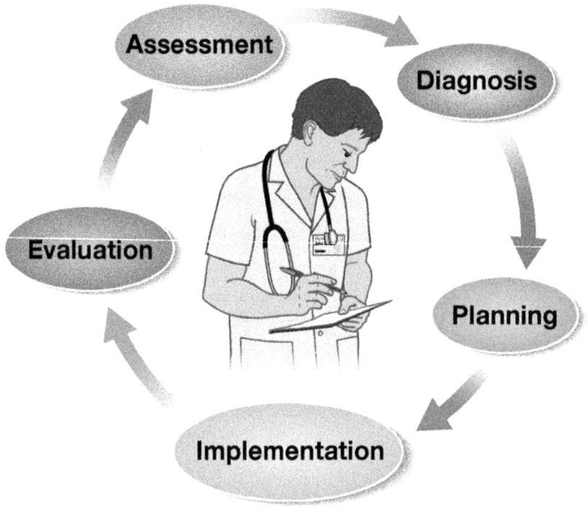

Communicating with others

- Patient
- 'No decision about me without me'[1]
- Relatives
- Multidisciplinary team
- Referring to other professionals
- Handovers/SBAR

Assessment — Diagnosis — Planning — Implementation — Evaluation

Assessment – subjective data

Collection of cues:
- patient history
- information from relatives
- symptom exploration
- review of systems
- review activities of living
- assess self-care ability
- lifestyle behaviours

Evaluation and reflection

- Self evaluation/self awareness
- Lifelong learning
- Reflection on decisions taken and care delivered

Knowledge underpinning practice

- Epidemiology
- Pathophysiology
- Social and behavioural sciences
- Pharmacology
- Ethics
- Law
- Nursing

Standardisation

- Assessment and interventions guided by evidence and policy help to reduce variation in delivery and patient outcomes e.g. National Institute for Health and Clinical Excellence (NICE) Quality Standards http://www.nice.org.uk/guidance/qualitystandards/qualitystandards.jsp
- NICE Pathways http://pathways.nice.org.uk/
- The Cochrane Collaboration http://www.cochrane.org/
- eGuidelines -http://www.eguidelines.co.uk/about_guidelines.php
- Scottish Intercollegiate Guidelines Network http://www.sign.ac.uk/guidelines/fulltext/129/index.html
- Evidence Based Nursing http://ebn.bmj.com/

Assessment – objective data

Collection of cues:
- vital signs
Physical examination:
- inspection
- palpation
- percussion
- auscultation
Diagnostic/laboratory data e.g. CXR/ECG/blood results/ABGs

Processing information

- Analysing data
- Synthesising data
- Selecting/rejecting cues
- Clustering cues
- Pattern recognition
- Identifying relationships
- Deductive reasoning
- Using experience and intuition

Acute and Critical Care Nursing at a Glance, First Edition. Edited by Helen Dutton and Jacqui Finch
© 2018 John Wiley & Sons, Ltd. Published 2018 by John Wiley & Sons, Ltd.
Companion website: www.ataglanceseries.com/nursing/acutecare

Clinical reasoning and decision making

Previous chapters have considered the challenge presented when caring for acutely unwell patients, and the many decisions made each day which impact on patient outcome. Patients who are acutely unwell present in a variety of healthcare settings and good clinical reasoning skills are needed in order to make sense of the care required in a range of different situations. Uncertainties exist in nursing practice; if the risk of patient deterioration is to be reduced, then the nurse must apply knowledge and make clinical judgements. An assessment is made, and then decisions as to the problem and required action. Planning follows and goals established to achieve the desired outcomes (Figure 53.1). This is a dynamic process and critical thinking is required so that the nurse is able to identify possible options based on evidence.

Assessment

Using a systematic approach in nursing, particularly in assessment, is important. The nursing process is familiar to all nurses but whilst this is useful in guiding problem solving, additional nursing frameworks and assessment tools are needed if assessment is to be effective. For the nurse to prioritise for the patient who is acutely unwell, physiologically based assessment tools such as the ABCDE approach (Figure 53.1) initially predominate. Once clinical stability is established, an appropriate nursing model (Figure 53.1) is a guide to ensure the patient's self-care ability is also assessed alongside lifestyle behaviours and coping ability. The patient's own experience and perceptions of critical illness/heath status (subjective data), gives insights into the individual's needs (Figure 53.1). Objective data through physical assessment can be obtained. Vital signs are recorded, as is data from a range of diagnostic tests (Figure 53.1). Using a systematic approach ensures that all relevant data is collected so that health needs/risks are identified and an accurate nursing diagnosis made.

The nurse must draw on a wide range of knowledge to process information (Figure 53.1) and inform the decision-making process. Patients bring risk with them into any healthcare encounter and whilst this may be linked to age, gender and lifestyle it may be influenced further by socioeconomic status, employment, education, gender and ethnicity, all interacting in complex ways. Social variations in health and illness are well documented and knowledge of life-course epidemiology will result in an awareness of the aetiology of disease and individual risk. An understanding of the pathophysiology of common disorders is important for all nurses as is knowledge of areas such as health psychology and pharmacology (Figure 53.1). With experience nurses are able to respond more speedily, often intuitively, in their decision making by recognising relevant cues and cue patterns, based on previous experiences. Identifying problems, developing plans of care and communicating these effectively (Figure 53.1) are essential elements to ensure coordinated care. The Government's aim is to give everyone more say over their care and treatment with more opportunity to make choices, with information and support, as outlined in 'No decision about me without me'.[1] Patients should be fully involved in decision making and nurses must ensure that informed consent is obtained at every stage of care.

Minimising risk

There are many risks which may impact adversely on patient outcome and whilst it is impossible to eliminate risk entirely, effective decision making minimises that risk. The Nursing and Midwifery Council require that all nurses are able to recognise and interpret signs of deteriorating mental and physical health and respond promptly.

Standardisation is seen as crucial due to the huge variations in healthcare delivery and patient outcomes. There is increasing evidence to show that when patterns of care are widely divergent, clinical outcomes suffer and safety may be compromised. Around one in 10 hospital admissions results in some form of harm.[2] There is excess mortality in hospital at weekends and more than half of acute hospitals inspected by the Care Quality Commissionin 2011 were non-compliant with standards of dignity and nutrition for older people.[3]

Evidence-based practice

Utilising the best evidence available to decide on the most appropriate course of action has been found to result in more consistent positive patient outcomes.Utilising evidence-based findings in healthcare practice is an important part of decision making and should involve nurses carrying out systematic searches and critical appraisal to improve patient care. The use of evidence-based findings in healthcare can be seen at a national level with the development of the NHS Outcomes Framework and the publishing of NICE Quality Standards (Figure 53.1), to drive commissioning as a result of the NHS Health and Social Care Act (2012).[4] At a more local level nurses may be involved in the use of structured multidisciplinary care plans outlining the essential steps in the care of patients with specific problems, e.g. clinical care pathways and enhanced recovery pathways. Care bundles have also been introduced as a way of improving specific care processes to improve patient outcomes. Care bundles consist of a group of evidence-based practices, that when performed together, consistently and reliably demonstrate an improvement in patient outcomes. Nurses are key players in reducing harm for patients in acute care through compliance to care bundles such as those for sepsis, catheter-associated urinary tract infection and care of central venous lines.

Ethical and legal issues

Nurses are accountable and must practise with confidence according to the Code: Standards of Conduct, Performance and Ethics for Nurses and Midwives[5] and within other recognised ethical and legal frameworks (also Chapter 54). Nurses need to be cognisant of how ethical principles relate to their practice, e.g.:
- Autonomy – informed consent/assumption of capacity.
- Beneficence – duty of care/promoting interests of patients.
- Non-maleficence – keeping up to date/evidence-based care/reducing risk/antidiscriminatory practice.
- Justice – human rights/dignity and respect (Figure 53.1).

All this must be accomplished with the nurse mindful of competing priorities and situational constraints such as time and resources available. On-going reflection is an important part of decision making (Figure 53.1) in order to learn, improving standards of care delivery.

54 Professional, legal and ethical considerations

Figure 54.1 Mental Capacity Act 2005. Best interest pathway – an example. Source: adapted from Mental Capacity Act, 2005.

Anything done for, or on behalf of a person who lacks capacity must be done in the person's best interests

Example: Kevin had a stroke 2 days ago
- At the moment his level of consciousness is reduced
- He is unable to communicate meaningfully with family or healthcare providers
- He is not able to cough effectively to remove purulent secretions, despite physiotherapy
- He does not understand the risks/benefits of having a mini-tracheostomy inserted, to remove secretions

Test for Capacity has found the person lacks the capacity to consent
Is a best interest meeting required?

Is it likely that the person may have capacity in the future?

Yes → It is possible that full capacity may be regained

No →

Can the decision or act wait until that time; consider if it is likely that the person will at some time have capacity to the matter in question

Capacity may not be regained in the timescale needed for this decision

Decision needed to consider 'ceiling of care' or whether to not actively resuscitate (DNAR status Chapter 56)

Does the decision involve serious medical treatment?

Decision needed to proceed with all active treatment: mini-tracheostomy insertion

Yes → No →

Delay the decision until that time

Can you identify when the person may have the capacity?

Document and discuss with relevant others

You will need to evidence your decision making

He may not recover from his chest infection if decision is delayed

The Mental Capacity Act 2005 introduced the role of the independent mental capacity advocate (IMCA). IMCAs are a legal safeguard for people who lack the capacity to make specific important decisions: including serious medical treatment options, if they have no relatives or close friends

No → Arrange the best interest meeting, invite all relevant parties and consider best interest for patient

Multidisciplinary meeting

Yes → Is there a relative/friend of individual nominated by the person to consult?

Yes → Involve relatives in all decisions made

No → Instruct IMCA

Box 54.1 The Mental Capacity Act Deprivation of Liberty safeguards

The MCA DOL safeguards apply to anyone:
- aged 18 and over
- who suffers from a mental disorder or disability of the mind, such as dementia or a profound learning disability
- who lacks the capacity to give informed consent to the arrangements made for their care and/or treatment and
- for whom deprivation of liberty (within the meaning of Article 5 of the ECHR) is considered after an independent assessment to be necessary in their best interests to protect them from harm

Box 54.2 The six 'C's

- Care
- Compassion
- Competence
- Communication
- Courage
- Commitment

Figure 54.2 A model for ethical decision making

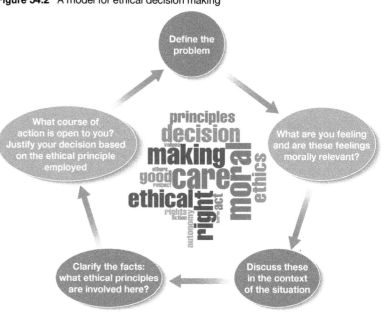

Define the problem

What are you feeling and are these feelings morally relevant?

Discuss these in the context of the situation

Clarify the facts: what ethical principles are involved here?

What course of action is open to you? Justify your decision based on the ethical principle employed

principles decision making good care ethical right moral ethics

Acute and Critical Care Nursing at a Glance, First Edition. Edited by Helen Dutton and Jacqui Finch
© 2018 John Wiley & Sons, Ltd. Published 2018 by John Wiley & Sons, Ltd.
Companion website: www.ataglanceseries.com/nursing/acutecare

Legal considerations

Mental Capacity Act (2005)

The issue of informed consent has long since been a challenge for critical care staff, particularly nurses who are caring for critically ill patients, may be with fluctuating levels of consciousness, too ill to make decisions. Informed consent may be assumed rather than explicit. The Mental Capacity Act (2005) came into practice in 2007 and exists to protect vulnerable people who cannot make decisions for themselves.[1] The Mental Capacity Act Best Interest Pathway (Figure 54.1) gives a practical guide to using the Act in practice, by asking a series of questions and providing the options and direction which clinical staff can then take.[2] Clinicians need to understand not only their duty in protecting vulnerable patients, but also need to 'have regard to' the Act's Code of Practice. In 2009 the Deprivation of Liberty safeguards (formally known as the Bournewood safeguards) came into being,[3] and apply to all organisations registered under the Care Standards Act (2000).[4] The standards clearly clarify the critical care nurse's responsibility to ensure these standards are adhered to for patients who cannot explicitly consent to their care (Box 54.1).

Ethical considerations

'Moral philosophy is the attempt to achieve a systematic understanding of the nature of morality and what it requires of us – in Socrates' words, of "how we ought to live", and why.' (UK Clinical Ethics Network, 2014)[5]

Ethical decision-making frameworks

All nurses face ethical dilemmas on a daily basis, and mostly can respond quickly and appropriately, making the right decision. But sometimes, ethical decisions create conflict, not least for critical care nurses working in high impact, high pressure areas where decisions have to be made quickly. Whether in the process of making the decision (reflection in action) or after the event (reflection on action) ethical decision-making frameworks are useful to help nurses understand and account for their decision-making process. A decision-making model will not tell you if you make the right decision (ethical decisions are rarely black and white) but it will give you an opportunity to check you make your decision for the right reason (Figure 54.2).

Deontology

From the Greek work Deos, meaning 'to do good', this theory comes from the philosophical work of Immanuel Kant, and is very focused on the individual, and the universal, unconditional and imperative requirement to adhere to all moral laws and principles. It is concerned with duty and obligation and is uniquely focused on the respect for the individual. For nursing, it is about making the right decision for that one patient at that time, regardless of the consequences.

Teleological theory

Based on the theories of John Stuart Mill, teleological theory focuses the consequences of one's actions. Unlike deontological theory, this approach considers what is likely to produce the greater outcome for the majority of the people affected by the decision. It is about producing the greatest good for the greater number. In critical care nursing, this approach can generate conflicts, for example with the closure of critical care beds and the redistribution of critical care services to specialist centres which can be several miles from the family home. Whilst this may help NHS managers rationalise resources, it does not take into account the needs of the individual family member who in addition to the stress of having a critically ill relative, may have to travel extensively or arrange local accommodation to be near loved ones.

Professional considerations

Nursing and Midwifery Council

The Code for Nurses and Midwives, effective from March 31, 2015, presents the professional standards that nurses and midwives must uphold in order to be registered with the NMC in order to practice in the UK. It is structured around four themes: prioritise people, practice effectively, preserve safety and promote professionalism and trust.[6] It was published with additional resources to explain what the Code means for patients. There is now clear and explicit detail regarding each registrant's requirement in respect of revalidation. For the first time, guidance on the use of social networking is now available.

Within the Code there is a clear focus on dignity and trust, both key elements of critical care nursing. The onus will be on both organisations and registrants to show that practice is transparent, and patient care is embedded with the 6 'Cs' (Box 54.2); six enduring values of nursing practice that were identified as priorities in the 2012 3-year strategy for nursing.[7] Following on from the reports into the Mid Staffordshire NHS Foundation Trust public enquiry (2013)[8] and others around the country, the 6 'Cs' have been widely used to support staff development and student nurse recruitment.

Record keeping

Accurate record keeping is both essential to good quality patient care, and good professional practice. Particularly when patients are not able to articulate their symptoms, the ability to detect trends and variation in a client's condition depends on the accuracy and completeness of the record. Meticulous completion of observation charts such as used in NEWS, with calculation of risk of deterioration are essential in the patient at risk of deterioration. The NMC (2015) have dedicated a complete section of the new Code to record keeping and this clearly outlines the registrants' obligation to keep clear and accurate records which identify risk and problems, shows all the steps that have been taken in response to a problem identified and how effective these have been.[6] Records should be completed at the time care has been provided or as soon as possible afterwards. The Code makes specific reference to the use of electronic records and stipulates that entries made must be attributable to the nurse making that entry.

Vulnerable adults

The NMC has issued guidance on caring for and safeguarding vulnerable adults (available from https://www.nmc.org.uk/standards/safeguarding/).[9] Critical care nurses need to be fully aware of both national guidance and their own local arrangements by reading their organisational policy on safeguarding and identify their local safeguarding champion. An excellent source and easy read version of the Government plan for safeguarding adults, is available from https://www.gov.uk/government/uploads/system/uploads/attachment_data/file/233284/Adult_Safeguarding_Statement_EasyRead.pdf.[10]

55 Mental health concerns

Figure 55.1 Top tips for nursing patients with dementia

Family
- Ask family for brief history to support conversations
- Show around the ward
- Have regular routines and staff
- Clocks visible to orientate to time

Eating and drinking
- Give regular prompts to eat and drink
- Offer finger foods to maintain independence
- Allow time to finish
- Have flexibility with meal times

Washing
- Ensure areas not being washed are covered to maintain dignity
- Warm room
- Showers may be frightening
- Don't wash hair if it increases distress

Box 55.2 Common signs of depression
- Poor concentration
- Fatigue, or energy loss
- Loss of appetite
- Low mood, feelings of guilt
- Loss of pleasure or interest in normally enjoyed activities
- Feelings of worthlessness
- Indecisiveness
- Disturbed sleep pattern

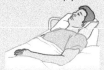

Interaction with patient
- Approach from the front
- Minimise distractions
- Maintain eye contact and be on the patient's level (sit if needed)
- Be patient
- Picture signs are more effective than words

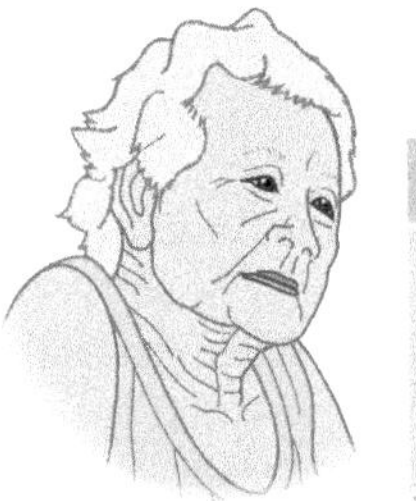

Toilet
- Show patient where the toilets are and ensure they are able to access them
- Give regular reminders
- Keep door open when not in use
- Easy to remove clothing

Activities
- Provide mental and physical activities to occupy
- When walking - ask them where they need to go and accompany them if possible
- Consider pain relief if walking being used to ease discomfort

Aggression
- Remember aggression is not deliberate
- Consider pain, thirst/hunger, need to toilet
- Stay calm, reassure, distract
- Give space, avoid closing in
- Look for warning signs and triggers

Figure 55.2 Risk factors and physiological mechanisms for delirium

Risk factors
- Anticholinergic drugs
- Age/dementia
- Hypoxia
- Anaemia
- Hypotension
- Poor nutrition
- Infection
- Surgery
- Alzheimer's disease

Physiological mechanism
↓ Acetylcholine
= neuronal excitability

Risk factors
- Benzodiazepines
- Alcohol withdrawal

Physiological mechanism
↓ Gamma-aminobutyric acid
= neuronal excitability

Risk factors
- Antidepressants
- Infection
- Hepatic encephalopathy

Physiological mechanism
↓ Serotonin

Risk factors
- Drugs, e.g. dopamine agonists
- Infection
- Trauma, especially fractured neck of femur
- Age/dementia

Physiological mechanism
↑ Dopamine
= ↓ release of acetylcholine

Risk factors
- Exogenous glucocorticoids
- Disruption of circadian rhythm

Physiological mechanism
↑ Cortisol and beta-endorphins

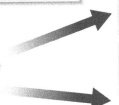
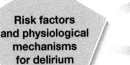

Risk factors and physiological mechanisms for delirium

Figure 55.3 Generalised Anxiety Disorder Assessment (GAD-7)

Over the **last 2 weeks**, how often have you been bothered by the following problems?	Not at all	Several days	More than half the days
1 Feeling nervous, anxious or on edge	0	1	2	3
2 Not being able to stop or control worrying	0	1	2	3
3 Worrying too much about different things	0	1	2	3
4 Trouble reading	0	1	2	3
5 Being so restless that it is hard to sit still	0	1	2	3
6 Becoming easily annoyed or irritable	0	1	2	3
7 Feeling afraid as if something awful might happen	0	1	2	3

GAD 7 total scores = column 1 + column 2 + column 3 + column 4
0–5 = mild, 6–10 = moderate, 11–15 = severe

Box 55.1 Screening for cognitive impairment – Abbreviated Mental Test Score (AMTS)

1 How old are you?
2 What time is it (nearest hour)?
3 Address for recall at the end – this should be repeated by the patient, e.g. 42 West Street
4 What year is it?
5 What is the name of this place?
6 Can the patient name two relevant persons (e.g. nurse/doctor)
7 What was the date of your birth?
8 When was the Second World War?
9 Who is the present Prime Minister?
10 Count down from 20 to 1 (no errors, no cues)

Scoring = 1 for each correct answer
Total less than 8 indicates cognitive impairment

Acute and Critical Care Nursing at a Glance, First Edition. Edited by Helen Dutton and Jacqui Finch
© 2018 John Wiley & Sons, Ltd. Published 2018 by John Wiley & Sons, Ltd.
Companion website: www.ataglanceseries.com/nursing/acutecare

Nurses working in acute and critical care areas frequently care for people with an enduring mental illness and/or long-term ailments as they are frequent users of acute hospital services. Mental health and physical health are indistinguishably interwoven, with chronic conditions such as diabetes and cancer associated with high rates of mental illness. Some 70% of NHS spend goes on the treatment of chronic illnesses including the assessment and treatments of psychosocial wellbeing in acute hospitals.[1] Physical illness increases the risk of mental illness, which may be exacerbated by admission into acute care. Mental health conditions account for 30% of acute inpatient bed occupancy and 30% of acute readmissions.[2] Older people occupy 66% of NHS beds and around 60% will have or develop a mental disorder during their admission.[3]

Patients admitted to acute care with an existing mental illness are likely to have received poorer quality healthcare prior to admission.[4] They are less likely to seek medical help, attend screening programmes, register with a GP, or may have difficulties in making and keeping appointments. The presence of a mental disorder may 'overshadow' the recognition and treatment of physical health problems. It is essential that acute care nurses are aware of the complexity of exploring patient problems, ensuring that physical problems are not missed in those experiencing mental illness. It is often overlooked how physical conditions can manifest as a deterioration in acute mental health status.

Recognising and assessing needs

Identifying important factors for mental wellbeing will influence patient care and management when acutely unwell. These include:

- dementia
- delirium
- depression

Older adults in particular may have elements of two or three of these conditions and it is important to understand each, in order to deliver immediate effective care and enable referral to appropriate services such as the Liaison Mental Health Service, or a psychiatrist.

Dementia

Dementia is caused by a group of conditions affecting the brain, most commonly Alzheimer's and vascular dementia. Symptoms include progressive problems with memory loss, problem solving and thinking. It affects over a half a million people in England alone, with many deaths directly attributable to the disease. A large proportion of people with dementia are undiagnosed and go into hospital with a physical problem. Detailed assessment of all patients therefore is required, recognising that a change in behaviour, or acute confusion, could be attributable to existing dementia. Understanding what is normal for that person often requires the assistance of family and carers. Cognitive impairment can be identified using simple tools such as the **Abbreviated Mental Test Score (AMTS)**, a quick screening tool that can be used on the hospital ward (Box 55.1). This aids in the delivery of appropriate care until a full assessment for dementia can be undertaken. Assessment for patients at risk should enable appropriate clinical actions to be utilised and improve the quality of care, reducing additional associated risks such as falls, poor nutrition and hydration. Potential environmental changes such as new admission to an acute care ward, new faces and alien clinical procedures can cause additional distress. Some top tips for nursing patients with dementia are been identified in Figure 55.1.

Delirium

Patients with delirium also experience disturbed cognitive function. Delirium features a sudden onset of either hypo- or hyperactivity, with significant changes from normal patterns of sleep and activity. Thinking is disorganised, perceptual disturbances, illusions or hallucinations may be present. Risk factors (identified in Figure 55.2) can lead to a number of physiological changes associated with delirium. NICE (2010)[5] recommend assessment and diagnosis using the Confusion Assessment Method (CAM) (Chapter 6), with treatment strategies to reduce harm, until delirium reduces. Patients with dementia and/or delirium require optimisation of nutrition and hydration status, strategies to reduce falls, the appropriate use of pain relief and regular reassurance suitable to their current mental state.

Depression

Depression is characterised by a history of low mood and a loss of pleasure in most activities, even those that were previously enjoyed. It is more common in those with a chronic physical illness; the risk is doubled for people with diabetes, hypertension, coronary artery disease and heart failure, and tripled in those with stroke and chronic obstructive pulmonary disease. As acute episodes for those with chronic physical illness precipitate acute care admission, nurses need to be aware of symptoms that suggest the patient may be depressed (Box 55.2). Formal screening tools such as the **Hospital Anxiety and Depression Scale (HADS)** and the **Generalised Anxiety Disorder Assessment (GAD-7)** are used to assist in providing insight into patients' psychological wellbeing, whether it is for a mental health diagnosis or hospital-induced anxiety and stress (Figure 55.3). Expert referral enables a treatment plan to be tailored to the individual's needs.

Liaison psychiatry services

Liaison psychiatry services are focused on the needs of people with dementia, substance misuse, anxiety and depression, the aim being that at least half of all Acute Trusts will deliver 'core 24' liaison psychiatry by 2020.[6] Access to mental health services within the acute setting should improve, with a range of strategies including psychosocial interventions, brief psychotherapeutic interventions, and pharmacotherapy. Services will follow the patient journey from primary care, to planned/unplanned hospital admission, to discharge, then back to primary care.[7]

56 Last days of life

Acute and Critical Care Nursing at a Glance, First Edition. Edited by Helen Dutton and Jacqui Finch
© 2018 John Wiley & Sons, Ltd. Published 2018 by John Wiley & Sons, Ltd.
Companion website: www.ataglanceseries.com/nursing/acutecare

Box 56.1 Decisions on ceilings of care. Source: RCP, 2013.

- Should involve the patient's consultant and be agreed by the whole team
- Should not be based on assumptions about age, disability or a professional's view on the patient's quality of life
- Should involve patients and their relatives or carers
- Should be clearly documented and reviewed periodically
- Should consider patient entry to end of life pathway

Figure 56.1 Advance care plan template

ACP

Step 3
- How should the agreed ACP outcome be operationalised?
- Communicate and document plan
- Prescribe end-of-life medications

Step 2
- What should be discussed and documented?
- Goals and ceilings of care
- Agreed management plan: medication and monitoring

Step 1
- Who is suitable?
- Does the patient have an advanced condition?
- Has the patient had three or more unplanned admissions in the last 6 months?
- Is a DNAR order in place?

Box 56.2 Five priorities of care. Source: LACDP, 2014.

'One chance to get it right'

- The possibility that a person may die within the coming days and hours is recognised and communicated clearly, decisions about care are made in accordance with the person's needs and wishes, and these are reviewed and revised regularly
- Sensitive communication takes place between staff and the person who is dying and those important to them
- The dying person, and those identified as important to them, are involved in decisions about treatment and care
- The needs of families and others identified as important to the dying person are actively explored, respected and met as far as possible
- An individual plan of care, which includes food and drink, symptom control and psychological, social and spiritual support, is agreed, coordinated and delivered with compassion

Figure 56.2 Care of the dying patient

Manage pain with:
- oral or subcutaneous morphine, or
- oral or subcutaneous oxycodone, or
- transdermal fentanyl or
- buprenorphine

Manage agitation and 'terminal restlessness' with midazolam or levomepromazine

Manage secretions with glycopyrronium bromide

Manage breathlessness with positional change. Oxygen may be prescribed for some patients

Ensure personal hygiene, oral and skin integrity

Manage GI disturbance:
- treat drug-induced nausea with metoclopramide, or cyclizine, or levomepromazine
- treat hiccups with baclofen or chlorpromazine
- treat constipation with co-danthramer or lactulose (rectal examination must be performed first)
- treat diarrhoea with loperamide (exclude infective cause first)

Manage hydration and nutritional support: offer sips of water and appropriate foods for as long as patient can swallow

Enable presence of loved ones providing privacy and support

Last days and hours of life

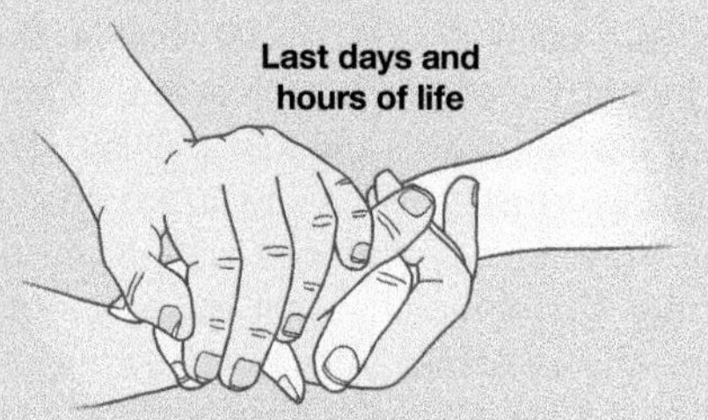

Deliver empathetic, compassionate care

Clinical decision making in the last days of life

It has been suggested that today we live in a 'death denying' society, even within healthcare settings. There is limited vocabulary for death; it is not a part of life with which people care to engage.[1] With the development of increased scientific knowledge and enhanced technological capability, expectations of the health service are high, especially within the critical care setting. Many patients and their relatives view a successful outcome only as survival from illness or injury, in spite of the immense physical and emotional distress that may be endured by patients and their families during the course of ill health. In contrast, healthcare professionals have been found to be more accepting of death and, during the last days of a patient's life, wish to see fewer therapeutic interventions.[2] In part, this can be attributed to repeated exposure to the sadness of end-of-life situations, but is also formulated by notions of what constitutes medical futility and whether or not a patient has currently, or will have in the future, any quality of life. Treatments may be viewed as prolonging the patient's suffering unnecessarily, whilst death is simultaneously seen as inevitable. However, whilst healthcare professionals must continually make decisions regarding the welfare of others, great care must be taken when making moral judgements about the quality of someone else's life. Conditions that some people would find unacceptable to live with, others might not.

Advance care planning

One of the challenges facing medical and nursing practitioners is that there is often uncertainty about the prognosis of acutely ill and deteriorating patients. Degree of responsiveness to treatment is unknown and, if a positive response is seen, in what time frame. Historically, this lack of recognition has been compounded by inadequate care planning for the last days of life.[3] The overall result, that quick transition from high interventional care to palliation has been problematic, with both patients and clinicians poorly prepared.[1,4] In the interests of patient-centred care, therefore, it is good practice (whenever possible) to ascertain the patient's wishes regarding the continuation or non-escalation of treatment in advance of severe deterioration. Discussion with the patient prior to the loss of capacity will greatly contribute to legally valid and ethically sound decision making. Treatment escalation strategies or ceilings of care (Box 56.1) should be debated.[5] For example, establishing time limits for response to non-invasive mechanical ventilation, or the decision made regarding whether or not to proceed to invasive ventilation should be initiated. A judgement on when a 'do not attempt resuscitation' (DNAR) status should be put in place can also be explored, as can the patient's wishes on organ/tissue donation.

Historically, some patients may have presented with advance directives (commonly known as living wills), but these have now been superseded by the notion of advance care planning. With their origins in the Mental Capacity Act (2005) an **Advance Care Plan** (ACP) or an '**Advance Decision to Refuse Treatment**' (ADRT) may be constructed with the patient prior to clinical deterioration or a '**lasting power of attorney for health**' (LPA) may be appointed. The latter will have the legal right to make choices on behalf of the patient when the capacity to self-determine is lost. In short, both the advance plans and the appointed attorneys will be able to identify patient preferences, when nearing the end of life.[6,7] Fortunately, advanced palliative care planning is becoming embedded across all healthcare settings and this is facilitating a more communicative and holistic approach to the care of dying patients.[1] Guidelines for the construction of an ACP are available and a three-step process is recommended (Figure 56.1).

Owing to the speed of their decline some patients will be unable to contribute to clinical decision making regarding their treatment. In fact, even if they were to request further or less intervention, if hypoxemia were a feature of their condition their capacity for sound reasoning could be legally challenged. In such cases it is incumbent upon the multidisciplinary team to make all decisions in the patient's best interests and the nurse in particular has a unique role to play. The close relationship that exists between nurses, patients and their families enables the former to act as a powerful advocate, articulating concerns and wishes to the medical staff on their behalf. The nurse is also able to effectively contribute to multidisciplinary clinical decision making, helping to ensure that actions taken are always in the patient's best interest. The nurse is primarily responsible for guaranteeing that whilst there may be '**futility of cure**', there will never be '**futility of care**'. The **Leadership Alliance for the Care of the Dying Patient**[8] published the '*One chance to get it right*' guidelines, replacing the previously controversial Liverpool Care pathway. These guidelines outline the approach to be taken when caring for patients in the last days and hours of their lives. Five key priorities are highlighted in Box 56.2.

Care of the dying patient in critical care

Critical care settings are generally very busy, noisy places. For this reason, whenever possible (and ward/unit geography allowing), the patient should be moved to a side room for peace and privacy. The patient's family will also benefit from this, allowing them proximity to their loved one independent of restrictive 'visiting hours' and the company of other patient's visitors who may not realise what is happening. If the use of a side room is not possible, the curtains around the bed space should be closed and treated as a closed door would be, with no unwanted intrusions. Seclusion of the patient will also facilitate delivery of all the physical care that is required, from removing unnecessary equipment such as cardiac monitoring, to effective symptom control. There are many unpleasant physical disturbances that the patient may experience in the last days of life; some of these symptoms will be primarily due to the dying process itself, others as a result of the pharmacology being used. Whatever the cause, they need to be carefully managed if the patient is to have a peaceful, dignified death[9] (Figure 56.2).

Immense psychological support is also required at this time and good communication is vital if all parties are to be kept well informed. The patient may not be aware of what is happening, but the family still requires reassurance, empathy and compassion. Culturally congruent care is important too, with any specific ethnic or religious requirements catered for wherever possible and spiritual representatives contacted to assist with this process. Finally, following death, the nurse is responsible for not only performing his or her last duties of care for the patient, but also caring for the relatives at this difficult time.

Appendix

Figure 45.5 Adult advanced life support algorithm. Source: RCUK, 2015. Reproduced with permission.

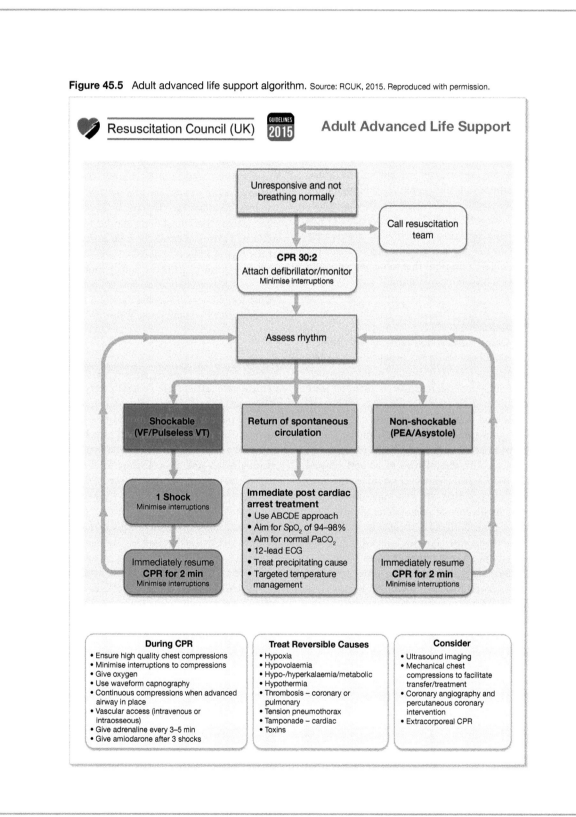

Acute and Critical Care Nursing at a Glance, First Edition. Edited by Helen Dutton and Jacqui Finch
© 2018 John Wiley & Sons, Ltd. Published 2018 by John Wiley & Sons, Ltd.
Companion website: www.ataglanceseries.com/nursing/acutecare

References and Further Reading

BTS, British Thoracic Society. DH, Department of Health. ICS, Intensive Care Society. NCEPOD, National Confidential Enquiry into Perioperative Deaths. NICE, The National Institute for Health and Care Excellence. NMC, Nursing and Midwifery Council. RCP, Royal College of Physicians. RCUK, Resuscitation Council UK. SIGN, Scottish Intercollegiate Guideline Network.

Part 1: Nursing in Acute and Critical Care

Chapter 1 Critical Care Without Walls

1. DH (2000) *Comprehensive Critical Care: A Review of Adult Critical Care Services*. The Stationery Office, London.
2. NICE (2014) Safer Staffing for Nursing in Adult inpatient Wards in Acute Hospitals. https://www.nice.org.uk/guidance/sg1 (accessed 12 April 2017).
3. Network National Nurse Leads (2015) National Competency Framework for Adult Critical Care Nurses. cc3n.org.uk/competency-framework/4577977310 (accessed 12 April 2017).
4. NMC (2015) The Code: Professional standards of practice and behaviour for nurses and midwives. http://www.nmc.org.uk/globalassets/sitedocuments/nmc-publications/revised-new-nmc-code.pdf (accessed 12 April 2017).
5. ICS (2013) Core Standards for Intensive Care Units. https://www.ficm.ac.uk/sites/default/files/Core%20Standards%20for%20ICUs%20Ed.1%20(2013).pdf (accessed 12 April 2017).
6. Francis R (2013) *Report of the Mid Staffordshire NHS Foundation Trust Public (Inquiry: Executive Summary)*. Stationery Office, London.
7. Findlay G *et al.* (2012) *Time to Intervene? A Review of Patients who Underwent Cardiopulmonary Resuscitation as a Result of an In-Hospital Cardiorespiratory Arrest*. NCEPOD, London.
8. NICE (2007) (CG50) Acute illness in adults in hospital: recognising and responding to deterioration. https://www.nice.org.uk/Guidance/CG50 (accessed 12 April 2017).
9. RCP (2012) National Early Warning Score (NEWS). Standardising the Assessment of Acute-Illness Severity in the NHS. https://www.rcplondon.ac.uk/sites/default/files/documents/national-early-warning-score-standardising-assessment-acute-illness-severity-nhs.pdf (accessed 12 April 2017).
10. The Shelford Group (2014) Safer Nursing Tool Implementation Resource Pack. Association of UK University Hospitals. http://shelfordgroup.org/library/documents/Shelford_Safer_Nursing_23May14a.pdf (accessed 1 April 2017).
11. http://sepsistrust.org (accessed 12 April 2017).

Chapter 2 Recognising Risk of Deterioration: ABCDE Assessment

1. RCUK (2015) The ABCDE approach. https://www.resus.org.uk/resuscitation-guidelines/abcde-approach/ (accessed 12 April 2017).
2. O'Driscoll BR, Howard LS and Davison AG on behalf of the British Thoracic Society (2008) BTS guideline for emergency oxygen use in adult patients. *Thorax*, **63** (Suppl VI) Vi1–vi68. https://www.brit-thoracic.org.uk/document-library/clinical-information/oxygen/emergency-oxygen-use-in-adult-patients-guideline/emergency-oxygen-use-in-adult-patients-guideline/ (accessed 12 April 2017).
3. Goldhill D, White S, and Sumner A (1999) Physiological values and procedures in the 24 h before ICU admission from the ward. *Anaesthesia*, **54**, 529–534. http://onlinelibrary.wiley.com/doi/10.1046/j.1365-2044.1999.00837.x/pdf (accessed 12 April 2017).

Chapter 3 Early Warning Tools and Care Escalation

1. NMC (2015) The Code: Professional Standards of Practice and Behaviour for Nurses and Midwives. http://www.nmc.org.uk/globalassets/sitedocuments/nmc-publications/revised-new-nmc-code.pdf (accessed 12 April 2017).
2. NICE (2007) (CG50) Acutely ill patients in hospital: recognising and responding to deterioration. https://www.nice.org.uk/guidance/cg50 (accessed 12 April 2017).
3. RCP (2012) National Early Warning Score (NEWS). Standardising the Assessment of Acute-Illness Severity in the NHS. https://www.rcplondon.ac.uk/sites/default/files/documents/national-early-warning-score-standardising-assessment-acute-illness-severity-nhs.pdf (accessed 12 April 2017).
4. RCP (2013) Acute care toolkit. The medical patient at risk: recognition and care of the seriously ill or deteriorating patient. https://www.rcplondon.ac.uk/resources/acute-care-toolkit-6-medical-patient-risk (accessed 12 April 2017).
5. O'Driscoll B, Bakerly N, Murphy P *et al.* (2013) Concerns regarding the design of the bedside monitoring chart for use with the NEWS (National Early Warning System). *Clinical Medicine*, **133**, 19–20.

Chapter 4 Hospital-Acquired Infection: Infection Prevention and Control

1. Hopkins S, Shaw K and Simpson L (2012) English national point prevalence survey on healthcare associated infections and antimicrobial use, 2011: preliminary data. Health Protection Agency.
2. Smyth ETM, McIlvenny G, Enstone JE *et al.* and Hospital Infection Society Prevalence Survey Steering Group (2008) Four country healthcare associated infection prevalence survey 2006: overview of the results. *Journal of Hospital Infection*, **69**, 230–248.
3. Loveday HP, Wilson J, Pratt R *et al.* (2014) Epic3: national evidence-based guidelines for preventing healthcare-associated infections in NHS hospitals in England. *Journal of Hospital Infection*, **86**, S1–S70.
4. WHO (2009) 'How to Handwash'. www.who.int/gpsc/5may/How_To_Handwash_ Poster_pdf (accessed 29 July 2017).
5. WHO (2009) 'How to Handrub'. www.who.int/gpsc/5may/How_To_Handrub_ poster_pdf (accessed 29 July 2017).
6. Blaine C, Pellowe C and Hodgkinson S (2012) Improving infection prevention practice in primary and community care. *Journal of Hospital Infection*, **82**, 274–276.
7. DH (2007) Saving lives: reducing infection, delivering clean and safe care. http://webarchive.nationalarchives.gov.

Acute and Critical Care Nursing at a Glance, First Edition. Edited by Helen Dutton and Jacqui Finch
© 2018 John Wiley & Sons, Ltd. Published 2018 by John Wiley & Sons, Ltd.
Companion website: www.ataglanceseries.com/nursing/acutecare

uk/20120118164404/hcai.dh.gov.uk/whatdoido/high-impact-interventions (accessed 12 April 2017).

8. Rowley S and Macqueen CS (2010) ANTTv2: an updated practice framework for aseptic technique. *British Journal of Nursing*, **19**(Suppl), S5–S11.

Chapter 5 Pain Management

1. Carr EC, Meredith P, Chumbley G *et al.* (2014) Pain: a quality of care issue during patients' admission to hospital. *Journal of Advanced Nursing*, **70**, 1391–1403.
2. Subramanian P, Allcock N, James V *et al.* (2011) Challenges faced by nurses in managing pain in a critical care setting. *Journal of Clinical Nursing*, **21**, 1254–1262.
3. Macintyre P and Schug S (2015) *Acute Pain Management: A Practical Guide* (4th edn). CRC Press, Boca Raton.
4. Paulson-Conger M, Leske J, Maidl C *et al.* (2011) Comparison of two pain assessment tools in non-verbal critical care patients. *Pain Management Nursing*, **12**, 218–224.
5. Smith J, Rockett M, Creanor S *et al.* (2015) Pain Solutions in the Emergency Setting (PASTIES) – patient controlled analgesia versus routine care in emergency department patients with non-traumatic abdominal pain: randomised trial *BMJ*, **350**, h3147.

Chapter 6 Psychosocial Issues

1. Yu J and Kahn J (2015) Creating a learning healthcare system in the ICU, in Annual update in *Intensive Care and Emergency Medicine* (ed. J. Vincent). Springer, Switzerland. pp. 587–596.
2. Ely E, Margolin R, Francis J *et al.* (2001) Evaluation of delirium in critically ill patients: validation of the Confusion Assessment Method for the Intensive Care Unit: CAM ICU. *Critical Care Medicine*, **29**, 1370–1379
3. NICE (2010) (CG103) Delirium: prevention, diagnosis and management (revalidated 2015). https://www.nice.org.uk/guidance/cg103 (accessed 12 April 2017).
4. Mental Capacity Act (2005) https://www.legislation.gov.uk (accessed 12 April 2017).
5. Mental Capacity Act Deprivation of Liberty Safeguards (2009) http://webarchive.nationalarchives.gov.uk/+/www.dh.gov.uk/en/socialcare/deliveringadultsocialcare/mentalcapacity/mentalcapacityactdeprivationoflibertysafeguards/index.htm (accessed 12 April 2017).

Chapter 7 Safe Transfer of the Acutely Unwell Patient

1. ICU (2011) Guidelines for the transport of the critically ill adult (3rd edn). http://www.ics.ac.uk/ICS/guidelines-and-standards.aspx
2. RCUK (2015) Advanced Life Support. https://www.resus.org.uk/resuscitation-guidelines/adult-advanced-life-support/ (accessed 12 April 2017).
3. O'Driscoll BR, Howard LS and Davison AG on behalf of the British Thoracic Society (2008) BTS guideline for emergency oxygen use in adult patients. *Thorax*, **63** (Suppl VI) Vi1–vi68. https://www.brit-thoracic.org.uk/document-library/clinical-information/oxygen/emergency-oxygen-use-in-adult-patients-guideline/emergency-oxygen-use-in-adult-patients-guideline/ (accessed 12 April 2017).
4. Handy J and Van Zwanenberg G (2009) Secondary transfer of the critically ill patient *Current Anaesthesia and Critical Care*, **18**, 303–310.

Further Reading
Finch J (2012) The safe transfer of acutely ill patients, in *Acute Nursing Care. Recognising and Responding to Medical Emergencies* (1st edn) (eds I Peate and H Dutton). Pearson, Harlow. pp. 313–325.

Part 2: Airways: Maintaining Airway Patency

Chapter 8 Upper Airway Assessment and Management

1. RCUK (2015) Adult basic life support. https://www.resus.org.uk/resuscitation-guidelines/adult-basic-life-support-and-automated-external-defibrillation/ (accessed 12 April 2017).
2. Peate I and Nair M (2011) *Fundamentals of Anatomy and Physiology for Student Nurses*. John Wiley & Sons, Ltd, Chichester.
3. Leach RM (2014) *Critical Care Medicine at a Glance* (3rd edn). John Wiley & Sons, Ltd, Chichester.

Further Reading
Elliot S (2012) Recognition and management of cardiopulmonary arrest, in *Acute Nursing Care. Recognising and Responding to Medical Emergencies* (1st edn) (eds I Peate and H Dutton). Pearson, Harlow. Chapter 7.

Chapter 9 Advanced Airway Management

1. RCUK (2015) Adult basic life support. https://www.resus.org.uk/resuscitation-guidelines/adult-basic-life-support-and-automated-external-defibrillation/ (accessed 12 April 2017).
2. Leach RM (2014) *Critical Care Medicine at a Glance* (3rd edn). John Wiley & Sons, Ltd, Chichester.

Further Reading
Elliot S (2012) Recognition and management of cardiopulmonary arrest, in *Acute Nursing Care. Recognising and Responding to Medical Emergencies* (1st edn) (eds I Peate and H Dutton). Pearson, Harlow. Chapter 7.

Chapter 10 Airway Management: Tracheostomy

1. ICS (2014) Standards for the care of adult patients with a tracheostomy: standards and guidelines. http://www.ics.ac.uk/ICS/guidelines-and-standards.aspx (accessed 12 April 2017).
2. NCEPOD (2014) On the right trach? A review of the care received by patients who underwent tracheostomy. http://www.ncepod.org.uk/2014report1/downloads/OnTheRightTrach_FullReport.pdf (accessed 12 April 2017).
3. McGrath BA, Bates L, Atkinson D *et al.* (2012) Multidisciplinary guidelines for the management of tracheostomy and laryngectomy airway emergencies. *Anaesthesia*, **67**, 1025–1041.

Part 3: Breathing: Patients with Breathing Problems

Chapter 11 Respiratory Physiology: Oxygenation

Further Reading
Margereson C and Withey S (2012) The patient with acute respiratory problems, in *Acute Nursing Care. Recognising and Responding to Medical Emergencies* (1st edn) (eds I Peate and H Dutton). Pearson, Harlow. pp. 82–106

Chapter 12 Respiratory Physiology: Ventilation

Further Reading

Margereson C and Withey S (2012) The patient with acute respiratory problems, in *Acute Nursing Care. Recognising and Responding to Medical Emergencies* (1st edn) (eds I Peate and H Dutton). Pearson, Harlow. pp. 82–106

Chapter 13 Assessment of Breathing

1. Goldhill DR, Worthington L, Mulcahy A *et al.* (1999) The patient-at-risk team: identifying and managing seriously ill ward patients. *Anaesthesia*, **54**, 853–860.
2. RCP (2012) National Early Warning Score (NEWS). Standardising the Assessment of Acute-Illness Severity in the NHS. https://www.rcplondon.ac.uk/sites/default/files/documents/national-early-warning-score-standardising-assessment-acute-illness-severity-nhs.pdf (accessed 12 April 2017).
3. O'Driscoll BR, Howard LS, Earis J, Mak V on behalf of the Oxygen Guidelines Development Group (2017). BTS Guideline for oxygen use in adults in healthcare and emergency settings. *Thorax*, **72**, (Suppl 1)i1–i90 https://www.brit-thoracic.org.uk/document-library/clinical-information/oxygen/2017-emergency-oxygen-guideline/bts-guideline-for-oxygen-use-in-adults-in-healthcare-and-emergency-settings/ (accessed 2 June 2017).

Chapter 14 Respiratory Investigations

1. BTS (2016): SIGN 153 British guideline on the management of asthma. A national clinical guideline. https://www.brit-thoracic.org.uk/document-library/clinical-information/asthma/btssign-asthma-guideline-2016/ (accessed 02 June 2017).
2. NICE (2010) (CG101) Chronic obstructive pulmonary disease in over 16s: diagnosis and management (partial update 2014). http://www.nice.org.uk/guidance/cg101 (accessed 12 April 2017).
3. Clarke C and Dux A (2011) *Chest X-rays for Medical Students*. John Wiley & Sons, Ltd, Chichester.
4. Leach RM (2014) *Critical Care Medicine at a Glance* (3rd edn). John Wiley & Sons, Ltd, Chichester.

Chapter 15 Oxygen Therapy

1. O'Driscoll B, Howard, L, Davidson (2011) Emergency oxygen use in adult patients: Concise guidance to good practice sheets Royal College of Physicians. https://www.rcplondon.ac.uk/guidelines-policy/emergency-oxygen-use-adult-patients (accessed 12 April 2017).
2. O'Driscoll B, Howard L, Earis J, *et al.* on behalf of the British Thoracic Society Emergency Oxygen Guideline Development Group (2017) BTS guideline for oxygen use in adults in healthcare and emergency settings. *Thorax* **72** Supplement i1-i89. https://www.brit-thoracic.org.uk/standards-of-care/guidelines/bts-guideline-for-emergency-oxygen-use-in-adult-patients/ (accessed 25 July 2017).
3. Davidson C, Banham S, Elliot M *et al.* BTS/ICS Acute Hypercapnic Respiratory Failure Guideline Development Group, On behalf of the BTS standards of Care Committee (2016) BTS/ICS Guidelines for the Ventilatory Management of Acute Hypercapnic Respiratory Failure in Adults. *Thorax*, **71**, ii1–ii35. https://www.brit-thoracic.org.uk/document-library/clinical-information/acute-hypercapnic-respiratory-failure/ventilatory-management-of-ahrf/ (accessed 12 April 2017).
4. Brill SE and Wedzicha JA (2014) Oxygen therapy in acute exacerbations of chronic obstructive pulmonary disease. *International Journal of COPD*, **9**, 1241–1252
5. Nishimura M (2015) High-flow nasal cannula oxygen therapy in adults. *Journal of Intensive Care*, **3**, 15. http://www.jintensivecare.com/content/3/1/15 (accessed 12 April 2017).

Chapter 16 Respiratory Failure

1. Davidson C, Banham S, Elliot M *et al.* BTS/ICS Acute Hypercapnic Respiratory Failure Guideline Development Group, On behalf of the BTS standards of Care Committee (2016) BTS/ICS Guidelines for the Ventilatory Management of Acute Hypercapnic Respiratory Failure in Adults. *Thorax*, **71**, ii1–ii35. https://www.brit-thoracic.org.uk/document-library/clinical-information/acute-hypercapnic-respiratory-failure/ventilatory-management-of-ahrf/ (accessed 12 April 2017).

Further Reading

Margereson C and Withey S (2012) The patient with acute respiratory problems in in *Acute Nursing Care. Recognising and Responding to Medical Emergencies* (1st edn) (eds I Peate and H Dutton). Pearson, Harlow. pp. 82–106.

Chapter 17 Breathing Problems: Obstructive Disorders

1. RCP (2014) Why asthma still kills. The National Review of Asthma Deaths (NRAD), Confidential Enquiry Report. https://www.rcplondon.ac.uk/sites/default/files/why-asthma-still-kills-full-report.pdf (accessed 12 April 2017).
2. BTS (2016): SIGN 153 British guideline on the management of asthma. A national clinical guideline. https://www.brit-thoracic.org.uk/document-library/clinical-information/asthma/btssign-asthma-guideline-2016/ (accessed 02 June 2017).
3. NICE (2010) (CG101) Chronic obstructive pulmonary disease in over 16s: diagnosis and management (partial update 2014). http://www.nice.org.uk/guidance/cg101 (accessed 12 April 2017).
4. Davidson C, Banham S, Elliot M *et al.* BTS/ICS Acute Hypercapnic Respiratory Failure Guideline Development Group, On behalf of the BTS standards of Care Committee (2016) BTS/ICS Guidelines for the Ventilatory Management of Acute Hypercapnic Respiratory Failure in Adults. *Thorax*, **71**, ii1–ii35. https://www.brit-thoracic.org.uk/document-library/clinical-information/acute-hypercapnic-respiratory-failure/ventilatory-management-of-ahrf/ (accessed 12 April 2017).
5. NCEPOD (2012) Time to Intervene? A review of patients who underwent cardiopulmonary resuscitation as a result of an in-hospital cardiorespiratory arrest. A report by the National Confidential Enquiry into Patient Outcome and Death (2012). http://www.ncepod.org.uk/2012report1/downloads/CAP_full-report.pdf (accessed 12 April 2017).
6. RCP (2008) (Updated 2013) Non-invasive ventilation in chronic obstructive pulmonary disease. 1 Concise Guideline. https://www.rcplondon.ac.uk/resources/concise-guidelines-non-invasive-ventilation-chronic-obstructive-pulmonary-disease (accessed 12 April 2017).

Chapter 18 Breathing Problems: Lung (Parenchymal) Disorders

1. World Health Organisation (2011) Pneumonia Fact Sheet No. 331. http://tinyurl.com/72u95la (accessed 12 April 2017).
2. Lim WS and Woodhead M (2011) British Thoracic Society adult community acquired pneumonia audit 2009/10. *Thorax*, **66**, 218–549.

3. NICE (2014) (CG191) Pneumonia in adults: diagnosis and management. http://www.nice.org.uk/guidance/cg191/resources/guidance-pneumonia-pdf (accessed 12 April 2017).
4. BTS and NHS Improvement (2012) BTS Community Acquired Pneumonia (CAP) Care Bundle 2012 CAP1. https://www.brit-thoracic.org.uk/document-library/audit-and-quality-improvement/care-bundles-project/care-bundle-data-collection-sheets/bts-cap-care-bundle-data-sheets/ (accessed 12 April 2017).
5. Leach RM (2014) *Critical Care Medicine at a Glance* (3rd edn). John Wiley & Sons, Ltd, Chichester.

Chapter 19 Breathing Problems: Pleural Disorders

1. BTS (2010) Pleural disease guideline. https://www.brit-thoracic.org.uk/document-library/clinical-information/pleural-disease/pleural-disease-guidelines-2010/pleural-disease-guideline/ (accessed 12 April 2017).
2. Myatt R (2014) Diagnosis and management of patients with pleural effusions. *Nursing Standard*, **28**, 51–58.
3. MacDuff A, Arnold A, Harvey J and the BTS Pleural Disease Guideline Group (2010) Management of spontaneous pneumothorax: British Thoracic Society Pleural Disease Guideline. *Thorax*, **65** (Suppl 2), ii8–ii31.
4. Woodrow P (2013) Intrapleural chest drainage. *Nursing Standard*, **5**, 49–56.
5. Hooper C, Lee YC, Maskell N and the BTS Pleural Guideline Group (2010) Investigation of a unilateral pleural effusion in adults: British Thoracic Society Pleural Disease Guideline. *Thorax*, **65** (Suppl 2), ii4–ii17.

Chapter 20 Respiratory Support: Non-invasive Ventilation

1. RCP (2015) COPD: Who Cares Matters. National COPD Audit Programme: clinical audit of COPD exacerbations admitted to acute units in England and Wales 2014. Executive summary. https://www.rcplondon.ac.uk/projects/outputs/copd-who-cares-matters-clinical-audit-2014 (accessed 12 April 2017).
2. Davidson C, Banham S, Elliot M *et al.* BTS/ICS Acute Hypercapnic Respiratory Failure Guideline Development Group, On behalf of the BTS standards of Care Committee (2016) BTS/ICS Guidelines for the Ventilatory Management of Acute Hypercapnic Respiratory Failure in Adults. *Thorax*, **71**, ii1–ii35. https://www.brit-thoracic.org.uk/document-library/clinical-information/acute-hypercapnic-respiratory-failure/ventilatory-management-of-ahrf/ (accessed 12 April 2017).
3. Nishimura M (2015) High flow nasal cannula oxygen therapy in adults. *Journal of Intensive Care*, **3**, 15. http://www.jintensive-care.com/content/3/1/15 (accessed 12 April 2017).
4. Moxon A and Lee G (2015) Non-invasive ventilation in the emergency department for patients in type II respiratory failure due to COPD exacerbations. *International Emergency Nursing*, **23**, 232–236.
5. NHS England (2015) Patient Safely Alert Stage One: Warning. Risk of severe harm and death from unintentional interruption of non-invasive ventilation NHS/PSA/W/2015/003. http://www.england.nhs.uk/wp-content/uploads/2015/02/psa-niv.pdf (accessed 12 April 2017).
6. Leach RM (2014) *Critical Care Medicine at a Glance* (3rd edn). John Wiley & Sons, Ltd, Chichester.

Chapter 21 Principles of Thoracic Surgery

There are no references or Further Reading for this chapter.

Part 4: Circulation: Patients with Circulatory Problems

Chapter 22 Circulatory Physiology 1: Circulation

1. Peate I, Wild K and Nair M (2014) *Nursing Practice: Knowledge and Care*. John Wiley & Sons, Ltd, Chichester.

Further Reading

Dutton H, Elliot S and Sargant A (2012) The patient with acute cardiovascular problems, in *Acute Nursing Care. Recognising and Responding to Medical Emergencies* (1st edn) (eds I Peate and H Dutton). Pearson, Harlow. pp. 108–182.

Chapter 23 Circulatory Physiology 2: The Heart and Cardiac Cycle

1. Ward JPT and Linden RWA (2013) *Physiology at a Glance* (3rd edn). John Wiley & Sons, Ltd, Chichester.
2. Aaronson PI, Ward JPT, Connolly MJ (2013) *The Cardiovascular System at a Glance* (4th edn). John Wiley & Sons, Ltd, Chichester.

Further Reading

Dutton H, Elliot S and Sargant A (2012) The patient with acute cardiovascular problems, in *Acute Nursing Care. Recognising and Responding to Medical Emergencies* (1st edn) (eds I Peate and H Dutton). Pearson, Harlow. pp. 108–182.

Chapter 24 Circulatory Physiology 3: Control of the Circulation

Further Reading

Dutton H, Elliot S and Sargant A (2012) The patient with acute cardiovascular problems, in *Acute Nursing Care. Recognising and Responding to Medical Emergencies* (1st edn) (eds I Peate and H Dutton). Pearson, Harlow. pp. 108–182.

Chapter 25 Assessment of Circulation

1. National Institute for Cardiovascular Outcomes Research (NICOR) (2013) National Heart Failure Audit April 2012–March 2013. https://www.ucl.ac.uk/nicor/audits/heartfailure/documents/annualreports/hfannual12-13.pdf (accessed 12 April 2017).
2. RCP (2013) Acute care toolkit 6 The medical patient at risk: recognition of the seriously ill or deteriorating medical patient May 2013). https://www.rcplondon.ac.uk/sites/default/files/acute_care_toolkit_6.pdf (accessed 12 April 2017).
3. Clark C, Taylor R, Shore A, Cambell J (2012) The difference in blood pressure readings between arms and survival: primary cohort study. *BMJ*, **344**, e1327.
4. NICE (2011) (CG127) Hypertension in adults: diagnosis and management (reviewed 2016). https://www.nice.org.uk/guidance/cg127 (accessed 12 April 2017).

Chapter 26 Cardiac Investigations

1. NICE (2014) (CG187) Acute heart failure: diagnosis and management. https://www.nice.org.uk/guidance/cg187 (accessed 12 April 2017).
2. NICE (2010) (CG108) Chronic heart failure in adults: management. https://www.nice.org.uk/guidance/cg108 (accessed 12 April 2017).

3. NICE (2013) (CG167) Myocardial infarction with ST-segment elevation. https://www.nice.org.uk/Guidance/CG167 (accessed 12 April 2017).
4. NICE (2010 updated 2016) (CG95) Chest pain of recent onset: assessment and diagnosis. https://www.nice.org.uk/guidance/cg95/chapter/Recommendations (accessed 22 July 2017).

Chapter 27 Fluid, Electrolytes and Intravenous Fluids

1. NCEPOD (2011) Knowing the risks: a review of the perioperative care of surgical patients. http://www.ncepod.org.uk/2011report2/downloads/POC_fullreport.pdf (accessed 12 April 2017).
2. NICE (2013) (CG174), Intravenous fluid therapy in adults in hospital. Update 2016. https://www.nice.org.uk/guidance/cg174 (accessed 12 April 2017).
3. Wunderlich R (2013) Principles in the selection of intravenous solution replacement: sodium and water balance. *Journal of Infusion Nursing*, **36**, 126–130.
4. Raghunathan K, Murray P, Beattie, W *et al.* (2014) Choice of fluid in acute illness: what should be given? An international consensus. *British Journal of Anaesthesia*, **113**, 722–783.

Chapter 28 Haemodynamic Monitoring

1. Lesle R, Gouldson S, Habib N *et al.* (2013) Management of arterial lines and blood sampling in intensive care: a threat to patient safety. *Anaesthesia*, **68**, 1114–1119.
2. NICE (2013) (CG174) Intravenous fluid therapy in adults in hospital. Update 2016. https://www.nice.org.uk/guidance/cg174 (accessed 12 April 2017).
3. Gordy S and Rowell S (2013) Vascular air embolism. *International Journal of Critical Illness and Injury Science*, **3**, 73–76.
4. Loveday H, Wilson J, Pratt R *et al.* (2014) Epic 3 National evidence-based guidelines for preventing healthcare associated infections in NHS hospitals in England. *Journal of Hospital Infection*, **8651**, S1–S70.

Chapter 29 Acute Chest Pain

1. Tagney J (2012) Clinical skills: history taking in cardiac patients. *British Journal of Cardiac Nursing*, **7**, 588–594.
2. Ambrose A and Singh M (2015) Pathophysiology of coronary artery disease leading to acute coronary syndromes. F1000Prime Reports 2015, 7:08 doi 10.12703/P7-08.
3. SIGN (2012) SIGN 93. Acute Coronary Syndromes. http://www.sign.ac.uk/pdf/qrgchd.pdf (accessed 12 April 2017).
4. NICE (2013) (CG167) Myocardial infarction with ST-segment elevation: acute management. https://www.nice.org.uk/guidance/cg167 (accessed 12 April 2017).
5. Roffi *et al.* (2016) 2015 ESC Guidelines for the management of acute coronary syndromes in patients presenting without persistent ST-segment elevation. *European Heart Journal*, **37**, 267–315.

Chapter 30 The 12-Lead Electrocardiogram

1. Aaronson PI, Ward JPT, Connolly MJ (2013) *The Cardiovascular System at a Glance* (4th edn). John Wiley & Sons, Ltd, Chichester.

Further Reading

Dutton H, Elliot S and Sargant A (2012) The patient with acute cardiovascular problems, in *Acute Nursing Care. Recognising and Responding to Medical Emergencies* (1st edn) (eds I Peate and H Dutton). Pearson, Harlow. pp. 108–182.

Hampton J (2013) *The ECG Made Easy* (8th edn). Churchill Livingstone, Edinburgh.

Chapter 31 Altered Heart Rhythm

1. NICE (2014) (CG180) Atrial fibrillation: management. https://www.nice.org.uk/guidance/cg180 (accessed 12 April 2017).
2. RCUK (2015) Resuscitation Guidelines. https://www.resus.org.uk/resuscitation-guidelines/in-hospital-resuscitation/ (accessed 12 April 2017).
3. Hughes T and Cruickshank J (2011) *Adult Emergency Medicine at a Glance* (1st edn). John Wiley & Sons, Ltd, Chichester.

Chapter 32 Physiology of the Immune System

1. Peate I and Nair M (2011) *Fundamentals of Anatomy and Physiology for Student Nurses*. John Wiley & Sons, Ltd, Chichester.

Further Reading

Blay A, Finch J and Dutton H (2012) The immune and lymphatic systems, infection and sepsis, in *Acute Nursing Care. Recognising and Responding to Medical Emergencies* (1st edn) (eds I Peate and H Dutton). Pearson, Harlow. pp. 283–312.

Chapter 33 Acute Circulatory Failure 1: Distributive (Sepsis)

1. NCEPOD (2015) Just say sepsis! A review of the process of care received by patient with sepsis. http://www.ncepod.org.uk/2015report2/downloads/JustSaySepsis_FullReport.pdf (accessed 12 April 2017).
2. Dellinger P, Levy M, Rhodes A *et al.* (2013) Surviving Sepsis Campaign: International guidelines for management of severe sepsis and septic shock: 2012. *Critical Care Medicine*, **41**, 580–637. http://www.sccm.org/Documents/SSC-Guidelines.pdf (accessed 12 April 2017).
3. Singer M, Deutschman CS, Seymour CW *et al.* (2016) The third international consensus definitions for sepsis and septic shock (Sepsis-3). *JAMA*, **315**, 801–810. http://jama.jamanetwork.com/article.aspx?articleID=2492881 (accessed 12 April 2017).
4. Russell J (2015) A positive future for novel sepsis candidates. *International Symposium on Intensive Care and Emergency Medicine News* March Issue 1, pp. 2–3.
5. NICE (2016) Sepsis: recognition, diagnosis and management NICE guidelines: short version. Draft for Consultation. https://www.nice.org.uk/guidance/GID-CGWAVE0686/documents/short-version-of-draft-guideline (accessed 12 April 2017).
6. Shankar-Hari M, Phillips G, Levy M *et al.* (2016) Assessment of definition and clinical criteria for septic shock. *JAMA* doi:10.1001/jama.2016.0289
7. UK Sepsis Trust, and The College of Emergency Medicine (2014) Sepsis: A Toolkit for Emergency Departments. http://sepsistrust.org/wp-content/uploads/2015/08/1409306451EMTLoolkit2014FINAL.compressed.pdf (accessed 12 April 2017).

Chapter 34 Acute Circulatory Failure 2: Distributive (Anaphylaxis and Neurogenic)

1. RCUK (2008, revalidated 2011) Emergency treatment of anaphylactic reactions: Guidelines for healthcare providers. https://www.resus.org.uk/anaphylaxis/emergency-treatment-of-anaphylactic-reactions/ (accessed 12 April 2017).
2. NICE (2011) (CG134) Anaphylaxis: assessment and referral after emergency treatment. https://www.nice.org.uk/guidance/cg134 (Reviewed 2014) (accessed 12 April 2017).

Chapter 35 Acute Circulatory Failure 3: Hypovolaemia

1. Resuscitation Council UK (2011) The ABCDE approach. https://www.resus.org.uk/resuscitation-guidelines/abcde-approach/ (accessed 12 April 2017).
2. NICE (2013 , updated 2017) (CG174) Intravenous fluid therapy in adults in hospital. https://www.nice.org.uk/guidance/cg174 (accessed 12 April 2017).
3. Ragahunathan K, Murray P, Beattie W *et al.* (2014) Choice of fluid in acute illness: what should be given? An international consensus. *British Journal of Anaesthesia*, **113**, 772–783.

Chapter 36 Acute Circulatory Failure 4: Obstructive

1. NICE 2012 (CG144) Venous thromboembolic diseases: diagnosis, management and thrombophilia testing http://www.nice.org.uk/guidance/cg144/chapter/1-recommendations (accessed 12 April 2017).
2. Roberts DJ, Leigh-Smith S, Faris PD *et al.* (2014) Clinical manifestation of tension pneumothorax: a protocol for a systematic review and meta-analysis. *Systematic Reviews*, **3**, 3.
3. Woodrow P (2013) Intrapleural chest drainage. *Nursing Standard*, **37**, 49–56.

Chapter 37 Acute Circulatory Failure 5: Heart Failure

1. Pearse S and Cowie M (2014) Heart failure: classification and pathophysiology. *Medicine*, **42**, 556–561.
2. NICE (2010) (CG108) Chronic heart failure in adults: management. http://www.nice.org.uk/guidance/cg108 (accessed 12 April 2017).
3. NICE 2014 (CG187) Acute heart failure: diagnosis and management. http://www.nice.org.uk/guidance/cg187/chapter/1-recommendations (accessed 12 April 2017).
4. Riley J (2013) Acute decompensated heart failure: diagnosis and management. *British Journal of Nursing*, **22**, 1290–1295.

Chapter 38 Principles of Cardiac Surgery

Further Reading

Danitsch D (2011) Cardiothoracic care, in *Nursing in Cardiac Care* (1st edn) (ed. M Humphreys). John Wiley & Sons, Ltd, Chichester. pp. 112–123.

Chapter 39 Anatomy and Physiology of the Gastro-intestinal Tract

1. Peate I and Nair M (2011) *Fundamentals of Anatomy and Physiology for Student Nurses*. John Wiley & Sons, Ltd, Chichester.

Chapter 40 Acute Medical and Surgical Gastro-intestinal Problems

1. NICE (2012) (CG141) Acute upper gastrointestinal bleeding in over 16s: management. https://www.nice.org.uk/guidance/cg141 (accessed 12 April 2017).

Further Reading

Howard J and Morgan A (2012) The patient with acute gastrointestinal problems, in *Acute Nursing Care. Recognising and Responding to Medical Emergencies* (1st edn) (eds I Peate and H Dutton). Pearson, Harlow. pp. 240–261.

Marini J and Wheeler A (2012) Hepatic failure, in *Critical Care Medicine* (4th edn). Lippincott Williams and Wilkins, Philadelphia. pp. 555–564.

Chapter 41 Physiology of the Renal System

1. Peate I and Nair M (2011) *Fundamentals of Anatomy and Physiology for Student Nurses*. John Wiley & Sons, Ltd, Chichester.

Further Reading

Finch J (2012) The patient with acute renal problems, in *Acute Nursing Care. Recognising and Responding to Medical Emergencies* (1st edn) (eds I Peate and H Dutton). Pearson, Harlow. pp. 184–205.

Chapter 42 Acute Kidney Injury

1. NCEPOD (2009) Acute Kidney Injury: Adding Insult to Injury available from http://www.ncepod.org.uk/2009report1/Downloads/AKI_report.pdf (accessed 12 April 2017).
2. NICE (2013) (CG169) Acute kidney injury: prevention, detection and management. https://www.nice.org.uk/guidance/cg169 (accessed 12 April 2017).
3. Bellomo R, Ronco C, Kellum JA, Palevsky P and ADQI Workgroup (2004) Acute renal failure – definition, outcome measures, animal models, fluid therapy and information technology needs: the Second International Consensus Conference of the Acute Dialysis Quality Initiative (ADQI) Group. *Critical Care*, **4**, 204–212.
4. Mehta RL, Kellum JA, Shah SV, Molitoris. B, Ronco. C, Warnock.D, Levin.A and the Acute Kidney Injury Network (2007) Acute Kidney Injury Network: report of an initiative to improve outcomes in acute kidney injury https://www.ncbi.nlm.nih.gov/pubmed/17331245 (accessed 12 April 2017).
5. Kidney Disease Improving Global Outcomes (KDIGO) (2012) Clinical practice guideline for acute kidney injury *Kidney International Supplement* 3.1. http://www.kdigo.org/clinical_practice_guidelines/pdf/KDIGO%20AKI%20Guideline.pdf (accessed 12 April 2017).

Further Reading

Finch J (2012) The patient with acute renal problems, in *Acute Nursing Care. Recognising and Responding to Medical Emergencies* (1st edn) (eds I Peate and H Dutton). Pearson, Harlow. pp. 184–205.

RCP (2015) Acute care toolkit 12. Acute kidney injury and intravenous fluid therapy. https://www.rcplondon.ac.uk/guidelines-policy/acute-care-toolkit-12-acute-kidney-injury-and-intravenous-fluid-therapy (accessed 12 April 2017).

Chapter 43 Burns: Immediate Care

1. Hettiraratchy S and Papini R (2004) Initial management of a major burn: assessment and resuscitation. *BMJ* **329**(7457), 101–103.

Chapter 44 Major Trauma

1. NICE (2016) (NG39) Major trauma: assessment and initial management. https://www.nice.org.uk/guidance/ng39/resources/major-trauma-assessment-and-initial-management-1837400761285 (accessed 12 April 2017).
2. NICE (2016) (NG41) Major trauma: service delivery. https://www.nice.org.uk/guidance/ng40/resources/major-trauma-service-delivery-1837446110917 (accessed 12 April 2017).
3. CEMS News (2014) Emergency medical journal. emj.bmj.com/content/suppl/2014/05/15/DCI/EMJSUPP-2014.S5.pdf (accessed 29 July 2017).
4. London HEMS medical student workbook (2014) Module 5: Breathing. www.uk.hems.co.uk (accessed 29 July 2017).

Chapter 45 Resuscitation

1. RCP (2012) National Early Warning Score (NEWS). Standardising the Assessment of Acute-Illness Severity in the NHS. https://www.rcplondon.ac.uk/sites/default/files/documents/national-early-warning-score-standardising-assessment-acute-illness-severity-nhs.pdf (accessed 12 April 2017).
2. Douw G, Schoonhoven L, Holwerda T *et al.* (2015) Nurses' worry or concern and early recognition of deteriorating patients on general wards in acute care hospitals: a systematic review *Critical Care*, **19**, 230.
3. RCUK (2015) Resuscitation Guidelines. https://www.resus.org.uk/resuscitation-guidelines/ (accessed 12 April 2017).
4. Dwyer T and Freil D (2016) Inviting family to be present during cardiopulmonary resuscitation. *Nurse Education in Practice*, **16**, 247–249.
5. Omar KS and Duran CR (2010) Health care providers' evaluations of family presence during resuscitation. *Journal of Emergency Nursing*, **36**, 524–533.
6. RCUK (1996) Should Relatives Witness Resuscitation? A report from a project team of the Resuscitation Council UK. https://www.resus.org.uk/archive/archived-cpr-information/should-relatives-witness-resuscitation/ (accessed 12 April 2017).
7. Nolan J, Soar J, Smith G, Gwinnutt C *et al.* on behalf of the National Cardiac Arrest Audit (2014) Incidence and outcome of in-hospital cardiac arrest in the United Kingdom. National Cardiac Arrest Audit. *Resuscitation,* **85**, 987–992.

Part 5: Disability: Patients with Neurological Impairment

Chapter 46 Physiology of the Brain

1. Peate I, Wild K and Nair M (2014) *Nursing Practice: Knowledge and Care.* John Wiley & Sons, Ltd, Chichester.

Further Reading

Scales K (2012) The patient with acute neurological problems, in *Acute Nursing Care. Recognising and Responding to Medical Emergencies* (1st edn) (eds I Peate and H Dutton). Pearson, Harlow. pp. 313–325.

Chapter 47 Neurological Assessment

1. RCUK (2015) The ABCDE approach. https://www.resus.org.uk/resuscitation-guidelines/abcde-approach/ (accessed 12 April 2017).
2. Rank W (2013) Performing a focused neurologic assessment. *Nursing* 43(12) 37-40
3. Jevon P, Ewens B, Singh Pooni J (2012) *Monitoring the Critically Ill Patient* (3rd edn). Wiley–Blackwell, Oxford. pp. 154–176.

Further Reading

Scales K (2012) The patient with acute neurological problems, in *Acute Nursing Care. Recognising and Responding to Medical Emergencies* (1st edn) (eds I Peate and H Dutton). Pearson, Harlow. pp. 313–325.

Chapter 48 Neurological Impairment

1. Marini J and Wheeler A (2012) Neurological emergencies in *Critical Care Medicine* (4th edn). Lippincott Williams and Wilkins, Philadelphia. pp. 595–629.
2. Scales K (2012) The patient with acute neurological problems, in *Acute Nursing Care. Recognising and Responding to Medical Emergencies* (1st edn) (eds I Peate and H Dutton). Pearson, Harlow. pp. 313–325.

3. NICE (2008, updated 2017) Stroke and transient ischaemic attack in over 16s: diagnosis and initial management CG 68. https://www.nice.org.uk/guidance/cg68/chapter/1Guidance#pharmacological-treatments-for-people-with-acute-stroke (accessed 29 July 2017).
4. NICE (2014, updated 2017) 'Head injury: assessment and early management. www.nice.org.uk/guidance/cg176 (accessed 29 July 2017).

Chapter 49 Drug Overdose and Poisoning

1. National Poisons Information Service Report 2013/2014. http://www.npis.org/NPISAnnualReport2013-14.pdf (accessed 12 April 2017).
2. Commission on human medicines (2012) Treating Paracetamol overdose with intravenous acetylcysteine: new guidance. www.gov.uk/government/organisations/commission-on-human-medicines (accessed 29 July 2017).

Further Reading

Marini J and Wheeler A (2012) Drug overdose and poisoning in *Critical Care Medicine* (4th edn). Lippincott Williams and Wilkins, Philadelphia. pp. 579–594.

Chapter 50 Acute Endocrine Problems

1. British National Formulary (2015) 64. BMJ Group, London.
2. Howard J and Morgan A (2012) The patient with acute endocrine problems, in *Acute Nursing Care. Recognising and Responding to Medical Emergencies* (1st edn) (eds I Peate and H Dutton). Pearson, Harlow. pp. 263–282.
3. NICE (2015, updated 2016) Type 1 Diabetes in adults: diagnosis and management. www.nice.org.uk/guidance/ng17 (accessed 29 July 2017).
4. Resuscitation Council (2015) The ABCDE Approach. www.resus.org.uk/resuscitation-guidelines/abcde-approach/ (accessed 29 July 2017).
5. NICE (2017) Safer Insulin prescribing. www.nice.org.uk/advice/ktt20/chapter/Evidence-context (accessed 29 July 2017).

Further Reading

1. Huether S (2006) Mechanisms of hormonal regulation, in *Pathophysiology. The Biologic Basis for Disease in Adults and Children* (5th edn) (eds K McCance and S Huether). Elsevier Mosby, Utah. pp. 655–679.
2. Jones R and Huether S (2006) Alterations in hormonal regulation in *Pathophysiology. The Biologic Basis for Disease in Adults and Children* (5th edn) (eds K McCance and S Huether). Elsevier Mosby, Utah. pp. 683–734.

Part 6: Exposure

Chapter 51 Skin Integrity

1. NICE (2014) (CG179) Pressure ulcers; prevention and management. https://www.nice.org.uk/guidance/cg179/resources/pressure-ulcers-prevention-and-management-35109760631749 (accessed 12 April 2017).
2. National Pressure Ulcer Advisory Panel (NPUAP) (2016) NPUAP Pressure injury stages http://www.npuap.org/resources/educational-and-clinical-resources/npuap-pressure-injury-stages/ (accessed 12 April 2017).
3. Visual Infusion Phlebitis (VIP) Score (1998). http://www.vipscore.net
4. Infusion Nursing Standards of Practice (INS) (2011) *Journal of Infusion Nursing.* Supplement. 34(1s)

5. Peate I, Wild K and Nair M (2014) *Nursing Practice: Knowledge and Care*. John Wiley & Sons, Ltd, Chichester.
6. Nice (2015) (KTT 14) Wound care products. https://www.nice .org.uk/advice/ktt14 (accessed 12 April 2017).

Chapter 52 Nutritional Assessment and Support

1. NHS Choices (2015) The eat well plate. www.nhs.uk/livewell/ goodfood/ (accessed 12 April 2017).
2. NICE Quality Standard QS24 (2012) Nutrition support in adults. https://www.nice.org.uk/Guidance/QS24 (accessed 12 April 2017).
3. Woodrow P (2012) *Intensive Care Nursing. A Framework for Practice* (3rd edn). Routledge, Abingdon. pp. 86–94.
4. Care Quality Commission (2010) Outcome 5: Meeting nutritional needs. http://moderngov.staffordshire.gov.uk/documents/ s14410/Appendix%20Two%20Outcome%205.pdf (accessed 12 April 2017).
5. National Patient Safety Agency (2011) Reducing the harm caused by misplaced nasogastric feeding tubes in adults, children and infants. http://www.npsa.nhs.uk/corporate/news/ reducing-the-harm-caused-by-misplaced-nasogastric-feeding-tubes-in-adults-children-and-infants/ (accessed 12 April 2017).
6. Wischmeyer P and San Millan I (2015) Winning the war against ICU-acquired weakness: new innovations in nutrition and exercise physiology. www.ccforum.com/content/19/S3/S6/ (accessed 12 April 2017).

Part 7: Decision Making in Acute and Critical Care

Chapter 53 Summary of Decision Making

1. DH (2012) Liberating the NHS: No Decision About Me, Without Me. https://consultations.dh.gov.uk/choice/choice-future-proposals/supporting_documents/Choice%20consultation%20% 20No%20decison%20about%20me%20without%20me.pdf (accessed 12 April 2017).
2. House of Commons Health Committee (2009) Patient Safety. Sixth Report of Session 2008–2009. http://www.publications .parliament.uk/pa/cm200809/cmselect/cmhealth/151/151i.pdf (accessed 12 April 2017).
3. Care Quality Commission (2011) Dignity and nutrition inspection programme. National Overview. http://www.cqc.org.uk/sites/ default/files/documents/20111007_dignity_and_nutrition_ inspection_report_final_update.pdf (accessed 12 April 2017).
4. Health and Social Care Act (2012) http://www.legislation.gov .uk/ukpga/2012/7/contents/enacted (accessed 12 April 2017).
5. NMC (2015) The Code: Professional standards of practice and behaviour for nurses and midwives. http://www.nmc.org.uk/ globalassets/sitedocuments/nmc-publications/revised-new-nmc-code.pdf (accessed 12 April 2017).
6. Roper N, Logan WW, Tierney AJ (1996) *The Elements of Nursing: A model for nursing based on a model for living* (4th edn). London: Churchill Livingstone.
7. Orem D (2001) *Nursing: Concepts of Practice* (6th Ed). Missouri: Mosby.

Chapter 54 Professional, Legal and Ethical Considerations

1. Mental Capacity Act (2005) http://www.legislation.gov.uk/ ukpga/2005/9/pdfs/ukpga_20050009_en.pdf (accessed 12 April 2017).
2. Kent A, Hood M and Johns S (2010) Mental Capacity Act (2005) Best Interest Pathway. http://www.rcgp.org.uk/~/media/ Files/CIRC/Learning%20disabilities/Best%20Interest%20Path-way.ashx (accessed 12 April 2017).
3. Mental Capacity Act Deprivation of Liberty Safeguards (2009) http://webarchive.nationalarchives.gov.uk/+/www.dh.gov .uk/en/socialcare/deliveringadultsocialcare/mentalcapacity/ mentalcapacityactdeprivationoflibertysafeguards/index.htm (accessed 12 April 2017).
4. Care Standards Act 2000 (summary) http://www.legislation.gov .uk/ukpga/2000/14/notes/division/2 (accessed 12 April 2017).
5. UK Clinical Ethics Network (2014) http://www.ukcen.net/index .php/education_resources/support_guide/section_c_ethical_ frameworks Accessed 21/5/2014 (accessed 12 April 2017).
6. NMC (2015) The Code: Professional standards of practice and behaviour for nurses and midwives. http://www.nmc.org.uk/ globalassets/sitedocuments/nmc-publications/revised-new-nmc-code.pdf (accessed 12 April 2017).
7. Cummings J. and Bennett V (2012) Compassion in Practice, Nursing, Midwifery and Care Staff. Our Vision and Strategy. http://www.england.nhs.uk/wp-content/uploads/2012/12/ compassion-in-practice.pdf (accessed 12 April 2017).
8. Francis R (2013) Report of the Mid Staffordshire NHS Foundation Trust Public Inquiry. The Stationary Office, London. http:// webarchive.nationalarchives.gov.uk/20130107105354/http:/ www.dh.gov.uk/en/Publicationsandstatistics/Publications/ PublicationsPolicyAndGuidance/DH_113018 (accessed 12 April 2017).
9. NMC (2015) Introduction to safeguarding for adults. https:// www.nmc.org.uk/standards/safeguarding/introduction-to-safeguarding-for-adults/ (accessed 12 April 2017).
10. DH (2013) The Government's plan for safeguarding adults. https://www.gov.uk/government/uploads/system/uploads/ attachment_data/file/233284/Adult_Safeguarding_Statement_ EasyRead.pdf (accessed 12 April 2017).

Chapter 55 Mental Health Concerns

1. Royal College of Psychiatrists (2007) *No Health Without Mental Health: The Supporting Evidence*. Academy of Medical Royal Colleges/Royal College of Psychiatrists, London.
2. NHS Confederation (2009) Healthy mind, healthy body: how liaison psychiatry services can transform quality and productivity in acute settings. NHS Confederation, London. http://www .nhsconfed.org/~/media/Confederation/Files/Publications/ Documents/Briefing_179_Healthy_mind_healthy_body_ MHN.pdf (accessed 12 April 2017).
3. NICE (2009) (CG91) Depression in adults with a chronic physical health problem: recognition and management. https://www .nice.org.uk/guidance/cg91/resources/depression-in-adults-with-chronic-physical-health-problem-recognition-and-management-975744316357 (accessed 12 April 2017).
4. Disability Rights Commission (2006) Equal Treatment: Closing the Gap. A formal investigation into physical health inequalities experienced by people with learning disabilities and/or mental health problems. http://disability-studies.leeds.ac.uk/files/ library/DRC-Health-FI-main.pdf (accessed 12 April 2017).
5. NICE (2010) (CG 103) Delirium: prevention, diagnosis and management (revalidated 2015). https://www.nice.org.uk/ guidance/cg103 (accessed 12 April 2017).
6. Royal College of Psychiatrists (2016) The Five Year Forward View For Mental Health; A Policy Unit briefing on the findings of the independent Mental Health Taskforce and the implications for psychiatrists and the wider NHS workforce. http://www.rcpsych.ac.uk/pdf/The_Five_Year_Forward_View_ for_Mental_Health_RCpsych_Policy_Briefing.pdf (accessed 12 April 2017).

7. Aitkin P, Robens S and Emmend T (2014) Liaison psychiatry Services – Guidance. http://mentalhealthpartnerships.com/wp-content/uploads/sites/3/1-liaison-psychiatry-services-guidance.pdf (accessed 12 April 2017).

Further Reading

Snaith RP (2003) The Hospital Anxiety Depression Scale. *Health and Quality of Life Outcomes*, **1**, 29. http://hqlo.biomedcentral.com/articles/10.1186/1477-7525-1-29 (accessed 12 April 2017).

Mental Health Taskforce (2016) The Five Year Forward View for Mental Health. NHS England. https://www.england.nhs.uk/wp-content/uploads/2016/02/Mental-Health-Taskforce-FYFV-final.pdf (accessed 12 April 2017).

Goldberg SE, Cooper J, Blundell A *et al.* (2016) Development of a curriculum for advanced nurse practitioners working with older people with frailty in the acute hospital through a modified Delphi process. *Age and Ageing*, **45**, 48–53.

The Commission to review the provision of acute inpatient psychiatric care for adults (2016) Old Problems, New Solutions: Improving Acute Psychiatric Care for Adults in England. http://www.rcpsych.ac.uk/pdf/Old_Problems_New_Solutions_CAAPC_Report_England.pdf (accessed 12 April 2017).

NHS Education for Scotland (2011) Acute Care Dementia Learning Resource. http://www.nes.scot.nhs.uk/media/350872/acute_dementia_interactive_2011.pdf (accessed 12 April 2017).

Chapter 56 Last Days of Life

1. Endacott R and Boyer C (2013) Preparing for the unavoidable: public and clinical expectations of death. *Nursing in Critical Care,* **18**, 112–113.

2. Sprung C, Carmel S, Sjokvist P *et al.* and ETHICATT study group (2007) Attitudes of European physicians, nurses, patients and families regarding end of life decisions: the ETHICATT stud *Intensive Care Medicine*, **33**, 104–110.

3. NCEPOD (2012) Time to intervene? A review of patients who underwent cardiopulmonary resuscitation as a result of an in-hospital cardiorespiratory arrest. http://www.ncepod.org.uk/2012report1/downloads/CAP_summary.pdf (accessed 12 April 2017).

4. Andrews T (2015) To cure sometimes, to relieve often and to comfort always: nurses' role in end of life decision making. *Nursing in Critical Care*, **20**, 227–228.

5. RCP (2013) Acute Care Toolkit 6: The medical patient at risk. https://www.rcplondon.ac.uk/guidelines-policy/acute-care-toolkit-6-medical-patient-risk (accessed 12 April 2017).

6. RCP (2009) Advance care planning. Concise Guidance to Good Practice. Available from: https://www.rcplondon.ac.uk/guidelines-policy/advance-care-planning (accessed 12 April 2017).

7. General Medical Council (2010) Advance Care Planning. http://www.gmc-uk.org/End_of_life.pdf_32486688.pdf (accessed 12 April 2017).

8. Leadership Alliance for Care of Dying People (2014) One chance to get it right. www.england.nhs.uk/ourwork/qual-clin-lead/lac (accessed 12 April 2017).

9. NICE (2015) Care of dying adults in the last days of life. www.nice.org.uk/guidance/ng31 (accessed 29 July 2017).

Glossary

Abbreviated Mental Test Score A quick screening tool that can be used on the hospital ward to screen for dementia or confusion

Abciximab Abciximab (ReoPro) is a platelet aggregation inhibitor, belonging to the group that antagonise the glycoprotein IIb/IIIa receptor on platelets. Glycoprotein IIb/IIIa inhibitors are used during percutaneous coronary interventions to inhibit clot formation. Others in this group include eptifibatide (Integrilin) and tirofiban (Aggrastat)

Accessory muscles The accessory muscles of respiration are used when the work of breathing increases; their use is a sign of respiratory distress. The accessory muscles include the sternomastoid and the scalene

Accountability Accountability is being responsible for one's actions, and the result of these actions. Registered healthcare professionals are accountable for their actions. Additionally, registered nurses have a duty to ensure that any activity delegated must be given within that person's competence, and must be adequately supervised to ensure that the task delegated reaches the required standard

Acetylcholine A neurotransmitter of the parasympathetic nervous system

Acquired immune system See specific immune system

Active transport Using energy in the form of adenosine triphosphate to move substances across a membrane

Acute coronary syndrome An umbrella term for problems that interfere with coronary artery perfusion, including unstable angina, NSTEMI and STEMI

Acute left ventricular failure This is a condition where the left ventricle of the heart fails to contract forcefully enough, leading to insufficient cardiac output and back pressure of accumulated blood causing pulmonary congestion and oedema

Adenosine Adenosine is an antiarrhythmic medication given to slow down the electrical conduction of the heart. It can be used to treat supraventricular tachycardias that require the atrioventricular node for re-entry (e.g. atrioventricular nodal re-entrant tachycardia)

Adenosine triphosphate This molecule stores and releases energy for the metabolic processes that occur within cells

Adrenal gland The small adrenal glands, about the size of a walnut, are situated on top of each kidney. The adrenal medulla secretes noradrenaline and adrenaline. The adrenal cortex secretes mineralocorticoids (control of sodium), glucocorticoids glucocorticoids (increases blood sugar) and gonadocorticoids (regulates sex hormones)

Adrenaline A neurotransmitter of the sympathetic nervous system, sometimes referred to as epinephrine. Adrenaline can also be used as a drug to support the circulation. It is given via a volumetric pump, via a central line and titrated to blood pressure in a level 2 or level 3 environment, where increased monitoring is available. Adrenaline is also given during a cardiac arrest, as per advanced life support algorithm

Adrenergic receptors Receptors of the sympathetic nervous system: subtypes alpha 1, alpha 2, beta 1 and beta 2. Adrenergic receptor agonists increase the effects of the sympathetic nervous system, increasing blood pressure and heart rate

Adrenocorticotrophic hormone A hormone produced by the anterior lobe of the pituitary gland that is responsible for the release of cortisol by the adrenal glands

Adult advanced life support algorithm An algorithm or step-by-step procedure for problem solving, published by the Resuscitation Council (UK), to guide healthcare professionals when giving advanced life support

Advance care plan A structured discussion with the patient and his/her family or carers about their wishes for the future

Aerobic metabolism The breakdown of carbohydrates to produce energy, CO_2 and water, in the presence of oxygen. This process occurs in the mitochondria of the cell. When the process occurs without oxygen, it is known as *anaerobic metabolism*.

Aetiology The cause or origin of a disease

Afterload The load (normally of the left ventricle) that has to be overcome, to open the aortic valve, in order to eject stroke volume

Air embolism Occurs when a bubble of air travels in the bloodstream of the vascular system

Air trapping An abnormal retention of air in the lungs at the end of expiration. This may occur in people with obstructive lung disease, such as asthma and chronic obstructive pulmonary disease, when constriction or collapse of the smaller airway can reduce air flow out of the lung

Airway adjuncts This is a medical device designed to open, or maintain a patient's airway. Examples include oropharyngeal airway (sometime known as a Guedel airway) or a nasopharyngeal airway

Airway hyperresponsiveness Twitchiness of the airway muscles

Airway obstruction A blockage or obstruction in the patient's upper airway, preventing inspiration. This is a medical emergency

Albumin Albumin is the main protein found in blood plasma. It is essential for creating colloidal osmotic pressure in the blood, then enabling fluids to move freely back into the vascular compartment from the interstitial spaces

Aldosterone A hormone produced by the adrenal cortex, increasing sodium and water reabsorption in the kidney, and increasing potassium excretion

Alpha adrenergic receptors Receptor of the sympathetic nervous system

Alpha-1 antitrypsin This protease inhibitor protects tissues from the effects of inflammatory cells that can damage elastin. Elastin enables the lungs to recoil during expiration. When alpha-1 antitrypsin is absent, the lungs tissue becomes damaged and elastic recoil is lost, as in emphysema

Alveolar capillary membrane A thin membrane between the alveolus and the capillary that surrounds it. Oxygen and CO_2 diffuse through the alveolar capillary membrane in different directions, thereby oxygenating the pulmonary capillary blood and allowing CO_2 to be removed from the pulmonary capillary to the alveolus, to be expired

Alveolar ventilation This is the amount of air that reaches the alveoli, usually over 1 min. To calculate, the physiological dead space (usually 150 mL) is taken away from the tidal volume (around 500 mL), then multiplied by the respiratory rate

Aminophylline This medication is used to dilate the bronchioles or airways. It is helpful for some patients with asthma or chronic obstructive pulmonary disease, but is not the initial treatment of choice. Side effects include profound tachycardia

Amiodarone A class 3 antiarrhythmic medication given to treat both atrial and ventricular tachyarrhythmias, such as fast atrial fibrillation or ventricular tachycardia

Amitriptyline A tricyclic antidepressant medication

Amniotic fluid embolism This is a very uncommon problem, when a bolus of amniotic fluid (or other substances related to childbirth) enters the bloodstream during the time of delivery. Cardiac and/or respiratory failure and/or arrest can follow.

Acute and Critical Care Nursing at a Glance, First Edition. Edited by Helen Dutton and Jacqui Finch
© 2018 John Wiley & Sons, Ltd. Published 2018 by John Wiley & Sons, Ltd.
Companion website: www.ataglanceseries.com/nursing/acutecare

Amniotic fluid embolism is often fatal within an hour of symptoms starting

Anaemia A reduced level of red blood cells, reducing the blood's capacity to transport oxygen

Anaerobic metabolism The breakdown of carbohydrates to produce energy in the absence of oxygen. This process occurs in the mitochondria of the cell. Lactic acid is produced as a by-product of anaerobic metabolism

Anaphylaxis A life-threatening allergic reaction, that rapidly develops in response to an allergen

Anatomical dead space Air in the lungs that remains in the conducting airways, and does not reach the respiratory bronchioles and alveoli to take part in gas exchange

Angiotensin II A hormone that has strong vasoconstrictive properties. It is formed from the conversion of angiotensin I, by angiotensin-converting enzyme, in the lung. Angiotensin II also stimulates aldosterone production, causing increased sodium, and therefore water reabsorption in the distal convoluted tubule of the nephron

Angiotensin-converting enzyme A hormone necessary for the conversion of angiotensin I to angiotensin II

Angiotensin-converting enzyme inhibitors A medication that is used for heart failure and as an antihypertensive. They inhibit the action of angiotensin- converting enzyme, then reducing the formation of angiotensin II. A reduction in angiotensin II, causes vasodilation, and reduced sodium and water reabsorption in the distal convoluted tubule of the nephron

Angiotensin receptor blockers This medication is used in the management of hypertension, when patients do not tolerate angiotensin-converting enzyme inhibitors. The receptor site for angiotensin II is blocked, thereby allowing vasodilation and reduction of blood pressure. Angiotensin receptor blockers may also be used in heart failure, when vasodilation reduces afterload, and therefore myocardial oxygen consumption

Antiarrhythmic Medication that treats cardiac arrhythmia

Antidiuretic hormone A hormone released from the posterior pituitary, it promotes water reabsorption in the nephron, increasing blood volume. It is also caused widespread vasoconstriction of arterioles, leading to an increased blood pressure

Antiemetic Medication that reduces vomiting and the feeling of nausea

Antihypertensives Medication that reduces blood pressure

Antigen A foreign substance in the body that can induce an immune response with the production of antibodies

Aortic aneurysm An enlargement of the aorta, such that the diameter is greater than 3 cm. Abdominal aortic aneurysms are the most common with many forming below the renal arteries

Aortic dissection This occurs when the lining of the aorta becomes torn and blood flows between the layers of the wall of the aorta. This is extremely painful and a medical emergency

Aortic stenosis A stiffening of the aortic valve leaflets often due to age- related progressive calcification

Aortic valve The semilunar valves which lie at the root of the aorta, preventing flow of blood back into the left ventricle during systole

Arterial blood gas A blood test on arterial blood, either drawn from an arterial line, or taken directly from the artery (usually the radial artery). This test can measure the amounts of gases, such as oxygen and CO_2 in the blood, as well as determining pH, concentration of bicarbonate, lactate and electrolytes

Arteriole A small branch of an artery, that leads into a capillary network

Aseptic non-touch technique This is a clinical practice framework that identifies the principles and safeguards for carrying out invasive clinical procedures or for using invasive medical devices aseptically

Aspiration Aspiration occurs when particles or material such as stomach contents, food or drink enter the respiratory tract

Aspiration pneumonia Inhalation of gastric or oropharyngeal contents into the lungs causing pneumonitis and extensive lung damage

Asthma A chronic inflammatory airways disorder is triggered by many factors, resulting in airflow obstruction that is variable and reversible

Atelectasis A collapse of a part of the lung, caused by blockage of the bronchioles, or pressure from the surrounding lung tissue

Atherosclerosis The narrowing of the arteries due to the build-up of plaques in the arterial wall, caused by build-up of fatty material

Atrial fibrillation A common cardiac arrhythmia, with a chaotic firing of ectopic foci in the atria at a rate >300/min causing the atria to quiver instead of contract. On palpation the pulse feels irregular. There are no P waves seen on the ECG

Atrial flutter Cardiac arrhythmia occurring above the ventricles (supraventricular). A single ectopic focus in the atria fires rapidly causing abnormal atrial conduction. This fast rhythm is usually regular, or regularly irregular, with 'saw tooth' waves replacing the P wave on the ECG

Atrioventricular heart block The conduction between the atria and the ventricles is impaired, disrupting the coordination of the heartbeat. Atrioventricular blocks can be seen on the ECG, as the time between the P wave and the QRS complex (P–R interval) becomes prolonged. Pacing may be required when there is no electrical communication between the atria and the ventricles

Atrioventricular node The atrioventricular node is a group of specialised cells on the floor of the right atrium, forming part of the electrical conduction system of the heart. It connects the atria and the ventricles, forming a conduit for the electrical impulse

Atrioventricular valves These valves are situation situated between the atria and ventricle of the heart. The right atrioventricular valve (tricuspid) prevents blood flowing back into the right atrium during ventricular systole, and the left atrioventricular (mitral) valve prevents blood flow back into the left atrium during ventricular systole

Atropine Atropine is an anticholinergic medication that competitively blocks the action of acetylcholine, a neurotransmitter of the parasympathetic nervous system. Atropine may be used to speed up the heart rate, or to reduce secretions

Atrovent The brand name for the anticholinergic bronchodilator medication ipratropium bromide, usually taken as a metred dose inhaler or nebulised

Auscultation Listening to sounds produced in the body with the use of a stethoscope. A useful tool to identify abnormalities, particularly of the respiratory and cardiovascular system

Autonomic nervous system Branch of the peripheral nervous system, containing two major subdivisions, the sympathetic and parasympathetic nervous systems

Autonomy The right of an individual to make their own decisions, with independence and freedom of choice. In healthcare this may refer to the patient's right to make a decision, without the healthcare provider unduly influencing the decision

Autorhythmic cells Cells that can generate their own impulses, and transmit electrical waves across the heart

AV nodal re-entry tachycardia Paroxysmal supraventricular tachycardia arises when a re-entry circuit forms within, or next to the atrioventricular node. Impulses travels down the normal atrioventricular pathway but return via the abnormal pathway. It circles round the two pathways repeatedly activating the atria and ventricle

Back-up rate Patients on bi-level positive airways pressure can breathe spontaneously, but each breath triggers the machine to deliver the inspiratory positive airways pressure. A back-up rate will deliver a breath if the patient does not breathe

Bariatric Relating to the causes, prevention and treatment of obesity

Baroreceptor Sensory nerve endings in the carotid bodies and aortic arch that detect stretch, and therefore changes in blood pressure

Basal metabolic rate This is the rate at which energy is used by the body at rest, usually expressed either as calories released per kilogram of body weight

Basophils A type of white blood cell that is active in allergic reactions and inflammation. They are able to leave the blood stream and enter sites of tissue damage as mast cells

Beneficence The act of doing good, and act of kindness

Benzodiazepine A type of tranquilliser that is used to treat anxiety and convulsions

Benzylpenicillin An antibiotic from the penicillin group used to treat a range of bacterial infections

Beta adrenergic receptors A receptor of the sympathetic nervous system: subtypes beta 1 (myocardium) and beta 2 (in smooth muscles)

Beta blockers A group of medications that blocks the beta adrenergic receptors of the sympathetic nervous system. They may prescribed in order to reduce heart work in heart failure and/or post myocardial infarction, as an antihypertensive, or to reduce heart rate

Bicarbonate (HCO_3^-) Bicarbonate is an important buffer in the blood that helps keep serum pH between 7.35 and 7.45

Bi-level positive airways pressure (BiPAP) Usually a form of non-invasive mechanical ventilation. Two levels of pressure are delivered: inspiratory positive airway pressure and expiratory positive airway pressure

Blood–brain barrier Tightly packed cells in brain capillaries that alters their permeability, allowing some substances to pass and others (such as certain drugs) not

Blood pressure The force the blood exerts on the walls of the arteries of the cardiovascular system. Blood pressure is measured clinically as systolic and diastolic pressure

B lymphocytes A type of white blood cell, part of the immune response. Sometimes known as B cells, they form part of the humoral or antibody-mediated immune response

Bradyarrhythmias A cardiac arrhythmia that is slower than 60 beats per minute

Bradycardia A heart rate <60 beats per minute

Bradykinin An inflammatory mediator associated with vasodilation and increased capillary permeability

Bronchial sounds Heard on lung auscultation over the trachea and large airway. A high-pitched harsh sound, with a short inspiratory phase

Bronchial pneumonia Infection involving bronchioles of the lung

Bronchodilators A substance or medication that enables the bronchioles to dilate. Medications that are bronchodilators include salbutamol, ipratropium bromide and aminophylline

Bronchospasm A constriction of the walls of the bronchioles, decreasing their lumen, and increasing resistance to air flow

B-type natriuretic peptide B-type natriuretic peptide (BNP) or brain natriuretic peptide is a marker for heart failure. BNP is released by the heart normally in very small quantities, but is it raised in the heart that is failing. Blood tests to ascertain BNP, proBNP and NT-proBNP levels are used to diagnose/evaluate extent of heart failure

Buffer A weak acid and its salt or a weak base and its salt that is resistant to changes in pH.

Bullectomy Surgical removal of dilated air spaces (bullae) in the lung

Bundle branches Branches of the bundle of His, which split into the left and right bundle branches. They run down the interventricular septum to the Purkinje fibres

Bundle of His Specialist conduction tissue in the heart that runs down the interventricular septum, to enable ventricular depolarisation. The bundle of His transmits electrical impulses down the ventricle to the Purkinje fibres

Calcium A chemical element with symbol Ca. It is abundant in bones and teeth

CAM ICU Confusion Assessment Method: Intensive Care Unit. A tool used to assess the development of delirium in those who are critically unwell. Though initially designed for ITU, this tool is also useful for patients receiving level 2 care

Candida albicans A parasitic fungus that can infect the mouth, intestines, skin and vagina

Capillary refill time Used to assess the amount of blood flow to peripheral tissue. The hand is raised to the level of the heart, gentle pressure is applied to the nailbed to cause blanching, for about 5 s. The time taken for colour to return on removal of pressure is normally about 2 s. This is known as the capillary refill time

Carbimazole A medication used to treat an overactive thyroid gland that is producing too much thyroxine. Carbimazole reduces the uptake of inorganic iodine by the thyroid, thus reducing thyroxine production

Cardiac biomarkers These are substances that are released in to the blood when myocardium is damaged. Usually a series of blood tests are done over several hours to assess heart damage. Troponin (either T or I) is the most specific and sensitive test for myocardial damage, being released within 2–4 h of myocardial injury. Creatinine kinase (CK-MB) is seen within 10–24 h of myocardial injury

Cardiac cycle The sequence of events that occur from one completed heartbeat to the next. There are two main phases: diastole, when ventricles are relaxed and fill with blood; and systole, when the left and right ventricles are contracting and blood is ejected into the pulmonary artery and aorta respectively

Cardiac output The amount of blood ejected by the heart in 1 min. Cardiac Output = Stroke Volume × Heart Rate

Cardiac tamponade The compression of the heart caused by fluid in the pericardial sac or increased pressure in the thoracic cavity. The heart is squeezed raising the pressure in the ventricle during diastole, preventing adequate filling. This reduces the stroke volume of the next systole, and cardiac output drops. Cardiac tamponade can be a life-threatening condition, requiring urgent medical intervention

Cardiopulmonary arrest The sudden cessation of breathing and effective cardiac output, causing loss of consciousness

Cardiopulmonary bypass machine Sometimes known as the 'heart–lung' machine, this takes over the function of the heart and lungs during surgery, maintaining the circulation of blood and supplying oxygen to organs and tissues

Cardiopulmonary resuscitation An emergency procedure undertaken in the event of a cardiac arrest. The aim is to provide sufficient cardiac output and oxygenation of vital organs to prevent irreversible brain damage caused by cerebral hypoxia. It consists of cardiac compressions and rescue breaths and may also be known as basic life support

Cardiovascular centre A part of the medulla in the brain stem that regulates the cardiovascular system. It responds to sensory information from the autonomic nervous system, and acts to regulate blood pressure, cardiac output and systemic vascular tone via the autonomic nervous system (sympathetic and parasympathetic branches)

Cardioversion A procedure whereby an abnormally fast heart rate is returned to normal heart rhythm. This can be done 'chemically' by appropriate medication, or 'electrically', using a defibrillator synchronised with the ECG, where an electric current is used to reset the heart's rhythm

Care bundle A care bundle is a tool to aid healthcare workers give the best possible care. A small set of evidenced-based procedures are grouped together. This group of about three to five actions, when performed together, consistently are proven to improve health outcomes

Care Quality Commission (CQC) Founded in 2009, this is the UK's health and social care regulator

Carina A ridge or section of cartilage at the bottom of the trachea at the division of the left and right main bronchus

Carrier protein Proteins that are embedded in the cell membrane and transport molecules across through channels. Carrier proteins can either transport molecules through the membrane as facilitated diffusion down a concentration gradient (no energy required) or actively (usually against a concentration gradient), using energy in the form of adenosine triphosphate

Catheter-related bloodstream infections Presence of systemic infection with the same organism is isolated from both blood cultures and an intravascular catheter

Cauda equina syndrome This is a lower motor neuron lesion with acute loss of function of the lumbar plexus. Red flag symptoms requiring urgent treatment are: sciatica, back pain, altered sensation over the saddle area and urinary retention or incontinence

Ceiling of care An agreed point by the multidisciplinary team at which no further treatment will be given to a patient, often used in the context of no further increase in the amount of a drug being given or a time limit on response to non-invasive ventilation

Cell-mediated immunity An immune response generated by activation of phagocytes, T lymphocytes and cytokines. It is mostly responsible for fighting foreign bodies that are inside the cells. This response does not involve antibodies, but the phagocytes recognise antigen-presenting cells

Central chemoreceptors Situated in the medulla of the brain stem, central chemoreceptors detect changes in the blood or extracellular fluid, in pH level, or increase in H^+ concentration, usually caused by a rise in CO_2/carbonic acid. This drop in pH stimulates the central chemoreceptors to increase respiratory depth and rate, expelling CO_2 until homeostasis is restored

Central cyanosis The appearance around the lips and oral mucosa of a bluish tinge. This is due to a low oxygen saturation, but may not be visible until oxygen saturations drop to around 80–85%. This is a late sign of hypoxaemia

Central venous pressure The pressure of blood in the central veins near the right atrium of the heart

Chest drain A flexible plastic tube that is inserted through the chest wall into the pleural space to drain air, fluid or pus that has collected

Chest X-ray Non-invasive painless investigation that gives images of the heart, lungs, airways, blood vessels and the bones of the spine and chest

Cheyne–Stokes breathing Periods of respirations during which the tidal volume is initially shallow, gets progressively deeper, and then progressively shallow again. Apnoea follows, which can continue for some time

Cholinergic receptors Receptors of the parasympathetic nervous system, divided into two subtypes, nicotinic and muscarinic

Chronic bronchitis Inflammation of the bronchioles, causing excessive mucus secretion. Chronic bronchitis occurs when there is a productive cough that lasts for at least 3 months for 2 years in a row

Chronic obstructive pulmonary disease (COPD) A chronic inflammatory disorder causing progressive airflow limitation that is not fully reversible. The main cause is smoking

Chyle A milky fluid consisting of emulsified fat and lymph. Ducts in the intestine called lacteals, absorb this fluid and convey it into the bloodstream via the lymphatic system

Circumflex artery A branch of the left coronary artery, which supplies the posterior surface of the heart

Claudication A decrease in arterial blood flow caused by blocked arteries, often in the leg. Symptoms include cramp-like pain in the lower leg whilst exercising

Clopidgrel A medication with an antiplatelet activity. It prevents platelets from clumping and forming clots

Clorphenamine An antihistamine medication that reduces the symptoms of allergy

Clubbing Deformity of the finger or toe nails associated with respiratory or cardiac diseases

Colloids A solution containing large insoluble molecules such as gelatine or albumin. Colloid preparations for IV use include Gelofusin and Voluven. Colloids can be used as a volume expander as they preserve a high colloid osmotic pressure in the blood that can replace blood plasma. There is no evidence of benefit of using colloids as fluid replacement over crystalloids

Community-acquired pneumonia Pneumonia that is not acquired in hospital, or after recent hospitalisation

Complement An inactive series of substances that can be triggered by the non-specific and specific immune systems to become active and enhance the destruction of pathogens, making the immune response much more effective

Compliance The ability to change volume when stretched. Lung compliance refers to the ease with which the lungs stretch to accommodate the inspired air. A stiff or poorly compliant lung will not stretch as easily, increasing the work of breathing

Computerised tomographic pulmonary angiography A CT scan in which a dye is inserted before taking a series of X-rays. It is used to diagnose pulmonary embolus, which can be seen as a reduction in blood flow in portions of the lung

Concentration gradient This occurs when the concentration of particles changes over a certain distance. For example, there is a greater partial pressure of oxygen in the alveolus as compared to the pulmonary capillary; this creates a concentration gradient from alveolus to capillary

Conducting zone Airway generations 0–16

Contiguous leads Leads on the ECG which look at areas of the heart that are next to each other. Contiguous leads look at the same general area of the heart, for example leads II, III and aVF all look at the inferior surface of the heart

Continuous positive airways pressure A non-invasive method or respiratory support, supplied via a face mask. A continuous high flow of gas (air and oxygen) generates a consistent positive pressure in the airways. A positive end expired pressure valve maintains a positive pressure during exhalation, thereby splinting the alveoli open for the whole respiratory cycle. This improves oxygenation, and reduces work of breathing

Contractility The ability of a muscle to shorten and contract. A highly contractile muscle will shorten effectively, a poorly contractile muscle will have a weak contraction only

Coronary angiogram An invasive procedure where a catheter is guided through the femoral or radial artery to the coronary arteries. A dye is inserted into the coronary arteries and X-ray images are taken to show the passage of the dye through the coronary arteries. Blockages or vessel narrowing can clearly be seen

Coronary artery Arteries (left and right coronary artery) arising from the root of the aorta, and travel across the heart to supply blood and nutrients to the myocardium

Coronary artery bypass grafting A surgical procedure, where a blocked coronary artery is bypassed, using a healthy artery or vein, to improve blood flow to the myocardium. Multiple coronary arteries can be bypassed in one surgical procedure

Cortisol A glucocorticoid hormone produced by the adrenal glands that regulates the metabolism of proteins, carbohydrates and lipids

Crackles Heard on lung auscultation. Discontinuous popping sounds heard from mid to late inspiration, caused by air moving through fluid in small airways or alveoli, or by alveoli opening at the end of inspiration. Crackles may be heard in the presence of problems such as a chest infection or pulmonary oedema

Craniectomy Excision of a portion of the skull without replacement of the bone

Craniotomy Surgical removal of part of the skull to remove a haematoma or tumour

C-reactive protein A protein manufactured in the liver, which rises in response to inflammation. A rise in serum C-reactive protein is associated with infection, and is quicker to rise than the white cell count

Creatinine kinase-MB A cardiac biomarker for myocardial injury rising within 10–24 h of infarction

Cricoid cartilage The only complete ring of cartilage around the trachea

Critical care outreach team (CCOT) A team, often multiprofessional, that provides support in the recognition and treatment for the patient who is experiencing deteriorating health, often identified by a rise in NEWS. They support the ward team until transfer to a higher level of care has been achieved

Crowing Abnormal noise made in the upper airway, related to airway obstruction

Crystalloid An aqueous solution that contains minerals salts and other water soluble molecules. Examples of intravenous crystalloid solutions include normal saline and plasmalyte

Cuff pressure The pressure inside the cuff of a tube placed in the trachea. The cuff pressure should normally be <25 cmH$_2$O (18 mmHg) to enable capillary filling and oxygenation of the tracheal tissue

Cuffed tracheostomy tube A tracheostomy tube with a cuff that provides a seal in the trachea, thereby preventing aspiration of gastric or oral fluids

CURB 65 A score used in the assessment of severity of community-acquired pneumonia. C, confusion; U, urea > 7 mmol/L; R, resp rate ≥30, B, systolic blood pressure <80 mmHg; age ≥ 65. Each scores 1 point. A score greater than 2 will result in a hospital admission, and 3–5 admission with high-dependency care

Cushing's syndrome A rare endocrine disorder resulting from excessive production of cortisol

Cushing's triad A decreased pulse, an increased blood pressure and a widened pulse pressure indicative of raised intracranial pressure with brain stem herniation. Respiratory changes may also occur

DDAVP Desmopressin acetate (1-deamino-8-D-arginine vasopressin): a synthetic analogue of vasopressin used to treat diabetes insipidus. It enhances water reabsorption by increasing the permeability of the renal collecting ducts, therefore reducing the urinary output and increasing the concentration of the urine

D-dimers Small fragments of fibrin that appear in the blood when a clot is being broken down by fibrinolysis. A positive D-dimer blood test is an indication of thromboembolic disease such as deep vein thrombosis and pulmonary embolus, but could also be due to other disorders

Decannulation (tracheostomy tube) Refers to the removal of the tracheostomy tube

Decannulation cap A cap that is placed on the proximal end of a tracheostomy tube, towards the end of the weaning process. It is essential that the cuff is deflated prior to the cap being placed. Air flow around the tracheostomy tube enables breathing through the upper airway. Respiratory status needs to be monitored closely during this time

Deep vein thrombosis A clot in the deep veins of the body, often in the leg

Defibrillation Delivering a therapeutic electric shock via a defibrillator. A significant mass of the myocardium becomes depolarised by the shock which may stop the arrhythmia and allow sinus rhythm to be restored. Defibrillation is the treatment of choice for cardiac arrest with ventricular fibrillation or ventricular tachycardia

Delirium An acute confusional state often accompanied by disorganised thinking

Dementia Dementia is caused by a group of conditions affecting the brain, most commonly Alzheimer's and vascular dementia. Symptoms include progressive problems with memory loss, problem solving and thinking

Deontology From the philosophical work of Immanuel Kant, it is very focused on the individual, and the universal, unconditional and imperative requirement to adhere to all moral laws and principles

Depolarisation A rapid movement of ions across the cell membrane causing a change in voltage, that leads to an action potential. In the cardiac muscle, action potentials initiate muscle contraction

Depression Depression is characterised by a history of low mood, and a loss of pleasure in most activities, even those that were previously enjoyed

Dermis The fibrous inner layer of the skin

Desmopressin See DDAVP

Diabetes insipidus A lack of antidiuretic hormone caused by insufficient production and release by the brain or failure of the kidneys to respond to it. The patient will have a large loss of water in their urine and may become severely dehydrated as a result

Diabetes mellitus An endocrine disorder caused by either the body producing no or insufficient amounts of insulin or body cells not responding to the insulin that is produced

Diabetic ketoacidosis This potentially life-threatening condition is most commonly seen in patients with type 1 diabetes mellitus and it is manifested by hyperglycaemia, dehydration as a result of increased urine output and the production of excess ketones secondary to the metabolism of fats as a source of energy

Diaphoresis An unusual amount of sweating

Diastole A stage in the cardiac cycle when the ventricles are relaxed and filling with blood

Diazemul An intravenous sedation medication, belonging to the benzodiazepine group

Diazepam See benzodiazepine

Diencephalon A section of the brain that includes the hypothalamus and the thalamus

Diffusion The movement of particles from an area of high concentration to an area of lower concentration of that particle. This passive movement may occur through a semipermeable membrane

Digoxin A cardiac glycoside medication that is used to treat cardiac arrhythmias and heart failure

DINAMAP Device for direct non-invasive automated arterial blood pressure measurement

Distal convoluted tubule A part of the nephron in the kidney, between the loop of Henle and the collecting duct

Diuretic A medication that increases urine output, such as furosemide or amiloride

DNAR 'Do not attempt to resuscitate'

DO$_2$ Oxygen delivery

Dopamine A neurotransmitter of the central and peripheral nervous system. Dopamine as a medication has vasopressor and inotropic properties, increasing the strength of heart contractions. Patients receiving this medication need level 2 or level 3 care, as continuous cardiovascular monitoring is required

Doppler ultrasound A non-invasive test that can evaluate blood flow, using the images gained from ultrasound

Dura mater The outer, fibrous meningeal layer covering the brain and spinal cord

Dyspnoea The sensation of breathlessness

Echocardiography A non-invasive investigation using ultrasound waves to create and image of the heart, and blood flow through the heart

Ecstasy 304 Methylenedioxymethamphetamine. A recreational drug of abuse that creates increased energy and euphoria, which even in small amounts can be toxic to neurons

Elastic recoil The recoil of the lungs after being stretched in inspiration. Elastic recoil enable the lungs to rebound to a resting position of exhalation

Electrocardiogram A recording of the electrical activity of the heart, using electrodes place on the limbs and/or chest. The trace can be shown on a monitor, or taken as a reading looking at 12 different views of the heart, the 12-lead ECG

Electrolyte A solution containing charged particles. Atoms or molecules become charged by either gaining or losing an electron

Emergency needle decompression Usually for a tension pneumothorax: inserting a tube in to the pleural space, with a one-way valve system allowing air to escape but not re-enter

Emphysema A chronic disease of the respiratory system where there is destruction of lung tissue. This affects the ability of the lung to retain its normal shape, with the small airway collapsing on expiration. The alveoli become damaged leading to problems with gaseous exchange

Empyema A collection of pus in the pleural cavity

Encephalopathy A generic term used to describe brain dysfunction originating from disease or damage.

Endocarditis Inflammation of the inner lining of the heart (endocardium) caused by infection. The valves of the heart are normally affected, and may become damaged

Endothelium A single cell layer that lines the blood vessels, that provides a smooth surface for blood flow

Endotracheal suction Suction through an endotracheal tube to remove secretions

Endotracheal tube A tube inserted into the trachea, to ensure a patent airway. An inflated cuff prevents inhalation of oropharyngeal or gastric contents

End positive airways pressure Positive pressure at the end of expiration applied during non-invasive ventilation. This helps prevent alveolar collapse, so increases the time for oxygen to diffuse from the alveoli to the pulmonary capillary blood

Eosinophil A white blood cell that deals with parasitic infections by spraying their chemicals onto larger microorganisms that are too big to engulf

Epidemiology Looking at the patterns of disease, causes and effects in populations

Epidural analgesia A highly effective method of pain relief where analgesic agents are given via a catheter in the epidural space

Epidural space The space between the dura mater and the lining of the spinal canal

Epiglottis A flap of cartilage covered with a mucous membrane that sits behind the tongue. The epiglottis closes during the act of swallowing, preventing fluid or oral contents from entering the trachea, and ensuring it goes down the oesophagus

Epinephrine A neurotransmitter of the sympathetic nervous system, also a catecholamine or a hormone, sometime called adrenaline

Eptifibatide A platelet aggregation inhibitor used in acute coronary syndrome

Ethanol CH_3CH_2OH: a colourless, flammable liquid that is the major ingredient of alcoholic beverages

Extracellular fluid Fluid in the interstitial space and plasma

Falx cerebri The fold of dura mater that separates the two cerebral hemispheres

Fascia A sheet of fibrous connective tissue

Fat embolism When fat tissue enters and travels in the bloodstream. Fat may be released from the bone marrow of long bone fractures

Fenestrated tracheostomy tube A tracheostomy tube that has openings (or fenestrations) in the outer cannula, just above the inflatable cuff. With the cuff deflated, a finger or speaking valve placed over the outer tracheostomy tube opening will allow vocalisation on expiration. The air passes through the fenestrations over the vocal chords. A fenestrated inner should be present

A non-fenestrated inner tube is placed when the fenestrated tracheostomy tube is not required for speaking. If required the cuff can be inflated and air passes through the tracheostomy tube

FEV_1/FVC Forced expiratory volume in one second/ forced vital capacity

Fondaparinux An anticoagulant (factor Xa inhibitor)

Forced expiratory volume in 1 second (FEV_1) The maximum amount of air to be expired in one second

Forced vital capacity The amount of gas that can be exhaled forcefully and rapidly following full inhalation

Frank–Starling Law Myocardial contraction is directly proportional to the length of myocardial fibres, therefore cardiac output will be determined by how much heart muscle fibres are stretched in diastole. However, the muscle fibres can be overstretched and this will lead to a fall in cardiac output

Functional residual capacity The amount of gas remaining at the end of normal quiet respiration

GABA Gamma amino butyric acid

Generalised Anxiety Disorder Assessment (GAD-7) Formal screening tools used to assist in providing insight into patients' psychological wellbeing, whether it is for a mental health diagnosis or hospital-induced anxiety and stress

Glasgow Coma Scale This is a standardised system for assessing the patient's neurological response. Three areas are assessed: eye opening, verbal response and motor response and then an overall score is calculated. The lowest score achievable is 3 and the highest is 15. Scores of 8 or less indicate coma

Glia Non-neuronal tissue of the central nervous system, consisting of oligodendroglia, astrocytes and microglia

Glomerular afferent arteriole A branch of an interlobular artery that supplies blood to the glomerulus in the nephron

Glomerular filtration rate (GFR) The flow rate of filtered fluid through the kidneys (usually > 90ml/min/1.73 m^2)

Glossopharyngeal nerve This is the ninth cranial nerve which supplies the muscles of the pharynx, soft palate and posterior third of the tongue. It is responsible for the swallowing reflex

Glottis This is the part of the larynx where the vocal chords are located. It has a slit type opening which affects tone and pitch of the voice.

Glucagon A hormone produced by pancreatic alpha cells in response to hypoglyacaemia

Glucometer A battery-powered device used to calculate blood glucose from a drop of blood

Gluconeogenesis A process occurring mainly in the liver whereby glucose is produced from non-carbohydrate sources

Glyceryl trinitrate spray A potent coronary vasodilator

Glycogen The chief carbohydrate source, largely produced and stored by the liver

Glycogenolysis The splitting of glycogen in the liver to produce glucose

Granulocyte A type of white blood cell

Group A streptococcus A group of bacteria that lives in the skin and oral cavity which can lead to widespread infection

Guedel airway Oropharyngeal airway

Haemoptysis Coughing up blood that has originated in the bronchial or lung tissue

Haemothorax This is when blood collects in the pleural cavity, due to trauma or disease

Hartman's solution A type of crystalloid containing sodium, potassium and calcium chloride as well as sodium lactate

Healthcare-associated infection An infection occurring as a result of hospital admission and/or medical and nursing intervention

Heat and moisture exchanger This device is used in artificial ventilation to heat and humidify the gas supplied to a patient

High flow nasal cannula A treatment for hypoxaemia, delivering heated humidified medical gas at up to 60 L/min. It is tolerated well by most patients, and its use in adult critical care is increasing. The high flow of gas creates a positive pressure environment, and 'washes out' gases in the nasopharynx, helping CO_2 clearance

Hippocampus An area of grey matter in the brain found on the floor of the lateral ventricle

Histamine This nitrogen-containing substance is a potent mediator of immediate hypersensitivity. It can cause capillary permeability and dilatation, contraction of smooth muscle, increased gastric secretion and an accelerated heart rate

Hospital-acquired pneumonia Pneumonia occurring after the first 48 h of admission

Hospital anxiety and depression scale (HADS) Formal screening tools (HADS) and GAD-7 (Generalised Anxiety Disorder Assessment) are used to assist in providing insight in to patients' psychological wellbeing, whether it is for a mental health diagnosis or hospital-induced anxiety and stress

Humoral immunity Extra cellular pathogens, once activated by the presence of an antigen, develop into large plasma cells that secrete antibodies or immunoglobulins

Hydrocortisone The steroid hormone cortisol

Hydrogen ions (H^+) The acid element in blood

Hydronephrosis When one or both kidneys are stretched and swollen due to excess urine

Hydrostatic pressure Pressure within the vascular system

Hyperalgesic Excessive sensitivity and an increased threshold to pain

Hypercapnia Excessive CO_2 in the blood

Hyperglycaemia Raised serum glucose level

Hyperkalaemia Raised serum potassium level

Hypernatraemia Raised serum sodium level

Hyperosmolar Increased concentration, as in increased concentration of the blood

Hyperthyroidism Overproduction of thyroid hormones

Hypoglycaemia Low blood glucose level

Hypokalaemia Low blood potassium level

Hyponatraemia Low blood sodium level

Hypothyroidism Underproduction of thyroid hormones

Hypovolaemia Reduced volume, as in reduced blood volume

Hypoxaemia Deficiency of oxygen in arterial blood (<8 kPa)

ICU Intensive Care Unit

I:E ratio The ratio of inspiration to expiration

Informed consent The doctrine of informed consent is a legal concept whereby the patient has reasonable knowledge of a procedure to be carried out and an understanding of the risks involved.

Healthcare professionals therefore have a duty of disclosure to ensure that the patient can make informed choices

In-hospital resuscitation algorithm The Resuscitation Council (UK) 2015 guidelines on the management sequence for a collapsed patient in hospital

Innate immune system See non-specific immune system

Inner cannula/inner tube The inner tube of a tracheostomy that can be removed for cleaning; it has a lock on it to prevent it from being coughed out

Inotropic agents These are drugs that alter the force or energy of myocardial contractility. Negative inotropes such as beta blockers weaken the force of contraction whilst positive inotropes for example dobutamine increase force of contraction

Inspiratory positive airways pressure Using bilevel positive airway pressure (commonly known as BiPAP or BIPAP) this is the peak pressure applied during patient-triggered breaths

Insulin A hormone produced by pancreatic beta cells that reduces the blood glucose level

Intercostal muscles These are several groups of muscles that run between the ribs and help to form and move the chest wall. Their main function is to assist with the mechanics of breathing

Interhospital transfer Transfer of a patient between hospitals

Interleukin A group of cytokines that control cellular behaviour (see cytokine) and activate lymphocytes

Internal mammary artery graft Also called the internal thoracic artery, this vessel, running on either side of the sternum, supplies the anterior chest wall and the breasts

Interstitial The fluid or space that lies between cells, as in 'interstitial fluid' or 'interstitial space'

Interstitial pneumonia This is pneumonia that affects the interstitial lining of the alveoli and the lung tissue

Intracellular fluid This is the fluid within cells and it accounts for two-thirds of the total body water

Intracranial pressure This is the pressure within the skull, including the brain tissue and cerebrospinal fluid

Intrahospital transfer Transfer of patient between departments within the same hospital

Intravascular Occurring within blood vessels or within the vascular system

Intravenous Within the vein, usually referring to fluids given directly into a vein

Invasive monitoring Monitoring of cardiac, abdominal or neurological function that requires insertion of cannula or catheters into the patient's body, thus enabling continuous, accurate assessment

Ipratropium bromide Known under the trade name Atrovent, this anticholinergic bronchodilator is used to treat bronchospasm

Ischaemia A restriction of blood supply to the tissues resulting in a lack of oxygen and glucose, both needed for cellular metabolism

Isovolumetric ventricular contraction An event occurring in systole when the ventricles contract with no volume change (owing to all the heart valves being closed at this point)

Jugular venous distension A sign of increased blood volume that may be indicative of heart failure

Justice In healthcare this refers to fair distribution of resources, entitlement and equality

Juxtaglomerular cells Cells in the kidney that produce, store and secrete the enzyme renin

Killer cells A type of lymphocyte that destroys infected or cancerous cells

Kussmaul breathing A very deep and rapid respiratory pattern, possibly a response to a severe metabolic acidosis caused by problems such as diabetic ketoacidosis

Lactate A product of metabolism $C_3H_5O_3$, formed when glucose is broken down in cellular respiration, in the absence of oxygen (see also lactic acid). Lactate and lactic acid are often used interchangeably, but have a different chemical structure

Lactic acid An organic acid $C_3H_6O_3$, produced as a product of anaerobic respiration. As an acid it can donate hydrogen ions, giving the conjugate lactate, plus a hydrogen ion

$$C_3H_6O_3 \text{ (lactic acid)} \rightarrow C_3H_5O_3 \text{ (lactate)} + H^+ \text{ (hydrogen ion)}$$

Lactate and lactic acid are often used interchangeably (but have a different chemical structure)

Laryngeal mask airway A type of supraglottic airway device that sits in the upper airway, isolating the trachea

Lasting power of attorney This is a designated person chosen by the patient, who can make decisions on his or her behalf. The lastin power of attorney may be in place for financial decisions, for healthcare decisions, or for both

Left anterior descending artery A branch of the left coronary artery. It travels down the front of the heart between the right and left ventricle, this is the main blood supply for the left ventricle

Left coronary artery Major coronary artery. The left main stem arises from the aorta, and branches into two vessels; left anterior descending artery travels down the front of the heart between the right and left ventricle; the circumflex runs round the back of the heart

Lifestyle behaviours Choices, beliefs, opinions and patterns of activity that patients have which may impact on their health

Light's criteria Distinguishes exudate from transudate in pleural fluid. Pleural fluid higher in protein is likely to be exudate, due to problems such as infection or malignancy

Lithium Psychiatric medication used to treat patients with bipolar disease

Lobar pneumonia Infection involving a lobe of the lung

Lobectomy Removal of a lobe of the lung

Lung failure Failure of the gaseous exchange mechanism at alveolar level

Lung resection Removal of part of, or the entire lung, often due to a tumour

Lung volume reduction Resection of severely emphysematous lung tissue

Lymphocytes A small leucocyte (white blood cell) found especially in the lymphatic system

Lymphoid cells Innate immune cells that can produce cytokines

Macrophages Fixed or wandering: fixed macrophages (found in tissues in the brain, liver, lungs, kidneys) and 'wandering macrophages' that are able to respond immediately to signs of infection. They have phagocytic properties and can act as scavengers destroying old cells and other debris

Magnesium (Mg^{++}) A mineral that has many functions including: energy production, contributing to the structural development of bone and acting as a cofactor in more than 300 enzyme systems (regulating protein synthesis, muscle and nerve function, blood glucose control and blood pressure regulation)

Magnesium sulphate (MgSO$_4$) Owing to its ability to inhibit smooth muscle contraction this is used in a variety of clinical situations and these include: as an antiarrhythmic agent, as a bronchodilator and as a first-line treatment for pre-eclampsia/eclampsia (either to prevent or treat seizures). MgSO$_4$ is also given as replacement therapy in cases of hypomagnesaemia

Magnetic resonance imaging A type of scan that uses strong magnetic fields and radio waves to produce detailed images

Malnutrition universal screening tool A five-step screening tool used to identify adults who are malnourished, at risk of malnutrition or obese

Mean arterial pressure Average perfusion pressure throughout the cardiac cycle

Mechanical ventilation This is a mechanical method to assist or replace spontaneous breathing

Medulla oblongata This is located in the lowest part of the brain stem and contains key centres for controlling autonomic activity like breathing and cardiac function

Melatonin A hormone made by the pineal gland that controls sleep and wake cycles

Mental Capacity Act (2005) Government legislation in England and Wales that addresses decision making for those who lack mental capacity and are unable to make choices for themselves

Metabolic acidosis When the pH of the blood drops below 7.35 due to too much acid being produced or when the kidneys are not removing sufficient amounts from the blood

Metabolic alkalosis When the pH of the blood rises above 7.45 as a result of an increased bicarbonate level or when there is a reduced hydrogen ion level

Metoclopramide A prokinetic medication used to treat nausea and vomiting

Mini-tracheostomy This is when a small tube is passed through the cricothyroid membrane to facilitate the suctioning of sputum. The procedure is also sometimes performed in emergency situations if intubation fails

Minute ventilation Expired total ventilation (V_E) per minute

Mitochondria Double membrane structures found in most cells that generate energy for the body

Mitral valve The valve between the left atrium and the left ventricle

Monro–Kellie hypothesis This doctrine states that the content within the cranial compartment (brain matter, cerebrospinal fluid and blood) is non-compressible and of fixed volume: therefore, if there is an increase in one of the components this must be compensated by a decrease in one of the other two

Morphine An opioid analgesic used to relieve severe pain

Multidimensional This is something that possesses many different parts or aspects

Multiparameter early warning score A track and trigger system that generates a score based on the assessment of multiple clinical parameters

Multiple organ dysfunction syndrome Previously known as multiple organ failure this is when there is altered organ function (of at least two major organs) that requires medical intervention to sustain life

Muscarinic receptors These are special proteins that respond to the neurotransmitter acetylcholine

Myocardial infarction Damage to heart muscle caused by an absence of perfusion, the most common cause of which is blockage of a coronary artery owing to rupture of an atherosclerotic plaque

Myocardium The muscular wall of the heart

Myoglobin A protein found in muscle tissue

Myxoedema The severest form of hypothyroidism (see hypothyroidism)

Naloxone A competitive opioid antagonist, used to block or reverse the effects of opioid medication

Necrotic This is when death of body tissue secondary to poor perfusion occurs and it is due to injury or disease

Necrotising fasciitis This is a rapid inflammatory bacterial infection of the fascia that also destroys subcutaneous tissue

Neuropathic pain This is a chronic, complex type of pain where the nerve fibres themselves may be damaged or dysfunctional and therefore send abnormal signals to other pain centres

Neuropathy Damage to or disease of the sensory nerves

Neurotransmitter A chemical messenger, sending signals between nerve cells

Neutrophils The largest subgroup of the granulocytes and are 'phagocytic' cells containing chemicals that 'eat' and break down microorganisms they ingest

NEWS The National Early Warning Score is used as part of a 'track and trigger' system whereby elevated scores in the acutely deteriorating patient escalate response

NICE The National Institute for Health and Care Excellence is a non-departmental public body of the UK Department of Health. It seeks to ensure that national clinical guidelines are consistent, of a high quality and evidence based

Nitrates Nitrogen compounds. In medicine, nitrates are used in heart disease to dilate blood vessels, for example, in angina when blood supply to the heart is restricted

Nitrogen This is a fundamental component of amino acid and therefore one of the building blocks of protein. Calculating a patient's nitrogen balance is useful to determine how much protein is required daily and how much is being metabolised

NIV Non-invasive ventilation, often used to support spontaneous respiratory function and thus preventing the need for intubation and mechanical ventilation (see BiPAP)

Nociceptive pain Sharp, aching or throbbing pain caused by damage to body tissue

Non-maleficence Do no harm or inflict the least possible harm to reach a beneficial outcome

Non-rebreathe mask This is a type of oxygen mask that delivers high flow rate and concentration of oxygen to the patient, whilst preventing the re-inhalation of CO_2

Non-specific immune system The innate set of defences the body has against infection, which includes the skin, the bronchomucociliary escalator and the pH of body fluids. Response through non-specific immunity is antigen dependent. There will be an immediate maximum response, but there will be no immunological memory of the exposure

Noradrenaline (norepinephrine) This catecholamine and hormone functions as the main neurotransmitter of the sympathetic autonomic nervous system. It causes vasoconstriction.
In critical care this drug can be given by continuous infusion via central line to treat life-threatening hypotension

NPA Nasopharyngeal airway

NSAIDs Non-steroidal anti-inflammatory drugs work by blocking cyclooxygenase enzymes and reducing prostaglandins throughout the body to relieve pain and inflammation

NSTEMI A myocardial infarction caused by a severely narrowed but not fully occluded coronary artery

N-terminal pro-B type natriuretic peptide A serum marker of congestive heart failure

Nursing model This is a framework for organising ideas about patients, health, nursing and the environment and for systematically assessing, planning, implementing and evaluating care

Objective data During patient assessment this is what the nurse actually sees (the signs)

Obstructive lung disorders Failure of the lung can be caused by impedance of airflow through the airways

Oculomotor nerve The third cranial nerve which assists with controlling ocular movement

Oedema Fluid retention in the body

Oncotic pressure Also known as the colloid osmotic pressure, this is the pressure generated by the plasma proteins (for example albumin), in a blood vessel. Owing to their large molecular weight these proteins can pull water into the intravascular space

OPA Oropharyngeal airway

Opiates (opioids) Substances that act on opioid receptors in the brain

Orthopnoea Difficulty in breathing when lying flat

Osmosis The movement of water molecules from an area of high concentration through a semipermeable membrane to an area of lower concentration

Oxygen capacity The maximum amount of oxygen that will combine with haemoglobin in a unit volume of blood

Oxygen content The amount of oxygen bound to haemoglobin, plus the amount dissolved in the blood

Oxygen haemoglobin dissociation curve A tool that illustrates the relationship between the partial pressure of oxygen and the oxygen saturation of the haemoglobin molecule, useful for understanding how blood carries and releases oxygen to the tissues

Oxyhaemoglobin Haemoglobin combined with oxygen

Oxytocin A hormone secreted by the posterior lobe of the pituitary gland, it can also be given as medication. The primary function is contraction of the uterus

PAINAD Pain Assessment in Advanced Dementia

PaO_2 The partial pressure of oxygen in arterial blood

PAO_2 The partial pressure of oxygen in the alveoli

Paracetamol An analgesic agent that blocks the production of prostaglandins

Paradoxical breathing A condition where the chest moves inwards during inspiration instead of moving out and this soon impairs gas exchange

Parasympathetic nervous system A division of the autonomic nervous system sometimes called the 'rest and digest' system

Paravertebral nerve block Administering analgesia/anaesthesia into the paravertebral space adjacent to where the spinal nerves emerge

Paroxysmal nocturnal dyspnoea Coughing and shortness of breath occurring in a recumbent position at night

Partial airway obstruction Semiblockage of the airway characterised by a 'crowing' noise as air passes through a narrowed passage

Partial pressure The pressure that a gas exerts in a mixture of gases

Passive transport mechanisms The movement of biochemical substances and other molecular molecules across cell membranes without energy

PCA (patient-controlled analgesia) This is where the patient can administer their own analgesia via a machine with a predetermined amount of analgesia available at different intervals. All infusion doses are programmed by the prescriber, so overdose is unlikely

PEEP (positive end expired pressure) This is airway pressure maintained above atmospheric pressure at the end of expiration. It increases the volume of gas in the lungs and decreases the shunting of blood, therefore improving gas exchange

PEFR (peak expiratory flow rate) Peak expiratory flow rate. Measures the rate that air is forcibly expelled from the lungs in litres per minute

Percutaneous tracheostomy The creation of a tracheostomy stoma using a Seldinger technique and dilatation of the trachea, between the tracheal rings

Pericardial sac A sac of fibrous tissue surrounding the heart and major blood vessels. When this sac becomes inflamed it is known as *pericarditis*.

Pericardiocentesis A skilled procedure in which a needle or drain is inserted into the pericardial space under ultrasound guidance, to aspirate/drain the fluid

Peripheral chemoreceptors Peripheral chemoreceptors are situated in the aortic arch and carotid bodies (at the bifurcation of the common carotid arteries). They are sensitive to changes in PaO_2, $PaCO_2$ and pH, contributing to the regulation of each of these. They have, however, a particularly important role in initiating responses to hypoxaemia

pH A measure of acidity and alkalinity

Phaechromocytoma A tumour of the adrenal gland secreting catecholamines

Phagocytosis When cells, mostly phagocytes, engulf and ingest other cells or particles

Phantom pain Unpleasant sensations that the patient perceives to have originated in a limb that has been removed

Phenytoin Antiseizure medication

Physiological dead space The volume of air that does not take part in gas exchange either because it is in the airways or because it is in contact with alveoli that are poorly perfused

Pia mater The delicate innermost layer of the meninges, in contact with the brain and the spinal cord

Plasmalyte A balanced crystalloid solution, meaning that it is designed to match the electrolyte concentrations of plasma

Plasma proteins Substances mostly produced in the liver that maintain oncotic pressure, help to regulate blood pressure and are essential for blood clotting

Pleura The pleura is a thin double-layered membrane covering the surface of the lungs (visceral layer), the inside of the chest wall and thoracic surface of the diaphragm (parietal)

Pleural effusion An excess of fluid in the pleural space

Pleural fluid A small amount of fluid in the pleural space to reduce friction, and keep the pleural layers together

Pleurectomy Resection of the pleura

Pleurisy Inflammation of the pleura

Pleurodesis Surgery for recurrent pneumothorax. Abrasion of the pleura, mechanical or chemical, to cause permanent adhesion, reducing pneumothorax risk

Pneumonia Inflammation of lung tissue

Pneumothorax Air in the pleural cavity

Poikilothermic Where normal temperature control is disrupted and the patient's temperature will correlate with the environment, for example if the ward is very hot the patient will become very hot. This condition is most commonly seen in spinal cord injury

Polycythaemia Red blood cell production is increased

Posterior pituitary The posterior lobe of the pituitary gland which develops as an extension of the hypothalamus

Potassium (K^+) The major intracellular cation, it is an electrolyte and mineral essential for maintaining normal cellular function. Key actions are nerve impulse transmission and muscle contraction

PPE Personal protective equipment

Prasugrel A drug that inhibits platelets and therefore prevents thrombosis

PR interval The flat segment of the PQRS complex that starts from the beginning of the P wave and ends at the beginning of the QRS complex. Normally less than< 0.2 s (or five small squares on the ECG paper)

Preload The stretching of cardiac myocytes prior to contraction (end diastolic volume)

Pressure support The difference between inspiratory positive airways pressure and end positive airways pressure

Primary percutaneous coronary intervention This is coronary angioplasty, whereby a small balloon is inserted into the body and directed to a blocked coronary artery where it pushes the occluding matter out of the way and stents the blood vessel open

Primary spontaneous pneumothorax A collection of air in the pleural space, not caused by disease or injury but by small sacs of air (blebs) rupturing

Prokinetic therapy Medication that strengthens the lower oesophageal sphincter causing the stomach to empty faster; this reduces nausea, vomiting and acid reflux. Metoclopramide is an example of this type of drug

Propranolol A drug that blocks beta 1 and beta 2 adrenoreceptors, thus reducing heart rate and blood pressure but also increasing airway resistance

Prostaglandins Lipid compounds that have hormone-like effects, controlling inflammation, blood flow, the formation of blood clots and the induction of labour

Pruritus Severe itching of the skin

Pulmonary artery The artery carrying deoxygenated blood from the right ventricle to the lungs

Pulmonary oedema Fluid that leaks from the pulmonary capillaries into the interstitial space and alveoli

Pulmonary valve The valve that lies between the right ventricle and the pulmonary artery

Pulmonary veins Large blood vessels that receive oxygenated blood from the lungs

Pulse oximetry A non-invasive method for monitoring oxygen saturation

Purkinje fibres Networks of fibres that activate the right and left ventricles

Purse-lipped breathing Exhaling through tightly pressed lips makes breathing easier because it reduces the workload of respiratory muscle and returns the inspiration/expiration ratio to the normal 1:2 (often disrupted in patients with chronic obstructive pulmonary disease)

P wave Trace on ECG reflecting atrial depolarisation. Should be symmetrically rounded and, except for the lead aVR, it should be positive (upright)

Pyrexia Fever, a febrile response

QRS complex Made up of the three waves, Q, R and S on the ECG. If the first deflection of the QRS complex is downward, it is called a Q wave and it represents septal depolarisation. A Q wave is not always present, but should be less than 1 mm. The R wave is the first +ve deflection after the P wave, and the S wave the first −ve deflection after the R wave. QRS complex reflects ventricular depolarisation

Radiofrequency catheter ablation A procedure that destroys the tissue in the heart that is causing abnormal electrical signals. Ablation can halt the pathways that cause rapid irregular heartbeats, and restore normal heart rhythm destroy abnormal pathway

Ramp time The amount of time taken to achieve the preset inspiratory positive airways pressure. A gradual change in pressure over about 10 min is often better tolerated by the patient

Red flag Red flag symptoms requiring urgent medical attention

Relocation anxiety See transfer anxiety

REM One of the five stages of sleep characterised by rapid movement of the eyes and near paralysis of the muscles

Renin An enzyme produced by the kidney that contributes to the control of blood volume and systemic vascular resistance

Renin-angiotensin-aldosterone-system (RAAS) A hormone system that regulates blood pressure and fluid balance

Repolarisation A change in membrane potential that returns it to a negative value (after depolarisation)

Resistance The degree to which something is opposed: for example, in the lung, airway resistance is the opposition to airflow caused by the forces of friction in the airway

Respiratory acidosis Ventilatory failure occurs when the lungs can't remove enough CO_2 leading to a decrease in the pH of the blood (acidity)

Respiratory alkalosis Increased ventilation reduces the arterial levels of CO_2 leading to an increase in the pH of the blood (alkalinity)

Respiratory centres These are located in the medulla oblongata and the pons, both of which are parts of the brain stem

Respiratory depression Hypoventilation

Respiratory zone Consists of airway generations 17–23

Restrictive lung disorders Changes in the lung that reduce the lung volumes

Return of spontaneous circulation Resumption of sustained perfusion as heartbeats and circulation returns following cardiac arrest

Rhythm control (AF) Chemical (drug) cardioversion to control atrial fibrillation

Right coronary artery A major coronary artery, supplies the right ventricle

Right to left shunt No ventilation with blood bypassing the lung unit

Rise time The time for the pressure to rise from EPAP to IPAP

Safeguarding An action taken to protect someone from harm

SBAR A standardised communication tool

Secondary pneumothorax A pneumothorax that occurs as a complication of an underlying lung disease

Semilunar valves Valves at the base of the aorta and the pulmonary artery preventing the back flow of blood into the heart

Semipermeable membrane A selectively permeable membrane that allows water and certain ions to pass through it

Sensory cortex The region of the cerebral cortex that controls the receiving and interpreting of information

Sepsis A life-threatening organ dysfunction caused by a dysregulated host response to infection. This arises when the body's response to infection injures its own tissues and organs

Sepsis Six The name given to a care bundle for the early management of sepsis

Septic screen A screening process whereby cultures of blood and stool, urinalysis (and culture if necessary), wound swabs and throat swabs are carried out looking for the source of an infection

Septic shock Severe sepsis with a lactate >2 mmol/L and persistently low blood pressure <100 mmHg in spite of fluid resuscitation

Serevent A long-acting bronchodilator

Serotonin A neurotransmitter that helps relay signals from one area of the brain to another

Shunt In respiration, this is when gas exchange fails to take place in the lungs because although there is perfusion, there is poor ventilation in the alveoli. Blood is returned to the heart deoxygenated

Sinoatrial node A region of specialised cells in the heart situated in the upper part of the right atrium of the heart. The node spontaneously depolarises at around 100 beats per minute, and is known as the pacemaker of the heart

Sinus bradycardia A heart rate below 60 beats per minute in an adult patient

Sinus tachycardia A heart rate above 100 beats per minute in an adult patient

Sleep apnoea Periodic cessation of breathing during sleep as a result of relaxation and narrowing of the airway

Sleep cycle A period of 90 min composed of two stages: non-rapid eye-movement sleep (NREM) and rapid eye-movement sleep (REM)

Sleep deprivation An acute or chronic condition where there is an insufficient amount of sleep resulting in physical and psychological complications

Socioeconomic status The total measure of a person's social and economic status in comparison with others, based on income, education and occupation

SOCRATES A mnemonic for assessing pain (Site, Onset, Character, Radiation, Associated symptoms, Time course, Exacerbating and relieving factors, Severity)

Sodium An essential electrolyte, it is the major extracellular cation (positively charged ion) and it has an important role in maintaining cellular stability and regulating fluid balance within the body

Somatostatin A hormone that inhibits the action of several other hormones, for example growth hormone, as well as blocking secretion of insulin and glucagon

Sotalol An antiarrhythmic agent

Speaking valve A connector that can fit on tracheostomy tubes to allow speech in an alert patient

Specific immune system The reaction of T and B cells to an antigen

Sphygmomanometer A non-invasive instrument for measuring blood pressure, involving a pressure cuff being wrapped round the arm

Spirometry A non-invasive method of assessing lung function by measuring the volume of air that the patient can expel from the lungs after maximal inspiration

SpO_2 A measurement of arterial oxygen saturation using a pulse oximeter

Stable angina Pain or tightness in the chest owing to reduced myocardial perfusion

Standard precautions A set of infection control practices used to prevent the transmission of diseases that can be contacted via blood and other body fluids

Statins Lipid-lowering medication used to lower the level of low density cholesterol in the blood

ST depression A sign of myocardial ischaemia

STEMI ST elevation myocardial infarction

Sternocleidomastoid A large paired muscle of the neck that is an accessory muscle of respiration

Steroids Substances (natural or in medication form) that reduce inflammation in the body

Stoma An surgical opening on the body, for example a tracheostomy stoma

Stridor A harsh vibrating noise caused by obstruction of the larynx

Stroke volume The amount of blood ejected in one contraction

ST segment elevation ST segment is above the isoelectric line by more than 1 mm in limb leads and 2 mm in precordial leads

Subdural The space between the inner layer of the dura mater but external to the brain and the arachnoid mater

Subjective data The patient's symptoms: what they report including feelings, perceptions and concerns

Substance P A neurotransmitter and a neuromodulator (able to regulate neuronal activity)

Supraglottic Above the level of the glottis

Suprasternal notch The large dip seen between the neck and the clavicle

Supraventricular The impulse is generated above the ventricles with narrow QRS complexes

Surgical emphysema This is when air or gas accumulates in the subcutaneous tissue beneath the skin and can be caused by disease or medical intervention

Surgical tracheostomy A tracheostomy performed in the operating theatre, with the creation of a Bjork flap that is sutured to the skin

Sympathetic nervous system A branch of the autonomic nervous system and the primary mechanism for the 'fight or flight' response

Syncope A faint: short-term loss of consciousness and muscle strength

Syndrome of inappropriate ADH Excessive release of ADH

Systemic inflammatory response syndrome A controlled and appropriate response to injury or infection

Systemic vascular resistance The resistance offered to flow, generated by the systemic vasculature

Systole Contraction phase of the cardiac cycle where blood is ejected into the next chamber or blood vessel

Tachyarrhythmia Abnormal heart rhythm over 100 beats per minute

Tachycardia A heart rate over 100 beats per minute

Target oxygen saturation The desired oxygen saturation level for a patient depending on whether or not there is a risk of hypercapnic respiratory failure

T cells A type of lymphocyte

Teleological theory A school of thought that focuses on the consequences of one's actions, a central tenet being doing the 'greatest good for the greatest number'

Tension pneumothorax A life-threatening condition where there is a progressive accumulation of intrapleural air leading to increased positive pressure within the mediastinal and intrathoracic cavities

Thoracentesis A surgical procedure to remove excess fluid from the pleural space

Thoracotomy An incision into the pleural space

Thromboembolic disease Excess clotting in the arterial or venous circulation

Thrombotic emboli The formation of blood clots (thrombi) which can be dislodged and travel in the circulation eventually causing a blockage in a blood vessel, for example, a blockage in the pulmonary artery due to pulmonary embolism

Thyroid stimulating hormone A pituitary hormone that stimulates the thyroid gland to produce T_4 and T_3 important for metabolism

Ticagrelor A platelet aggregation inhibitor used in acute coronary syndrome

Tidal volume At rest the volume inhaled with each breath is approximately 500 mL and is called the tidal volume (V_T)

Ti inspiratory time The time set for the inspiratory phase on non-invasive ventilation, normally one-third of respiratory cycle

TIMI risk score The 'thrombolysis in myocardial infarction' (TIMI) score is a mortality scoring system for patients with unstable angina and non-ST elevation myocardial infarction (NSTEMI)

Tirofabin An antiplatelet medication

Tissue hypoxia Lack of oxygen in the tissues

Tracheostomy An opening created in the trachea so that a tube can be inserted to facilitate breathing and clearance of secretions

Tracheostomy tube Small, curved tube placed into the trachea to facilitate breathing and clearance of secretions

Transfer anxiety Patient anxiety (and sometimes that of their relatives too) about being moved from an area of high dependency such as the ICU or the HDU to a general ward area. Concern usually focuses around a perceived lack of safety following the reduction in nursing staff accessibility and the amount of intensive monitoring available

Transfer bag A checked bag containing all necessary equipment for the inter- or intrahospital transfer of an acutely ill patient

Transient ischaemic attack A 'mini stroke', usually lasting no longer than 24 h, caused by a temporary disruption to the blood supply to the brain

Transmission-based precautions Infection control precautions covering spread of infection by direct or indirect contact, droplet exposure and airborne transmission

Transtentorial herniation Protrusion of brain structures through the tentorial notch putting pressure on the brain stem beneath. This is caused by raised intracranial pressure

Trapezius squeeze The squeezing of the trapezius muscle to induce a pain response

Traumatic pneumothorax Caused by a penetrating chest trauma such as a stab wound, or blunt trauma causing a fractured rib. May be open, or closed. A closed traumatic pneumothorax is at risk of developing into a tension pneumothorax

Tricuspid valve The valve between the right atrium and the right ventricle

Trigeminal neuralgia Severe facial pain caused by irritation of the fifth cranial nerve, the trigeminal nerve

Trigger threshold The sensitivity of the trigger when a patient-initiated breath is detected

Tripod position When the patient is bent forward hands on knees, because it is easier to breath in this position

Troponin (I and T) Proteins used to regulate cardiac muscle contraction. They have been found to be excellent markers of cardiac damage in acute coronary syndrome because when raised they are indicative of myocardial necrosis

Tumour necrosis factor A cytokine involved in systemic inflammation

Tunica externa The outermost layer of an artery or vein

Tunica intima The innermost layer of an artery or vein

Tunica media The middle, muscular layer of an artery or vein

T wave Ventricular repolarisation, should follow the same direction as the QRS complex

Type 1 respiratory failure Profound hypoxaemia, identified by an SpO_2 <90% (or PaO_2 <8.0 kPa), with a normal or low $PaCO_2$ of <6.0 kPa

Type 2 respiratory failure Hypoxaemia, identified by an SpO_2 <90% (or PaO_2 <8.0 kPa), with an elevated $PaCO_2$ of >6.0 kPa

Uncuffed tracheostomy tube Used for patients who require airway maintenance for suctioning purposes, not for those who still require mechanical ventilation

Unstable angina An acute coronary syndrome, with chest pain that occurs even at rest and maybe lasting for more than 15 minutes

Urticarial rash Small raised blisters (wheals) appear on the skin and cause the patient extreme irritation

Vagus nerve The tenth cranial nerve, supplying the organs of the chest and abdomen

Vasoconstriction Narrowing of the blood vessels as a result of muscular contraction in their walls

Vasodilatation Widening of the blood vessels as a result of muscular relaxation in their walls

Vasopressin The antidiuretic hormone released from the posterior lobe of the pituitary gland and working on the kidneys to retain water in the body

Vasopressor An agent that produces vasoconstriction and therefore a rise in blood pressure

VATS (video-assisted thoracoscopic surgery) Uses video cameras and endoscopic instruments, to perform thoracic surgery, through two to three small incisions

VBG Venous blood gas

Venous thromboembolism When a blood clot forms in a vein, with a portion (embolus) breaking off and travelling in the venous system

Ventilatory failure Failure of ventilation, limiting the flow of gases through the respiratory system

Ventricular ejection The forceful ejection of blood from the right ventricle into the pulmonary artery and from the left ventricle into the aorta

Ventricular fibrillation A series of rapid, uncoordinated muscular contractions throughout the lower chambers of the heart. This is one type of cardiac arrest as no cardiac output can be achieved when the ventricles are 'quivering' in this fashion

Ventricular tachycardia This is a life-threatening arrhythmia where a fast heart rate originating from the left or right ventricle severely impairs the cardiac output if sustained

Venturi masks A type of oxygen mask that by carefully regulating how much air is inhaled can ensure delivery of a precise, concentrated amount of oxygen to the patient

Venule A small blood vessel that collects blood from the capillary

Verapamil A calcium channel blocking agent

Vertical plane Upright, as in being in an upright position

Vesicular A soft and low-pitched sound with a long inspiratory phase

Visual infusion phlebitis (VIP) score Used for assessing the site of an intravenous cannula

V/Q The ventilation/perfusion ratio is a measurement used to determine how well alveoli are ventilated and how well they are perfused

V/Q mismatch This occurs when alveolar ventilation is not well matched to alveolar perfusion. Different V/Q relationships exist:

an area of lung may be perfused with no ventilation (shunt) or it may be ventilated with no perfusion (dead space)

VTE (encompasses both PE and DVT) Venous thromboembolism, an umbrella term encompassing deep vein thrombosis and pulmonary embolism

Vulnerable adult A person over the age of 18 years who is in receipt of care for physical or mental health reasons and who is unable to care for his or herself

WCC White cell count

Wheeze This is a polyphonic musical sound, heard most clearly on expiration as a result of air flowing through narrowed airways

Wide-bore suction device A Yankuer suction catheter

Work of breathing The work expended to overcome the resistance to airflow through the airways and the resistance from the chest wall. In short, the effort required to inspire air into the lungs, which in respiratory difficulty will be increased

Yankeur sucker A wide-bore suction device

Index

The Glossary (Pp. 136–147) has not been indexed.
Page numbers in *italic* refer to figures.
Page numbers in **bold** refer to tables or boxes.

ABCDE assessment, 4–5
abdominal thrust, *18*, 19
acute coronary syndrome, *64*, 65, 59
acute tubular necrosis, 91
adrenaline, **54**, 55, *74, 75, 76, 108*
adult advanced life support algorithm, 97, *126*
advance care plans, *124*, 125
afterload, 53, 81
air embolism, 63
airway, *4*, 5, 15, 17–23, 93, 95, *14, 74, 75, 77, 86, 94, 104, 106, 108*
AKIN classification, **90**, 91
aldosterone, **54**, 55, 89, 109
allergy, 75
alveolar ventilation, 27, 29, 37
AMPLE history, major trauma, **94**
analgesics, *10*, 11, 65
anaphylaxis, **74**, 75
angina, 65
angiotensin II, **54**, 55
angiotensin-converting enzyme inhibitors, 55
angiotensin receptor blockers, 55
antidiuretic hormone, 55, *76, 80*
antiplatelet therapy, 65
anxiety, 11, 13, 55, 57, **64**
aorta, *50*, 51, *64*, 65
aortic valve, 51, *82*
arrhythmias, 67, 68–69
arterial blood gases, *32*, 33, **36**, 37, **38**, 39, *30, 34*, 35, 45
arterial pressure, 62–63
aspirin, 65, 107
asthma, 31, 33, *38*, 39
ATOM-FC mnemonic, *94*
atrial fibrillation, *68*, 69, 105
atrial flutter, *68*, 69
atrioventricular block, *68*, 69
atrioventricular valves, 51, *52*
Atrovent, 39, **44**
atypical pneumonia, **40**
auscultation, *30*, 31, 57
autonomic nervous system, **54**, 55, 101
AV nodal re-entry tachycardia, *68*, 69
AVPU assessment, 5, **102**, 103

baroreceptors, *54*, 55, *76*
basophils, **70**, 71
Beck's triad, 79
best interest pathways, *120*, 121
beta blockers, 55, 107
bicarbonate (HCO₃), *32*, 33, **36**, **38**, 89, 37
bile, **84**, 85
bi-level positive airways pressure (BiPAP), **44**, 45, 35
blood pressure, 5, 53, *54, 55*, **56**, 57, 63, *64, see also* arterial pressure
B lymphocytes, 71
bradyarrhythmias, 69
brain, 100–101
brain stem, *100*
breathing, *4*, 5, 19, 25–47, 103, *see also* airway
    after cardiac surgery, 83
    hypovolaemia, 77
    transfer of patient, 15
bronchial pneumonia, *40*, 41
Brudzinski's sign, 105

B-type natriuretic peptide, 59
buffering, 89
burns, 77, 92–93
calcium, **60**
calcium channel blockers, 107
CAM ICU (Confusion Assessment Method), *12*, 13, 123
capacity, mental, *120*
capillary refill time (CRT), **56**, 57, 77, 113
carbimazole, 109
carbon dioxide, 26, 27, *28, 29*, 31
carbon monoxide poisoning, **106**
cardiac arrest, 3, 69, 96–97
cardiac output, 53, 55, *80*
cardiac surgery, 82–83
cardiac tamponade, *78*, 79, *94, 96, 126*
cardiopulmonary bypass circuit, *82, 83*
cardiopulmonary resuscitation, 96–97
carotid arteries, *58*, 105
catecholamines, 109
catheter-related bloodstream infections, 63
ceilings of care, 7, **124**
central venous pressure, 51, *62*, 63
cerebral salt wasting, 103
cerebrospinal fluid, 101
cervical spine, major trauma, 95, **94**
chain of survival, cardiac arrest, 97
chemoreceptors, *28, 29, 54, 39*
chest, 5, *30, 42*
    drainage, *42*, 43, 47
    trauma, *78, 94*
    X-rays, *32*, 33, *58*, 59, 115, *40, 39, 41, 63*
chest pain, 64–65
Cheyne-Stokes breathing, *30*, 31, 103
chin lift, *18*, 19
choking, *18*, 19
cholinergic receptors, **54**, 55, 101
chronic obstructive pulmonary disease (COPD), 31, 33, *34, 38*, 39, **44**
circulation, *4*, 5, 49–97
    acute failure, 72–81
    transfer of patient, 15
clotting tests, **58**
clubbing, *30*, 31
coagulopathy, major trauma, 95
Code for Nurses and Midwives, 121
cognitive impairment, *122*, 123
collars, **94**
colloids, **60**, 61, 77
colon, 85
community-acquired pneumonia, 41
compensation, respiratory acidosis, 33
complement, *70*, 71
compliance, 29, **36**
conduction system, heart, *52*, 53
Confusion Assessment Method for the Intensive Care Unit (CAM ICU),
    12, 13
congestive cardiac failure (CCF), *80*, 81
consciousness, level of, 5, **102**, 103
contiguous leads, ECG, 67
continuous positive airways pressure (CPAP), 44–45
coronary angiography, *58*, 59
coronary arteries, *52*, 53, *66, see also* acute coronary syndrome
coronary artery bypass grafting, *82*, 83

Acute and Critical Care Nursing at a Glance, First Edition. Edited by Helen Dutton and Jacqui Finch.
© 2018 John Wiley & Sons, Ltd. Published 2018 by John Wiley & Sons, Ltd.
Companion website: www.ataglanceseries.com/nursing/acutecare

cor pulmonale, 81
cortisol, 109
coughing, 23, 31
crackles, 57, 31
cranial nerves, origins, *100*, 101
craniosacral outflow, 75
C-reactive protein, 71, *72*
creatinine, **58**, **90**
creatinine kinase-MB, 59
cricothyroid/mini-tracheostomy, 23
critical care outreach teams (CCOT), 3
crystalloid solutions, **60**, 61, 77
CURB 65 score, **40**, 41
Cushing's syndrome, 109
Cushing's triad, 103
cyanosis, 57, *30*, 77
cytokines, **70**, 71

DDAVP, 109
death, 124–125, 97
decannulation caps, 23
decerebrate rigidity, **102**
decompensated heart failure, 81
decorticate rigidity, **102**
deep vein thrombosis, 59, *78*, 79
defibrillation, *96*, 97
delirium, *12*, 13, *122*, 123
dementia, 11, *122*, 123
deontology, 121
dependency, 3
depolarisation, *66*, *52*, *53*
depression, *122*, 123
Deprivation of Liberty safeguards, **120**, 121, 13
diabetes insipidus, 103, 109
diabetes mellitus, **108**, 109
diastole, *52*, 53
diastolic heart failure, 81
digoxin, 107
diltiazem, 107
DINAMAP device, **56**
diuresis, forced, **106**
dopamine, 55
Doppler ultrasound, *58*, 59
dressings, **112**
drug overdose, 106–107
dyspnoea, 57

Early Warning Scores, 3, 6, 7
echocardiography, *58*, 59
echocardiogram, **80**
ejection fraction, 81
electrocardiography (ECG), *52*, 57, 59, **60**, *62*, **64**, 65–67, 81
electrolytes, 59–61, 69, 89
emphysema, 39
empyema, 43
encephalitis, 105
endocrine system, 108–109
end positive airways pressure, 45
enteral feeding, *114*, 115
eosinophils, **70**, 71
epidural analgesia, *10*, 11
epinephrine (adrenaline), **54**, 55, *74*, 75, *76*, *108*
escalation of care, 6–7, 45
ethics, 13, 119, *120*, 121
Evidence-Based Guidelines (Epic 3), infection control, 9
evidence-based practice, 119
exercise tolerance test, *58*, 59
expiratory reserve volume, *28*
expired total ventilation (V_E), 29
exposure, *4*, 5, 15, 95
exudate pleural fluids, **42**

FAST mnemonic, *102*
fenestrated tracheostomy tubes, *22*, 23
FEV$_1$/FVC, 33, *38*
five Rs, 61
flail chest, *94*
fluids, 60–61, 77
    burns, 93
    central venous pressure monitoring, 63

loss, **76**, 77
    major trauma, 95
    neurological impairment, 103
forced expiratory volume in 1 second (FEV$_1$), *32*, *38*, 39
forced vital capacity (FVC), *32*, *38*
fractures, 95
Frank-Starling Law, 53, *80*
functional residual capacity, *28*, 29, 35, 45

gallbladder, 85
gas exchange, *26*
gastrointestinal system, 84–87
gastrostomies, **114**
Generalised Anxiety Disorder Assessment (GAD-7), *122*, 123
Glasgow Coma Scale, **102**, 103, 5
glial cells, 101
glomerular filtration rate (GFR), 89
glomeruli, *88*, 89
glucagon, 85
glucose levels, 65, 85, 103, **104**, *4*

haemoglobin Hb, *26*, 27, **36**, **58**, **59**, 27
haemorrhage, **76**, 77
    gastrointestinal, 87
    intracranial, 105
    major trauma, 95
haemorrhagic stroke, *104*, 105
haemothorax, 43, *94*
handovers, major trauma, **94**
handwashing, *8*, 9
Hartman's solution, **60**
head tilt, *18*, 19
healthcare-associated infection, 8–9
heart, *50*, 51, *52*, 53, 58–59, *82*, 83
heart block, 67, *68*, 69
heart failure, 39, 59, 80–81
Helicobacter pylori, 87
hepatocytes, 85
high flow nasal cannulae, 35, 45
High Impact Intervention Care Bundles, 9
hospital-acquired infection, 8–9, 41
humidification
    oxygen therapy, 35
    tracheostomy, 23
hydrocortisone, 39, *74*, 75
hydrogen ions (H$^+$), *26* 29, *32*, 33, 89
hydronephrosis, 91
hydrostatic pressure, *60*, 61
hypercalcaemia, **60**
hypercapnia, *30*, 35, 37, 39
hyperglycaemia, *4*, 103, 109
hyperglycaemic hyperosmolar syndrome, **108**, 109
hyperkalaemia, **60**
hypernatraemia, **60**
hypersensitivity, 75
hypertension, 57
hyperthyroidism, 109
hyperventilation, **34**
hypocalcaemia, **60**
hypoglycaemia, *4*, 103, **108**, 109
hypokalaemia, **60**
hyponatraemia, **60**
hypotension, 5, 57
hypothalamus, *108*, 109
hypothyroidism, 109
hypovolaemia, 76–77
hypoxaemia, *34*, 35, 37

I:E ratio (breathing), *30*, 31
immobilisation, major trauma, **94**, 95
immune system, 70–71
incontinence, 113
independent mental capacity advocates, *120*
infection, *see also* sepsis
    central nervous system, 105
    hospital-acquired, 8–9, 41
    pneumonia, *32*, 40–41
    skin, 113
informed consent, 121
inhalation injuries, 93

inspiratory reserve volume, *28*
interstitial pneumonia, *40*, 41
intestinal obstruction, **86**, 87
intestines, **84**, 85
intracranial haemorrhage, 105
intracranial pressure, 15, 103, **104**, 105
intravenous fluids, **60**, 61, 77, 91
ipratropium bromide, 39, **44**
iron, overdose, 107
ischaemic stroke, *104*, 105
islets of Langerhans, 85

jaw thrust, *18*, 19
justice, 119
juxtaglomerular cells, 55

KDIGO criteria, acute kidney injury, **90**, 91
Kernig's sign, 105
ketoacidosis, **108**, 109
kidneys, 55, 88–91
Kupffer cells, 85
Kussmaul breathing, *30*, 31

lactate, **72**, 77, **86**, **95**
laparoscopy, *86*
laparotomy, *86*
lasting power of attorney, 125
left ventricular failure (LVF), *80*, 81
lethal triad, major trauma, 95
liaison psychiatry services, 123
Light's criteria, **42**
lithium, 107
liver, 84, 85, 87
lobar pneumonia, *40*, 41
Lund and Browder chart, *92*, 93
lung failure, *36*, 37
lung resection, *46*
lung volumes, *28*, 29
lymphocytes, **70**, 71

macrophages, 71
magnesium (Mg^{++}), **58**, 59, **60**
magnesium sulphate, 39
major trauma, 94–95
malnutrition, 115
mast cells, 75
mean arterial pressure, 53, 57
meningitis, 105
Mental Capacity Act (2005), **120**, 121
mental health, 122–123
mental status, *12*
metabolic acidosis, *32*, 33, 109
metabolic alkalosis, *32, 33*
minute volume, 29, **36**
monitoring
    BiPAP, 45
    blood pressure, **56**
    haemodynamic, 62–63
    thoracic surgery, 47
    transfer of patient, *14*
monocytes, **70**, 71
Monro-Kellie hypothesis, 105
myocardium, 53, 65
myxoedema, 109

N-acetylcysteine, **106**
nasal cannulae, oxygen therapy, 35
nasogastric tubes, *114*, 115
National Early Warning Score (NEWS), 3, *6*, 7, 35, 41, **42**, 43, 37, 63, *72*, 73, **76**, 81, 92, 97
NATMIST handover, major trauma, **94**
natural killer cells, 71
nebulisers, *34*, 35
necrotising fasciitis, 113
negative pressure wound therapy, **112**
nephrons, *88*, 89
neurogenic shock, **74**, 75
neurological assessment, 102–103
neurological impairment, 103–105

neurons, *100*, 101
neuropathic pain, **10**, 11
neurotransmitters, 101
neutrophils, **70**, 71
NEWS (National Early Warning Score), 3, *6*, 7, 35, 41, **42**, 43, 37, 63, *72*, 73, **76**, 81, 92, 97
New York Heart Association classification, **80**
nitrogen balance, 115
nociceptive pain, **10**, 11
non-invasive ventilation, 44–45, 81
non-steroidal anti-inflammatory drugs, 11
noradrenaline (norepinephrine), **54**, 55
nosocomial pneumonia, 8–9, 41
NSAIDs, 11, 47
N-terminal pro-B type natriuretic peptide, 59
nursing models, **118**, 119
nutrition, 113, 114–115

obstructive lung disorders, 31, 33, *34*, **36**, 37, 38–39, **44**
oedema, 61, 113
oliguria, 91
oncotic pressure, *60*, 61
one chance to get it right (guidelines), 125
opioids, *10*, 11
organ failure, sepsis, *72*
orthopnoea, 57
osmosis, 61
oxygen, 7, 26, 27
    SpO$_2$, 5, 7, **14**, 27, 29, *30*, 31, 35, 37, 39, *72*, **74**, **76**, *86*, *104*, *106*, *108*
Oxygen Alert cards, *34*
oxygen haemoglobin dissociation curve, **36**
oxygen therapy, 7, *14*, 15, 34–35, *34*, 45, 95

PaCO$_2$, 29, 31, *32*, 33, 35, **36**, 37, **38**
pain, *4*, 10–11, 47, 83
pain sensation, *102*
palmer method, *92*, 93
pancreas, **84**, 85
pancreatitis, 87
PAO$_2$, *26*
PaO$_2$, *26*, 33, **36**, 37, **38**
paracetamol, **106**, 107
parasympathetic nervous system, **54**, 55, 75, 101
parenteral feeding, **114**, 115
Parkland formula, 93
paroxysmal nocturnal dyspnoea, 57
paroxysmal supraventricular tachycardia, *68*, 69
partial pressures, *26*, 27
passive leg raise, *76*, 77
patient-controlled analgesia (PCA), *10*, 11
peak flow meters, *32*, 33
PEFR (peak expiratory flow rate), *32*, 33
percutaneous tracheostomy, 23
peritoneum, 85
pesticides, poisoning, **106**
phaechromocytoma, 109
phagocytosis, *70*, 71
pH (blood), 33, **36**, **38**, 89
pH (gastric aspirate), *114*, 115
pituitary gland, *108*, 109
Plasmalyte, **60**
pleural disorders, 42–43
pneumonia, 32, 40–41
pneumothorax, *42*, 43, 63, *94*
    tension pneumothorax, 31, *78*, 79, *94*
poisoning, 106–107
portal hypertension, 87
positive end expired pressure (PEEP), 45
postoperative pain, thoracic surgery, 47
posture
    air embolism, 63
    breathing, 29, 35
    hypovolaemic shock, *76*, 77
    neurological impairment, **104**
potassium (K$^+$), **58**, 59, **60**
PQRST (mnemonic), **64**
prednisolone, 39, **44**
preload, 53, *80*, 81
pressure ulcers, *112*, 113

primary percutaneous coronary intervention, 65
PR interval, 53, *66*, 67
propranolol, 107
prostaglandins, 11
psychosocial issues, 12–13, *see also* mental health
    cardiac arrest, 97
    cardiac surgery, 83
    thoracic surgery, 47
pulmonary artery, 51
pulmonary embolism (PE), *78*, 79
pulmonary oedema, *32*, 57, *80*, 81, 103
pulse oximetry, 31
pulse pressure, 53
pulses, *56*, 57
pupils, *102*, 103
purse-lipped breathing, 31
$PvCO_2$, *32*
PvO_2, *26*, *32*
P wave, *52*, 53, *66*, 67
pyrexia, 5, *56*

QRS complex, *52*, 53, *66*, 67
qSOFA (sepsis screening), 73
QT interval, *66*, 67

record keeping, 121
recovery position, *18*, 19
red flags, *6*, *22*, *40*, *56*, *72*, 73, *76*, 90
re-entry tachycardia, *68*, 69
re-feeding syndrome, 115
rehabilitation, 115
relatives
    best interest pathways, *120*
    dying patient, 125
    presence at cardiac arrest, 97
relocation anxiety, 13
renal system, 55, 88–91
renin-angiotensin-aldosterone-system (RAAS), 55, *76*
repolarisation, *52*, *66*
reservoir bags, oxygen therapy, *34*
residual volume, *28*
resistance, breathing, *29*, **36**
respiratory acidosis, *32*, 33
respiratory alkalosis, *32*
respiratory depression, *10*
respiratory distress, 5, 31, *56*
respiratory failure, 36–37, 47
    hypercapnia, *30*, 35
    hypoxaemia, *34*, 35, 37
respiratory rate, 5, 7, 31, 77
respiratory tract, *18*, 19, 26–29, *28*
restrictive lung disorders, **36**, 37
resuscitation, 96–97
Resuscitation Council (RCUK) choking algorithm, *18*, 19
rhythm strip, ECG, 67
RIFLE classification, acute kidney injury, **90**, 91
right to left shunts, 27
right ventricle, heart failure, 81
Ringer's lactate, **60**

safeguarding, 121
Safer Nursing Care Tool (NICE), **2**, 3
salbutamol, 39, **44**
saline (intravenous), **60**, 77
saliva, **84**
SaO_2, *34*, **36**, **38**
SBAR, 6, 7
seizures, 105
sepsis, 72–83, *see also* wounds
    catheter-related, 63
Sepsis Six, **2**
septic shock, *72*, 73
selective serotonin re-uptake inhibitors, 107
serotonin syndrome, 107
shock, *72*, 73, 74–75, *76*–77, *78*–79, 95
shockable rhythms, 96
sinoatrial node, 53
sinus bradycardia, 69
sinus rhythm, 67

sinus tachycardia, *68*, 69
six C's, 121
skin, 112–113
sleep cycle, *12*, 13
sleep deprivation, 13
SOCRATES, *10*
sodium, **60**
qSOFA (risk of sepsis), *72*, 73
somatostatin, 85
sotalol, 107
speaking valves, 23
specific immune system, 71
sphygmomanometers, **56**
spinal cord, 75, **94**, 95, *100*, 101
spirometry, *32*, 33, *38*
SpO_2, 5, *30*, 31, 35, 37, 39, 27, 29, 31, **36**, *38*, 41, 45,
staffing levels, **2**, 3
standardisation, decision making, **118**, 119
Starling's law, capillaries, *60*
ST depression, 65
stomach, **84**, 85
stroke, 5, *102*, *104*, 105
stroke volume, 3, 51
ST segment, 67
supraorbital ridge, testing for pain, *102*
supraventricular tachyarrhythmias, *68*, 69
sympathetic nervous system, *54*, 55, 57, 75, *76*, 101
synapses, *100*, 101
syndrome of inappropriate ADH, 103, 109
syringes, enteral feeding, *114*
systemic vascular resistance, 53
systole, *52*
systolic heart failure, 81

tachycardia, *68*, 69
teleological theory, 121
tension pneumothorax, 31, *78*, 79, *94*
thoracic surgery, 46–47
thoracolumbar outflow, 75
thrombotic emboli, 63, *78*, 79
thyroid crisis, 109
thyroid stimulating hormone, 109
thyroxine, 109
tidal volume, *28*, 29
TIME principle, wounds, **112**
TIMI risk score, **64**
T lymphocytes, 71
tongue, airway obstruction, 19
total body surface area, 93
tourniquets, 95
trachea, displacement, 5, 79
tracheostomy, 22–23
tranexamic acid, 95
transfer anxiety, 13
transfer bags, 15
transfer of patient, 14–15
transient ischaemic attacks, *104*, 105
transmission-based precautions, *8*, 9
transtentorial herniation, 105
transudates, **42**, 43
trapezius squeeze, *4*, *102*
trauma
    chest, *78*, *94*
    major, 94–95
    neurological, 105
trigger thresholds, 6, 7
tri-iodothyronine, 109
troponin (I and T), 59, **64**, 65
tubules (renal), *88*, 89
T wave, *52*, 53, 65, *66*, 67

ultrasound, 58, 59, 95
unstable angina, 65
upper airway obstruction, *18*, 19
urea, **58**, **90**
urinary tract, 88–91
urine, *88*, 89
urine output, 5, **56**, 57, 91

vacuum-assisted wound closure, **112**
valve surgery, heart, *82*, 83
varices, 87
VATS (video-assisted thoracoscopic surgery), 47
veins, *50*, 51
venous blood gases, *32*, 33
venous thromboembolism, *78*, 79
ventilation, 28–29
ventilation failure, *36*, 37
ventilation perfusion relationships, *26*, 27
ventilation (therapeutic), 44–45
ventricular ejection, *52*
ventricular fibrillation, *68*, 69, *96*
ventricular tachycardia, *68*, 69, *96*
Venturi masks, *34*, 35
verapamil, 107
video-assisted thoracoscopic surgery (VATS), 47

viral pneumonia, 41
visual infusion phlebitis (VIP) score, *112*, 113
vital capacity, *28*
volume resuscitation, 95
V/Q mismatch, 27
vulnerable adults, 121

weaning
    BiPAP, 45
    tracheostomy, 23
wheeze, 31
white blood cells, **70**, 71
work of breathing, 29, **36**, 37
wounds, 112
    after cardiac surgery, 83
    vacuum-assisted closure, **112**

Notes

Notes

Notes

Notes